THE COMPLETE BOOK OF PILATES FOR MEN

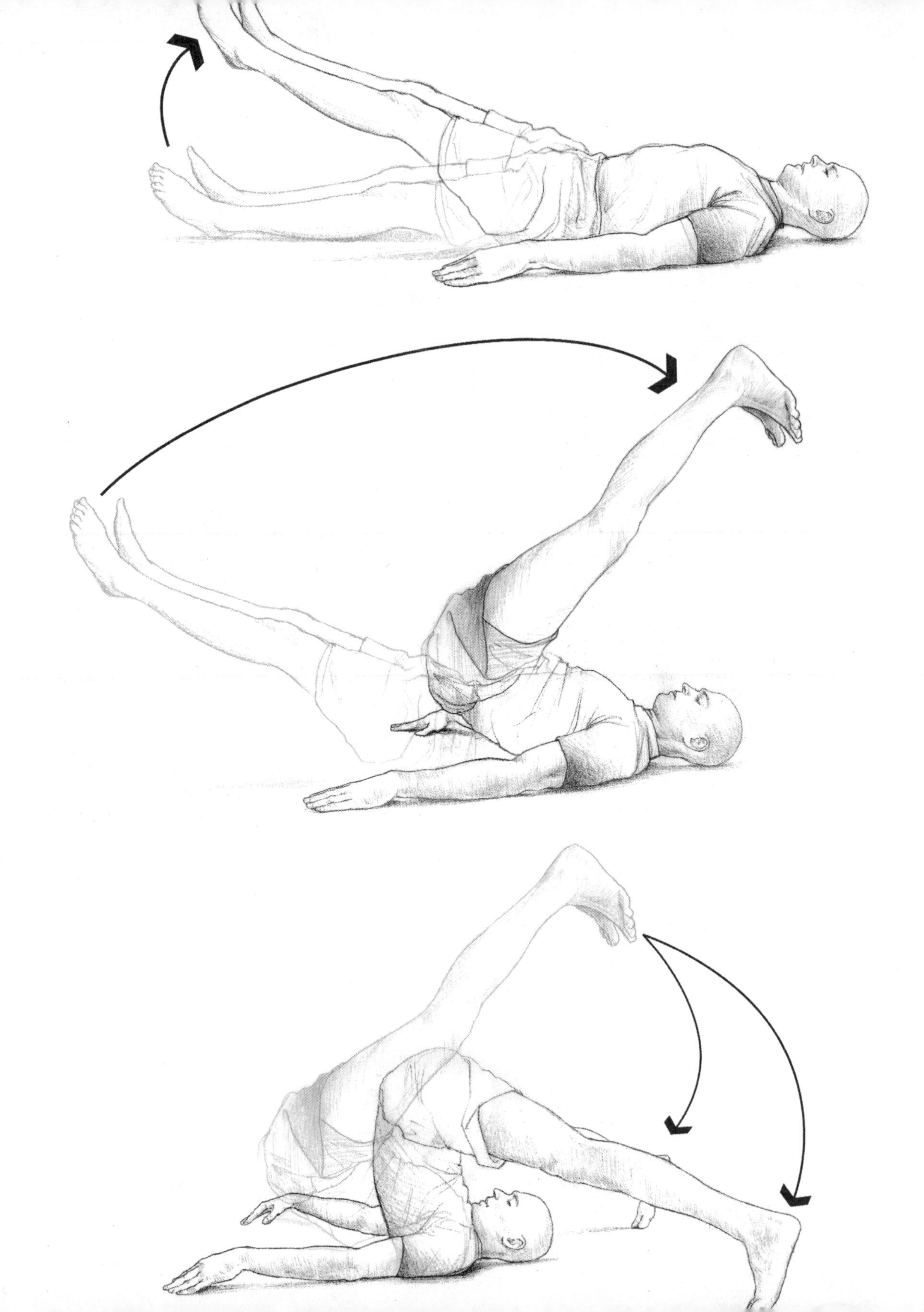

THE COMPLETE BOOK OF PILATES FOR MEN

THE LIFETIME PLAN FOR STRENGTH, POWER, AND PEAK PERFORMANCE

DANIEL LYON JR.

ILLUSTRATIONS BY WILLIAM A. ARBIZU

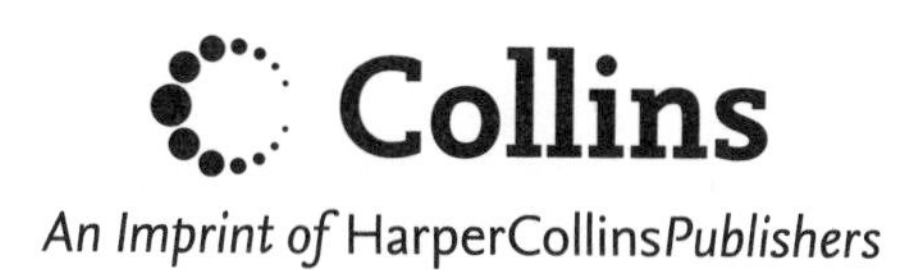

An Imprint of HarperCollins*Publishers*

This book is written as a source of information only. The information contained in this book should by no means be considered a substitute for the advice of a qualified medical professional, who should always be consulted before beginning any new exercise or other health program. The author and the publisher expressly disclaim responsibility for any adverse effects arising from the use or application of the information contained herein.

HarperCollins books may be purchased for educational, business, or sales promotional use. For information please write: Special Markets Department, HarperCollins Publishers Inc., 10 East 53rd Street, New York, NY 10022.

FIRST EDITION

Designer: Kris Tobiassen
Illustrations by William A. Arbizu

Printed on acid-free paper

Library of Congress Cataloging-in-Publication Data
Lyon, Daniel.
The complete book of Pilates for men : the lifetime plan for strength, power, and peak performance / Daniel Lyon, Jr. ; illustrations by Willam A. Arbizu.-- 1st ed.
p. cm.
Includes bibliographical references.
ISBN 0-06-082077-2
1. Pilates method. 2. Exercise for men. 3. Physical fitness for men. I. Title.

RA781.4L965 2005
613.7'1--dc22 2005046599

ISBN 0-06-082077-2

12 CG/RRDC 16 15 14

WITH LOVING GRATITUDE FOR
NORMAN AND FRANCES,
MY GRANDPARENTS

CONTENTS

PART I

PART II

PART III

PART IV

PART I

PILATES: THE MAN'S WORKOUT

This book offers the best exercise system available to practice on your own, wherever you are. Why is it the best? Simply put, Pilates works. It addresses exactly what we men need, especially as we grow older: overall health, long balanced muscles, strength from our centers, and control of our bodies.

You've probably come across Pilates in various places over the past few years. Your significant other may have taken a private lesson or mat class. You may have picked up a woman's magazine in the waiting room of anywhere, U.S.A. Or you may have seen a commercial on television showing a roomful of buff women performing leg raises as if they were the Rockettes. The fact that women and their networks have dominated the world of Pilates in recent years has bred the misconception that Pilates is a female-only activity. This couldn't be further from the truth. Joseph Pilates was a cigar smoking boxer, acrobat, and gymnast, and he developed his exercise program from that background first and foremost for men.

This book is designed for *all* men—including the athlete or jock, the sedentary man with little or no exercise history, and the injured man. If you're an active athlete, you will discover that Pilates is a natural cross-training resource. It will heighten your coordination, balance your strength, and sharpen your focus.

If you're a sedentary man, you will find Pilates to be a welcoming challenge because it feels natural. You will improve your strength and flexibility with each passing day, and within a short time you will see dramatic results in the mirror. In Joseph Pilates's own words: "In ten lessons you'll feel a difference, in twenty you'll see a difference, and in thirty you'll have a whole new body." His words continue to ring amazingly true.

If you're a man with an injury, you will realize that Pilates offers a logical method of working out while your body is healing. Pilates doesn't aggravate the body; the exercises are always to be performed with control. If ever an exercise hurts, then you simply stop, temporarily or permanently remove it from your practice, and move on to the next exercise. Each body is different. Chances are, you will not be able to perform every exercise from the outset. But eventually, as you gain more control over your body, you will be able to perform all or most of the exercises. Pilates works in this methodical manner, offering new challenges with healing and practice.

I speak from experience. When I hurt my lower back in a power-lifting contest in college, the injury plagued me on and off for ten years. Eight years of jiu-jitsu yielded me a right AC joint sprain, a migration of the left shoulder's clavicle and scapulae, multiple ankle and wrist strains, sprains, and bruises. I have used the Pilates method to rehabilitate my own body. My back no longer hurts; the pain is simply gone. My shoulder no longer "pops" out. I have a full range of motion in both of my shoulder joints. My wrists and ankles—formerly weakened by repetitive overstretching—now have new strength. My own body was breaking down during my full-time jiu-jitsu practice. Pilates has reversed the damage.

During and after my years in jiu-jitsu, I had a desk job. As a trader, I watched the markets from 7:30 A.M. to 4:00 P.M. My upper back began to take on that slumped, rounded look. My gut was far from lean, and, if I had not had such a vigorous workout in jiu-jitsu, I would have been rapidly accelerating the aging process. Such bad posture, when either seated or standing, places undue strains on our joints and organs. Just as our brain will stop working if it's deprived of oxygen, our organs won't function optimally if the blood flow to them is hindered or our joints aren't properly aligned. As Dr. Andrew Taylor Still, the founder of Osteopathic Medicine, states, "If the body structure is altered or abnormal, then proper body function is altered and can cause pain and illness."[1] Pilates counteracts the damaging effects of work-related repetitive postures and motions. My posture today is upright, like a sentry standing guard. I have the stomach of a lean twenty year old, and people routinely underestimate my age by seven or eight years. In my own body, I have seen the powerful benefits of Pilates from the vantage of both an injured athlete and a man with a sedentary job.

How does Pilates work for men? It integrates the body by focusing on activating and connecting the strongest parts of the body first—your core, or what we in Pilates refer to as the "powerhouse." For example, Pilates does not address arm weakness with the thought, "isolate the biceps and strengthen them with curls." Pilates approaches arm weakness and all other body imbalances with the conviction that you must first strengthen your powerhouse. From your powerhouse, you work your body with integrated movement, connecting all the weaker body parts to your strong core. The whole body becomes stronger as a result. In other words, you must strengthen the trunk of the tree and then integrate—not isolate—the branches. Through this process, the spine returns to its naturally supple condition.

Think of an aged person. What areas of his body lack the pliability of youth? Typically, they are the hips and spine. The center or core of the body is usually the last area to fail as a consequence of aging. A relatively young person with a rigid spine or immobile hips will appear to be older than his years. Inversely, an older person with a lean, strong powerhouse and a flexible spine will appear years younger than he actually is. This is how Pilates works. I know a man in his late sixties who has been practicing Pilates for thirty years. His workouts aren't as regular as they were when he was younger, but you would never know it by watching him exercise. He is lean and moves throughout the studio as if he were thirty. He embodies the success of the Pilates method as a long-term health and fitness practice. The first time I worked with him, while I was adjusting his body position, I was amazed to find that his stomach was as hard as steel.

Now, as controversial as this next statement may be, I must make an important point: *Men and women are different.* There, I've said it. There are certain tendencies that I see on a daily basis—tendencies that apply to women as well but seem to manifest more in men. Men tend to have more body strength but not necessarily integrated strength, whereas women usually demonstrate more flexibility. Men tend to be tighter in the shoulders, back, legs, and throughout the hips, whereas women tend to have better ranges of motion. The biological origins of these differences—like how flexible hips facilitate child bearing, or the genetic predisposition of testosterone levels, or gender specific daily habits—are not that important for our purposes. Simply know this: Men and women are different, and this book targets men's bodies and what they require within the Pilates method.

In addition to developing strength and flexibility, Pilates improves posture. Good posture is a subject of paramount importance to men, on many levels. Good posture yields more energy because it means we're not fighting gravity. Poor posture, on the other hand, results in a vicious cycle of deteriorating health due to unnecessary strains on our joints and organs. You have probably considered the physical benefits of good posture before. But also take a moment to think about how your posture affects the way others perceive you, and how you perceive yourself. The man who carries himself effortlessly conveys to those around him that he is confident, attractive, and intelligent. Improving your posture with Pilates has the potential to enhance everything from your personal relationships to your career.

What distinguishes the Pilates method from the rest of the world of fitness are six fundamental principles and the use of the powerhouse. The six principles of Pilates are: control, center, concentration, precision, flow, and breath. Moving with *control* from your *center* with *concentration* and *precision* while using proper *breathing* to create a natural *flow* from one exercise to the next is Pilates in action. While other exercise methods—like Yoga, the martial arts, and dance—follow these principles and crosscurrents, only at the heart of every movement in Pilates will you find all six principles working together in harmony.

The powerhouse is the workhorse in the Pilates method, comprised of the abdominal muscles, hips, lower back muscles, and buttocks. It begins at the base of the pelvic floor and continues upward to the bottom of the diaphragm. The transverses abdominus is the preeminent powerhouse muscle. It is the deepest of the abdominal muscles and surrounds the entire powerhouse. You feel it tighten your waist when you cough. When an exercise instructs you to engage the powerhouse, you must activate this muscle. All movement in each exercise is initiated from and connected to the powerhouse. In the modern day, Pilates instructors use expressions like "scoop your stomach" and "navel to spine" to teach practitioners how to activate the powerhouse. In my mat classes, I like to say "pull your stomach in" or "pull your navel in"—a variation of Joseph Pilates's "keep the abdomen drawn in."[2] For now, it is most important to know what a powerhouse is, recognize that you have one, and reconcile that it may take a little time to shake the rust off of it.

A third Pilates distinction, secondary to the powerhouse and the six principles, is what is called "the Box." If you draw imaginary lines connecting the two shoulders to each other, the two hip bones to each other, and finally the hip bones to the shoulders, then you'll have drawn a rectangle on your torso. The image of a superimposed box (or rectangle) on your body will help you keep your hips square and away from your ribcage, your tailbone anchored to the mat, and your shoulders aligned and pulled down away from your ears. The practice of maintaining your box during many of the Pilates exercises will help you develop a symmetrically strong torso (a stabilized box), and therefore an even stronger powerhouse.

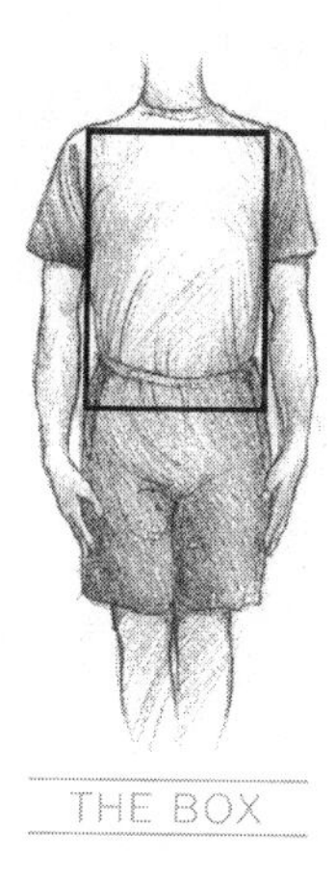

THE BOX

The Pilates method uses a minimum amount of time and resources to produce superior results. The time it takes to perform the Pilates mat exercises ranges from twenty minutes to one hour, three to four times a week. Pilates easily fits into a busy schedule and can be performed anywhere that has floor space—in homes, offices, hotels, you name it. All you will need, apart from this book, is an exercise mat in case your floor is too hard or slippery.

Men frequently ask me what other workouts they should follow to supplement or complement their Pilates practice. My answer is typically "What are your goals?" Pilates in and of itself was designed as a complete system and is alone enough to get in shape, maintain a healthy fitness level, and excel to higher standards of fitness. I have trained triathletes whose goals are drastically different from those of clients who simply want to have better posture. Simply put, Pilates goes with everything and is extraordinary by itself. If you are a frequent weight lifter, Pilates will help you integrate your strength and increase your flexibility. If you play golf, tennis, or baseball (or other sports and activities that require asymmetrical motions), Pilates will even out your posture and strength. I cannot think of one sport or physical hobby that Pilates doesn't make better. Can you practice Pilates *and* run? Can you spin? Can you continue playing with your weekly adult hockey league? The answer for all these questions is a resounding *yes.* Go run, spin, and skate your heart out. Use Pilates by itself or in tandem with anything you already do. One of my male clients, whose tennis game has improved tremendously, wishes he had practiced Pilates twenty years ago when he was a collegiate football player and shot-putter.

Athletes, actors, businessmen, and dancers all over the world have used Pilates for decades. Why? Pilates practitioners are forward thinkers who want to be at the top of their games. They know which resources give them an edge in a competitive world. Pilates has revolutionized their lives and mine. With this book, I aim to revolutionize yours. You will look and feel younger, stronger, more resilient, and powerful in every aspect of your life.

JOSEPH H. PILATES: A BRIEF HISTORY

Joseph H. Pilates was born in Germany in 1880 and began his career in the circus. He arrived in England in 1914. During this time he was also a successful middleweight boxer. When World War I broke out, he was interned along with thousands of other aliens on the Isle of Man. At the internment camp during wartime, Pilates took on the role of a physical instructor. The camp became a laboratory for his health and fitness beliefs. The men who were physically sound performed his floor exercises. For the bedridden, Pilates attached springs to the beds to rehabilitate them.

In 1919 Pilates returned to Hamburg, Germany, and took a job as a physical education instructor with the military police. From his experiences, he concluded that the common characteristic that yielded strong bodies—among boxers, acrobats, as well as ordinary people—was a flexible spine with a strong center and system-wide integrated strength. He also based the principles of his method on his observations of nature: "I soon discovered the animals had the best system of all for keeping fit. You never see a big cat out of shape. With just a little daily stretching and balancing on rocks and benches in a cage, a lion, tiger, or a panther will keep in condition."[3]

His life's work was now set. When seized again with wanderlust and an offer to train the German boxing champion, Max Schmelling, in 1925, Joseph left for America. He settled in New York City and opened a studio at 939 Eighth Avenue. His clients were among New York's A-list. In the early days of his New York studio, most of his clients were men, many of them boxers, wrestlers, and skiers of varying sizes and builds. But when choreographer George Balanchine and dancer Martha Graham caught onto his method, their influence led many dancers and artists to Joe's studio. Writers, athletes, actors, and dancers—eventually—all came to Joseph Pilates. When he died in 1967 at the age of eighty-seven, he left a legacy that has continued to flourish well into the twenty-first century. Although women have come to dominate the practice of Pilates in recent years, men are rediscovering it for their own distinct goals. These exercises are as formidable today as they were in Joseph Pilates's day.

YOUR PILATES UNIVERSE

This book is designed for your self-guided practice of the Pilates method at home or practically wherever you want. Pilates is also taught in studios with the use of various apparatuses that Joseph Pilates invented during his lifetime. He didn't call his inventions machines: "A machine does something to you; with the apparatus, you do the work."[4] Studio practice and home practice differ in a few distinct ways. But the goal, in both cases, is to lengthen, strengthen, and gain control of your body.

In a studio, you may take either a private session or group mat classes led by a certified Pilates instructor. The private hour-long sessions may have anywhere from one to three people, while the mat classes are limited to whatever amount of floor space is available in a given studio. Within a private session, the instructor uses the various apparatuses to personalize a workout that addresses the client's needs. The mat classes lead practitioners through a selection of the mat exercises, and each person works within his or her own ability. In private or shared private sessions, you get individual attention and guidance from the teacher, whereas a mat class offers you less individual attention but costs a third to a quarter less than a private session. In most cases, studio exposure will expedite the learning curve of how quickly your body absorbs the Pilates method.

In private sessions, the instructor will also address your specific needs and injuries. The apparatuses help provide both spring resistance and structural stability to facilitate the healing and "evening-out" processes. If you've ever broken your arm or leg, then you know how the broken limb is weaker than the non-broken limb when the cast is removed. Spring tension coupled with proper alignment works to even out this and other structural imbalances.

Available within a Pilates studio is exposure to all 500-plus exercises of the Pilates method. Many of the exercises can be practiced in various ways. For example, the Teaser exercise can be done on the mat or on any of the following apparatuses: the Universal Reformer, the Cadillac, the Wundachair, the Guillotine, the Spine Corrector, and—for the daring or partially insane—the Ladder Barrel. By offering structure to the exercise, an apparatus will effectively teach you how to move the body through the exercise. Performing an exercise on the various apparatuses can help put the movement in your body. Generally speaking, if you can do the exercise properly on the mat, then you'll be able to do it on an apparatus.

Would it benefit you to visit a studio and take a few private lessons or mat classes? The answer is both yes and not necessarily. The studio environment can help establish the ritual; you are there for a specific reason at a specific time. A certified Pilates instructor who is worth his or her mettle will teach you to integrate and control your body, as well as personalize the method to your needs. World-class athletes have coaches. Proper coaching in life is always beneficial, and a few lessons in a studio would serve to better your game. If you are not in shape—that is, if you haven't worked out in years, are overweight, or have limited mobility due to stiffness or old injuries—then I strongly suggest you visit a studio for a few private sessions in order to learn to move safely.

On the other hand, it's not strictly necessary for you to visit a studio. Why? My mentor, Joseph Pilates's oldest living protégé, who has been teaching Pilates for sixty-four years, says it best: "The apparatus are good, but the mat work is everything. If you can do the mat work perfectly, you don't need the apparatus."[5] The benefits of home practice are fairly straightforward: You plan the time. You learn at your own discretion. You create a distraction-free environment. As the famous Japanese swordsman Miyamoto Musashi put it centuries ago, "warriors must train alone to get more in touch with themselves."[6] By practicing alone at home, in your office, or wherever you choose, you will gain a deeper understanding of yourself; you will discover the connection between your mind and your body. You will develop the self-motivation and focus necessary to learn these exercises and take control of your body—without depending on anyone else. This approach to the Pilates method is thoroughly empowering.

MAT WORK NECESSITIES

In the mat work you will often see references to the Pilates stance, which is simply our way of standing. If you were to hang from a chin-up bar, your feet would rotate slightly outward. This is the natural rotation of the legs from the hips. It is also the basis of the Pilates stance. The easiest way to get into Pilates stance is to follow these steps:

PILATES STANCE

- Begin with your heels together and your toes about one to two inches apart. Imagine fitting half of a pizza slice between your feet to find the proper distance. (Dancers have a larger "turnout." Since I am not a dancer and neither are most men, it's necessary to separate your toes only a little bit.) Your knees should be aligned with your toes.
- Press your legs together, as if they were a zipper, right into the pelvic girdle. You want to minimize the amount of light that can be seen coming through your legs.
- Please pardon this next image: Imagine you have to go to the bathroom. Engage the muscles of the pelvic region to cut off the flow of urine. Squeeze your bottom and hold your abdominals in firmly.

- Keep the arms alongside the body with the fingers reaching long toward the floor. This helps to keep the shoulders down and back.

- Reach the crown of the head up toward the ceiling to keep the spine long.

- Finally, feel your body weight distributed evenly in your feet. Once the weight is distributed evenly, you may then—and only ever so slightly—pitch forward so that the weight of your body is leaning just a touch more onto the balls of your feet rather than on your heels. You may also stand with the weight evenly distributed, without the slight forward pitch. Just be sure that you're not putting the majority of your body's weight onto your heels. This is important so that you don't risk losing your balance. (If you have any grappling or martial arts experience, you know that once you get your opponent's weight onto his heels, it's easy to take him down.) Your entire body should feel strong and tight, like an ancient Roman soldier standing before Caesar's throne! But you should be able to stand like this in a relaxed fashion as well.

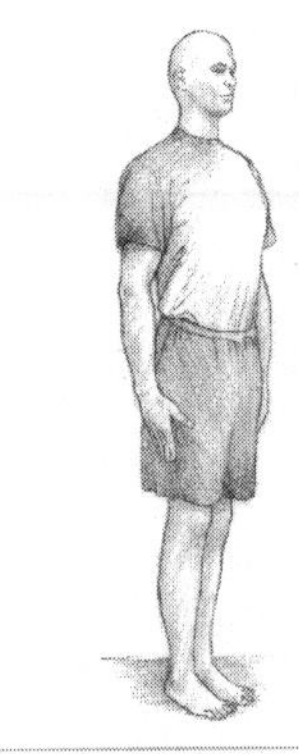

PILATES STANCE

Another common instruction during the mat work is "chin to chest." When you are lying down, it may also appear as "lift your head off the mat and look into your stomach." The purpose of chin to chest is both to involve the upper spine in the movements of the Pilates method and to lengthen the neck—which is part of lengthening the spine. The proper way to do this is to imagine lengthening the back of your neck as you draw your chin in. It will look like a slight nod. Standing helps to make the distinction between a long upper neck and spine and an incorrect collapsed shorter one.

CHIN TO CHEST

INCORRECT Stand in Pilates stance and drop your head so that your chin rests on your chest. Your neck will feel the weight of your head rather than the desired lengthening. This is not a long neck and is incorrect. If you were able to peer to your side into a nearby mirror without changing this position, the mirror would confirm this.

CORRECT Now stand tall in Pilates stance and draw your chin in toward the hollow of your throat as you lengthen your neck toward the ceiling. Don't strain the muscles in the front of the neck. You may also attain this position with the chin and head by tilting your head backward as far as comfortably possible—in effect, reaching your chin upward. Follow this movement with a nod of the chin into the hollow of your throat until the back of your neck feels long. (It helps to imagine that you are holding a small piece of fruit under your chin against your body.) Practice this a few times to get the feel.

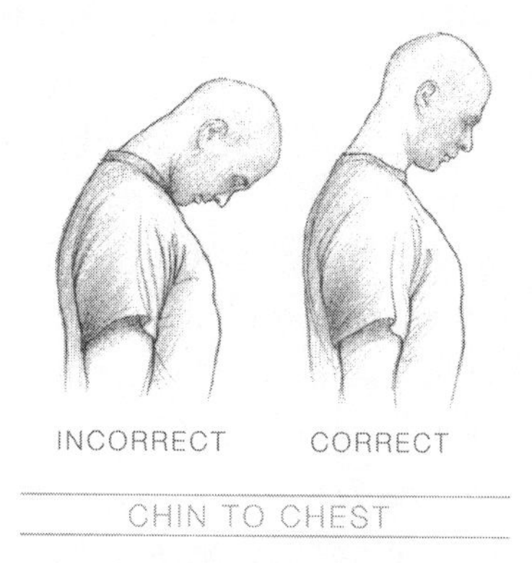

INCORRECT CORRECT

CHIN TO CHEST

Pilates instructors are an obsessive bunch. We are methodical both in our training and in our body movements throughout the day. Precision, one of the six principles of the method, is partly what attracts us to Pilates in the first place. However it is possible to overemphasize the precision element. Here's an example from my own training. Some instructors I worked with repeatedly reinstructed me to "pull in my ribs." Some people do flair their ribcage out, especially when they are incorrectly "sucking in" their gut or their back is arched at an incorrect moment. While they should learn to bring their ribs in, in my case, it was incorrect to keep repeating the point. I am barrel-chested; my ribs may look "out" when they really aren't. It is simply the shape of my body.

If you have some difficulty learning, say, to pull your ribs in, or pull your shoulders down, or lengthen your neck, remember this: Too much precision is a bad thing; it kills the dynamic of the movement, and movement *is* Pilates. Pilates is not a snapshot, but a moving picture. As my mentor has said, "I am tired of seeing people poking the ribs and shoulders. Just pull the stomach in and everything else will work out." Keep your Pilates simple. It was designed to be natural. In your mat work, move as instructed, pull the stomach in, and your precision will follow.

This brings us to the principle of breathing, which Joseph Pilates emphasized a great deal. "Above all else learn how to breathe properly. Squeeze every atom of air from your lungs until they are almost as free of air as is a vacuum," he wrote.[7] But first, a caution: When drawing your navel to the spine (a.k.a. pulling in your powerhouse) during to an exercise, sucking in your stomach in such a way that makes you hold your breath will only weaken your powerhouse. Do not hollow out your midsection. Instead, hold the abdominals in so that the stomach doesn't expand on the inhale but rather remains firm and—depending on your girth and powerhouse strength—hourglass-shaped at the waistline. Think of lying on the floor and tightening up your stomach because someone is about to stand on it. This will help you fully breathe into the sides and back of the ribcage while maintaining a strongly engaged powerhouse. Keep your stomach firm on the exhale (this will be easier to do on the exhale than on the inhale) as you pull your navel to the spine. Anything that hinders your breathing, such as sucking in your gut, will consequently slow or stop your movement. This will affect the third principle: flow.

Flow is continuous and easy movement. As you become more familiar with the exercises, you should move from one exercise to another smoothly and with a minimum of extraneous movement. Flow combines grace and rhythm. Grace occurs between the exercises, connecting them seamlessly. Rhythm occurs within each exercise. Flow will begin to manifest itself as you become more advanced. And with flow, Pilates becomes quite aerobic. If you are flowing well, you will find that your connection to your center, or powerhouse, comes naturally.

All movement in Pilates mat work is connected to your center. You will move more easily with awareness of your center as you become more proficient in the mat work exercises. Simply contract the muscles of the powerhouse. With practice, practice, and more practice, you will gain control over your body—which brings us to the next principle of mat work.

"Contrology" was Joseph Pilates's name for his method of physical conditioning. In practicing the exercises in this book, you will be practicing a science of control. Control has a dual purpose: It will prevent injury, and it will give you command over the greatest vessel you have—your body. Control will come with attention and diligence. After all, you control your body movements with your mind.

All of the mat principles are equally important. Sometimes, though, one principle permeates the work more than others do. This is how I regard concentration, which is usually the first of the principles discussed: Concentration is everything. Concentration will develop control. Concentration will train your breathing. Concentration will yield flow. Concentration results in precision. Concentration will find your center. When performing the mat exercises, always concentrate.

HOW TO USE THIS BOOK

Each exercise is titled and depicted with illustrations and text. The illustrations are drawn from photographs of yours truly. To keep things simple, the text corresponding to the illustrations describes body position, movement, and breathing alone. Following each exercise's illustrated instructions is a section called the "The Beast Within" which includes further guidance on "Body Position," "The Mind in Motion," and "Cautions." Each exercise yields a particular set of benefits, which I identify right after the title, but remember that the Pilates method is an integrated physical practice. If an exercise targets the flexibility of the spine, for example, it typically benefits many portions of the back and other areas of the body as well. We don't isolate a rhomboid or trapezius muscle. All of the exercises work many body zones simultaneously. Don't be intimidated or overwhelmed by all of my detailed instructions. They are there as guidelines, and over time you'll absorb the whole of each exercise.

This book accommodates different skill levels: beginner, intermediate, and advanced. Of course, to consider Pilates in terms of three stages can be limiting. In archival footage, I've seen Joseph Pilates give a man who was suffering from stiffness and working out for the first time exercises that many modern day instructors would never consider. My guiding question as a Pilates instructor is "What does this body need?" Let your body's intelligence guide you. If an exercise makes something hurt or you can't control your body throughout a movement, leave that exercise out. Progression in Pilates works like this: First we strengthen the powerhouse and stabilize the box, then we move toward exercises that change the body weight distribution, alter the leverage, change the spine's movement, and demand more control. Joseph Pilates defined "Contrology" as the science of lengthening, strengthening, and control. If you apply this paradigm to your own training, your mind will lead you intelligently through your Pilates practice.

The exercises are illustrated in the sequential order of a complete advanced mat workout. To begin, you'll perform the beginner exercises three times a week. A chart showing the beginner, intermediate, and advanced curriculums is available at the beginning of each exercise section. When you have become strong in the beginner exercises, simply refer to the curriculum to see which intermediate exercise to learn next and add it to your practice where it belongs sequentially. As you continue to gain more control over your body, you'll add on intermediate and advanced exercises to your routine until you can perform all or nearly all of the mat exercises. Remember, as you listen to your body and add on exercises, you will find that some exercises will not feel as easy or fluid as others. Try another exercise as long as it's not painful. If you must leave an exercise out, then do so and proceed to the next one.

This book is results driven. It will provide short term changes and long-term results. I am the model illustrated in the pictures. I have put the Pilates method into my body and have written this book to guide others to this same end. Now I pass the gift of Pilates on to you.

NOTE TO READER

These exercises can be challenging. It will take time for you to perform them correctly. Be patient. With each session, you will discover that you are getting closer and closer to being able to complete the exercise as shown in each diagram. Don't worry, for example, if you are not able to reach your head all the way to your knees in the Roll Up, or your legs over your head and onto the floor in the Roll Over. Remember, your range of motion in an exercise is a function of your control. (Range is for the ego, and control is for the soul!) If you practice control, range will eventually follow.

Within the exercises, there are many breathing cues to help you align your breathing with your movement. This will take time to accomplish, so don't worry if you are not able to breathe as perfectly as instructed. As you continue to practice, the breathing will come more naturally.

Many of the exercises throughout the book will instruct you to squeeze or flex your buttocks. If doing so causes tightness or pain in your lower back, then disregard this guideline. Do not force yourself to follow any instructions that do not suit your body specifically.

In Pilates, we do not believe that pain does your body any good. The German/Austrian expression "Von nichts kommt nichts," which translates to "no pain no gain," never applies to Pilates. Again, not every exercise is for every person. If you encounter pain, stop, omit the exercise, and go to the next exercise. It will take time for you to develop control. Your strength will grow each day. Work intelligently and steadily, and you will soon be astonished at how well you feel, look, and move.

PART II

TRADITIONAL PILATES MAT WORK

TRADITIONAL MAT CURRICULUM

BEGINNER

INTERMEDIATE

ADVANCED

THE HUNDRED

BENEFITS: EXERCISES THE HEART, LUNGS, AND POWERHOUSE

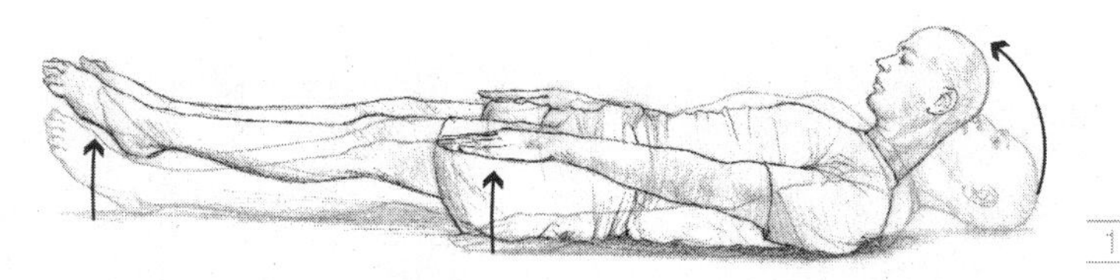

Lie on the floor with your arms alongside your body. Keep your feet turned out in Pilates stance. Draw your powerhouse in. In one motion, raise your feet 2 inches off the mat, lift your hands alongside the top of your thighs, and bring your head off the mat with your eyes focused on your toes.

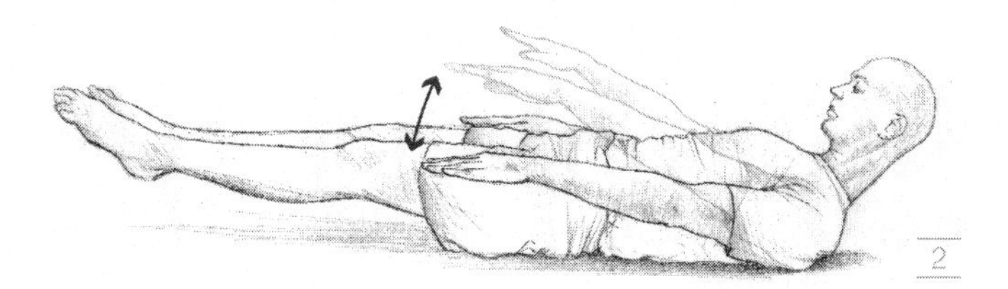

Begin pumping the arms up and down within a 4 to 8-inch range of motion. As you pump, inhale for 5 counts and exhale for 5 counts. This is 1 set. (1 set of 5 pumps inhaling and 5 pumps exhaling should take about 4 to 5 seconds.)

Perform 10 sets.

THE BEAST WITHIN

BODY POSITION When you first begin, lift your head and upper back so that just the tips of your shoulder blades are still touching the floor. Keep your tailbone flat on the floor. Also keep your spine straight and flat, but do not press it down so hard that your back hurts. Keep it down with your powerhouse. Imagine someone is trying to lift your feet from underneath your toes, and you are pressing down and forward through the toes to resist him. This will engage the muscles in your buttocks. Keep your shoulders away from your ears, your neck long, and your feet in Pilates stance.

THE MIND IN MOTION Don't release your powerhouse as you pump. Keep it drawn in. On each exhalation, squeeze the muscles of your inner thighs and pull your navel into your spine. If engaging your buttocks hurts your back, then only engage your abdominals and inner thighs to keep your legs lifted. Keep your arms hard like steel as you pump. If you feel your lower back tighten when you lift your legs, your tight hip flexors are probably doing the work and, consequently, your back is reacting. Men tend to have tight backs and hip flexors. If this applies to you, avoid a sore back by doing the Hundred with bent knees until you become a little more advanced. If your neck gets fatigued, then lower it to the mat and continue. If the pumping aggravates your shoulders, try a smaller pumping range. The Hundred is a fine example of working with the Pilates box. Even though your shoulders are lifted, your shoulders and hips should still maintain the right angles that form a rectangle—or the box. For an additional challenge, you may also shorten the inhalations and lengthen the exhalations (i.e., inhale for three counts and exhale for seven).

CAUTIONS If you are a smoker or have lung issues, perform only 4 to 6 sets and build up your endurance to 10 sets (a hundred pumps) over time. The Hundred is rarely omitted in a Pilates exercise sequence, but if the above modifications don't help, skip this exercise.

THE ROLL UP

BENEFITS: STRENGTHENS THE POWERHOUSE WHILE LENGTHENING THE SPINE AND LEGS

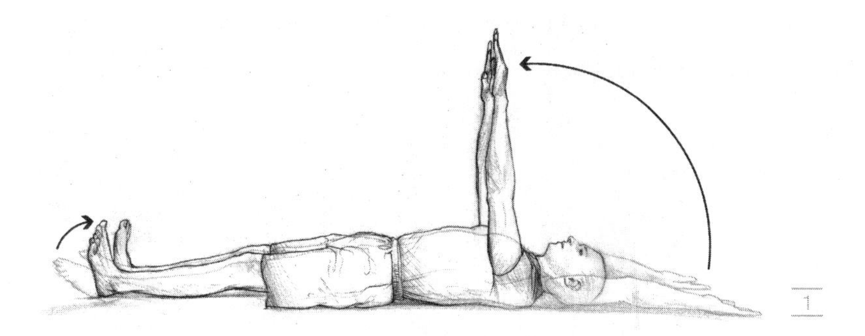
1

After completing the Hundred, you should be lying down on your back with your feet pointed. Raise your arms overhead and reach them away from your feet. Pull your powerhouse in. Inhale and bring your straight arms over the shoulders until they are perpendicular to the floor while simultaneously flexing the ankles.

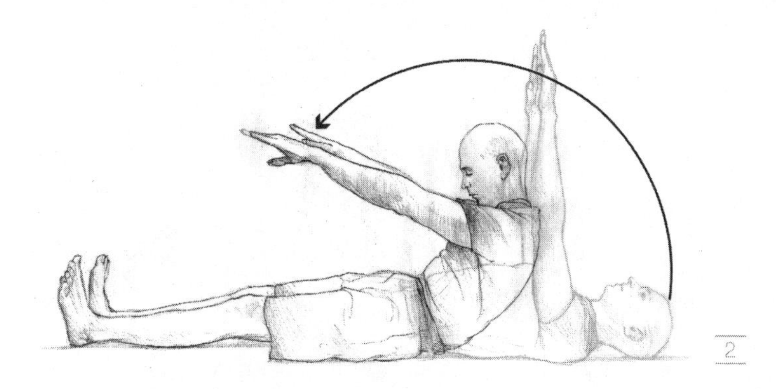
2

Bring your chin to your chest and begin to exhale as you roll your spine off the mat one vertebra at a time. Keep pulling your powerhouse in as you continue your Roll Up.

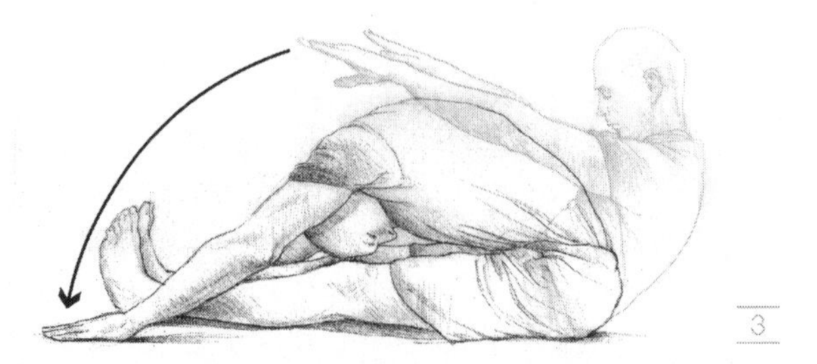

Continue rolling up with the eventual goal of placing your forehead onto your legs and your hands on either side of your heels.

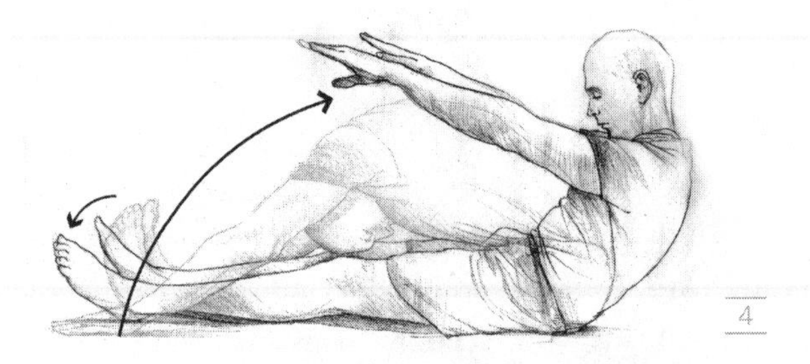

Keep your powerhouse in as you reverse the exercise. Point your toes and inhale as you roll back down, one vertebra at a time, onto the floor.

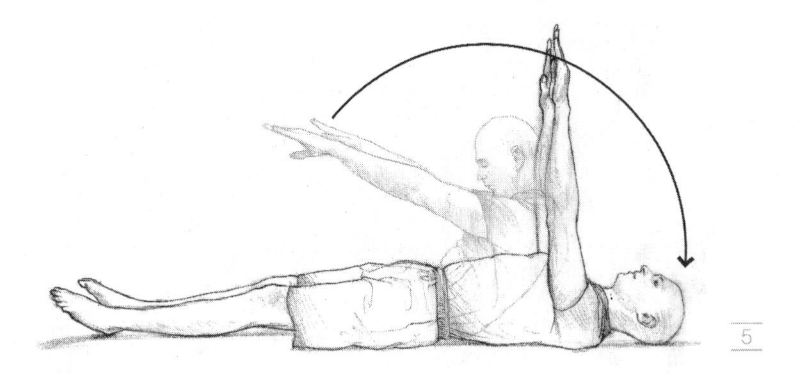

Begin exhaling about halfway down.

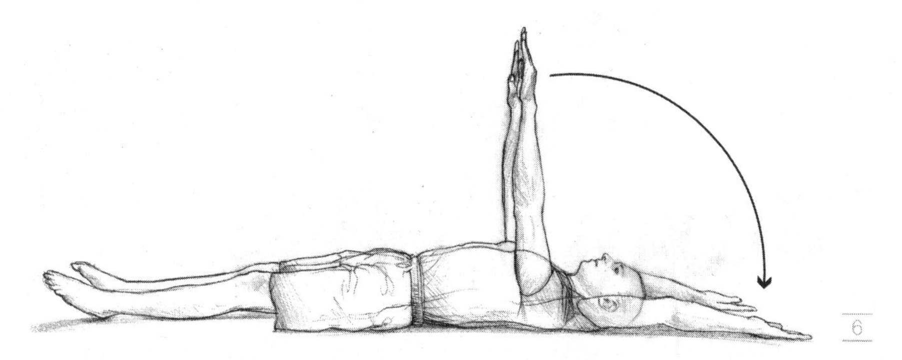

Finish exhaling and roll down as you extend your arms back over your head.

Perform 3 to 5 times.

THE BEAST WITHIN

BODY POSITION Keep your legs together. Don't arch your lower back when you are outstretched (see illustrations 1 and 6). I keep my knees locked throughout this exercise, as Joseph Pilates originally instructed, because it lengthens the backs of the legs and the spine.

THE MIND IN MOTION Roll up with control. Don't throw your body or arms. Press your legs into the mat. Make certain when you bring your arms up (see illustration 1) that your shoulders are pulled down and not shrugged up to your ears. When you reach illustration 3, keep your rib cage lifted off your legs by continuing to pull your powerhouse in and up. If rolling up is difficult or hurts your neck, shoulders and/or lower back, try hooking your ankles under a strap or convenient piece of furniture and bend your knees. With bent knees sit up tall and roll your spine down only as far as you can control. You may assist yourself by walking your hands down and up the backs of your legs as you lower and lift your spine. With this bent leg variation, keep the range of motion small and progressively increase it until you have rolled your entire spine down onto the floor. Articulate your spine in all variations. As you roll up your body, your shoulders should remain squared with your sides and equidistantly away from your hips, thus maintaining the box through the movement. This is a fantastic exercise!

CAUTIONS If the above modifications don't work to alleviate pain, then leave this exercise out.

THE ROLL OVER

BENEFITS: STRENGTHENS THE POWERHOUSE AND UPPER BODY WHILE LENGTHENING THE SPINE

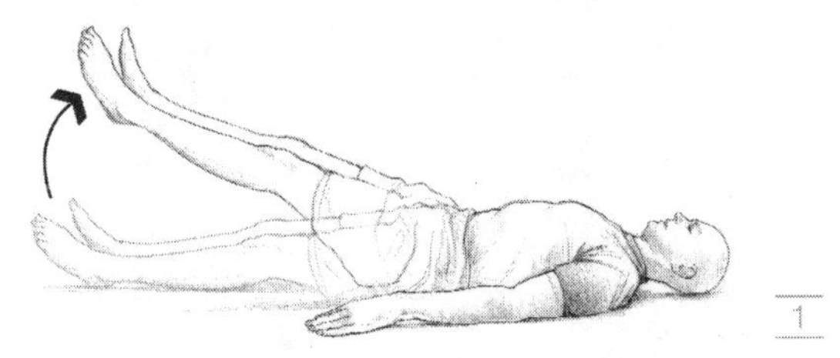

Following the Roll Up, bring the arms back alongside the body. Press your arms into the floor. Keep your neck long and shoulders down, away from your ears. With your heels together and toes slightly apart (Pilates stance) pull your powerhouse in, inhale, and lift your legs up.

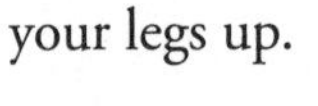

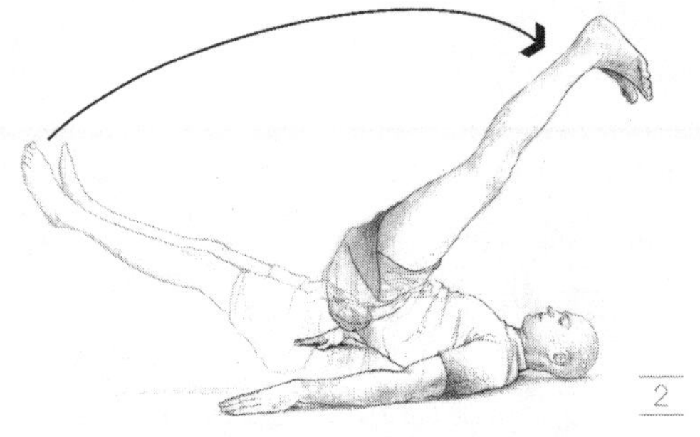

Begin exhaling and peel your hips and spine off the floor.

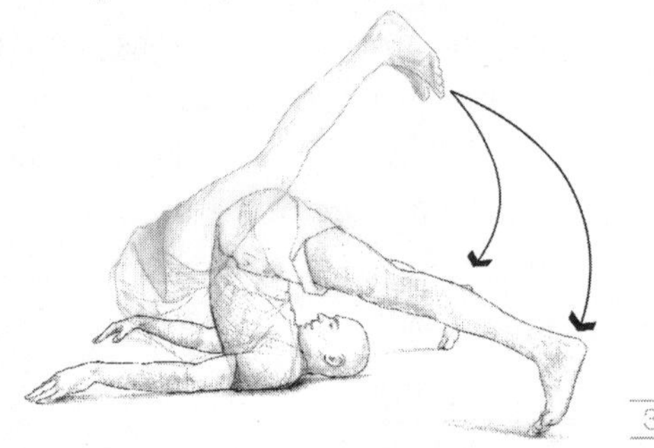

Bring your feet overhead all the way to the floor. Spread your legs in a range from shoulder width to as far as possible.

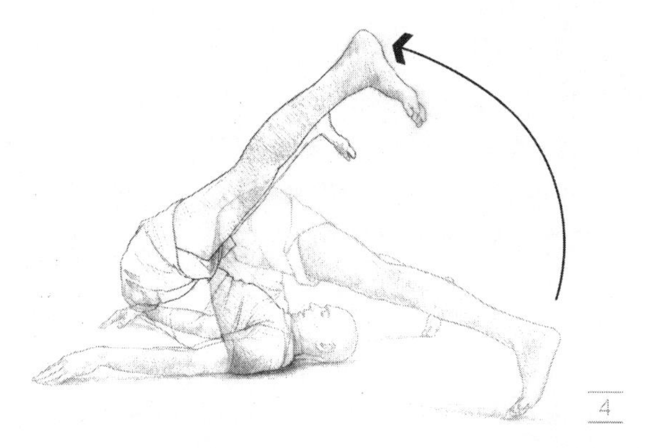

Pull your powerhouse in. Inhale as you begin to roll your spine back down to the floor. Press your arms and shoulders into the mat.

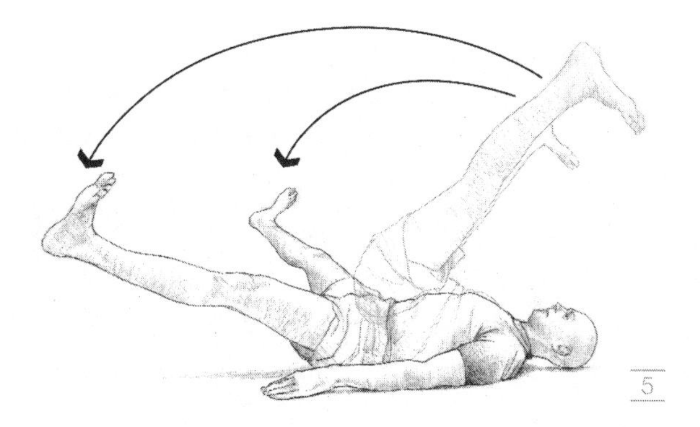

When your spine is all the way back down on the floor, continue to lower your legs and begin exhaling.

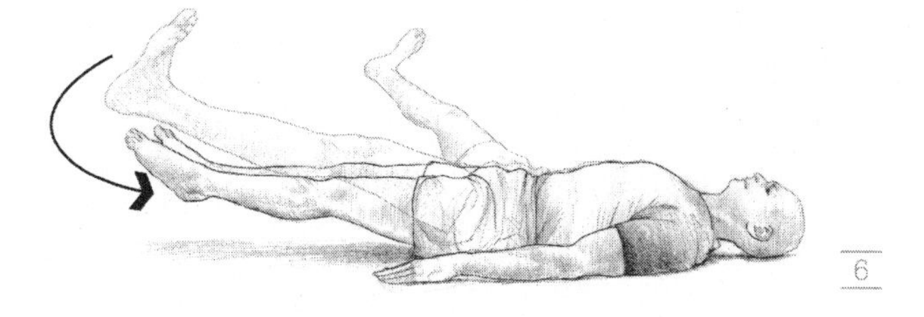

Bring your legs back together in Pilates stance when your feet are two inches off the mat.

Perform five times.

Then perform the exercise 5 more times, but begin with your legs apart, bringing them overhead apart. Bring them together when your toes are on the floor behind your head (see illustration 3), then roll your spine back down with your legs together. (Note: This is the same exact exercise but with the leg positions reversed in each step.)

THE BEAST WITHIN

BODY POSITION Think of lengthening your spine throughout the exercise. Press and lengthen your arms and shoulders down onto the mat. Reach your arms toward your feet to keep your shoulders away from your ears.

THE MIND IN MOTION Do not rush through. Control the exercise entirely. Articulate each vertebra both up and down to the mat. Do not push out your abdominals. Do not let the weight of your legs collapse onto your chest when you bring your legs over. Keep your knees locked. Once your legs are perpendicular to the floor, as your tailbone begins to peel off the mat, try to keep the same 80- to 90-degree angle between your legs and your torso. Keep your hips lifted when your legs are overhead and your feet are on the floor (see illustration 3). Bring your legs overhead only as far as you can comfortably control them. Your range of motion will increase over time. Don't press the back of your head into the floor, or your neck will become sore. As you roll your spine, keep your hips evenly aligned and distanced from each shoulder. Do not micromanage your breathing. Allow your breath to occur with the movement.

CAUTIONS Men have a tendency to forget about the powerhouse and muscle their legs over the bodies with momentum and upper body strength. Leave this exercise out if you are overweight or have neck, shoulder, elbow, back, or hip problems.

THE SINGLE LEG CIRCLES

BENEFITS: WORKS THE LEGS, HIPS, LOWER BACK, AND THE POWERHOUSE

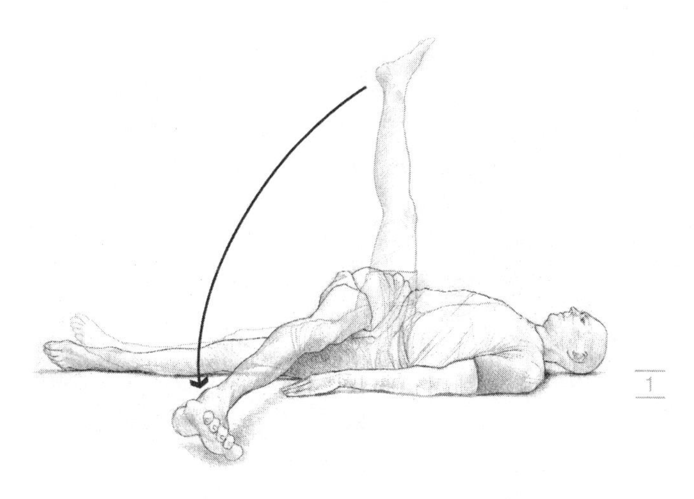

Lying on the floor, raise your right leg to the ceiling with your toes pointed and turned out from your hip; however, you don't have to turn out in this version. Keep the left ankle flexed or extended. We will call the non-circling leg the stable leg. Begin exhaling as you bring your right leg across your left leg until it's parallel to the floor. This will bring your right hip off the mat, but keep both shoulders on the mat, square and away from your ears.

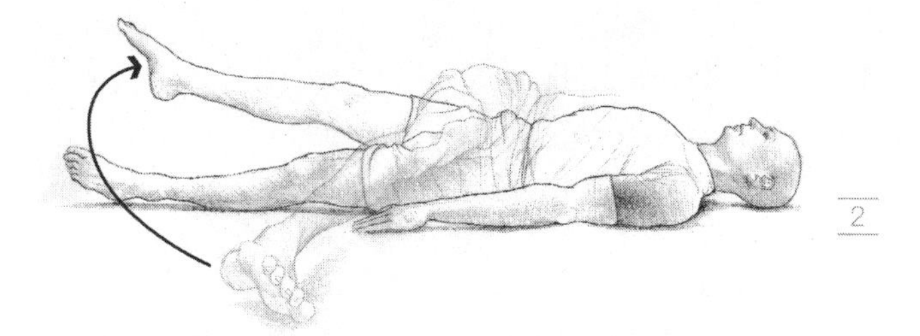

Circle your right foot toward your left foot and finish your exhalation.

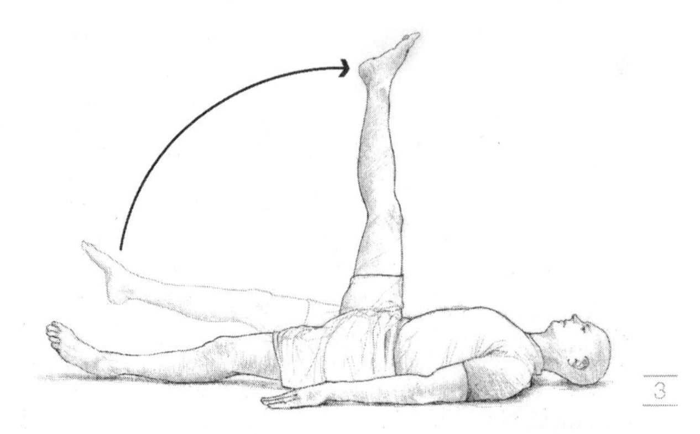

When your right leg passes over your stable leg, begin to inhale. Keeping your powerhouse in, circle your leg back up to the starting position.

Perform this 5 times, then reverse the circle's direction for another 5 repetitions. Then perform 5 forward and 5 reverse repetitions with the left leg as well.

THE BEAST WITHIN

BODY POSITION In modern day Pilates, both hips are kept down on the mat at all times. You may do the exercise with either your hip lifted, as illustrated, or down. This older variation of lifting the hip helps to stretch the entire region around the hip and lower back. For my own body, I do both. Keep your arms, shoulders, and head on the floor with your shoulders down and away from your ears. Keep your upper body relaxed but anchored. Think of lengthening in three directions: toward your two feet and your head.

THE MIND IN MOTION Rotate your leg as widely as you can control it. Start with a small circle and gradually enlarge it as you become stronger. If you feel tightness or discomfort in either your lower back or behind your leg, you may bend the knee on one or both legs. If you bend the knee of your stable leg, make sure the sole of your foot is flat on the ground and keep both hips down while you circle the leg. With this foot flat on the ground and your knee bent upward, your range of motion will be smaller.

CAUTIONS Men tend to have difficulty with this exercise because of tightness in their lower back, hips, and legs. Leave this out if you have any hip problems or if it aggravates your lower back.

ROLLING LIKE A BALL

BENEFITS: MASSAGES THE SPINE, STRENGTHENS THE POWERHOUSE, DEVELOPS YOUR SENSE OF BALANCE—AND, LIKE ALL THE OTHER ROLLING EXERCISES TO COME, WORKS THE LUNGS

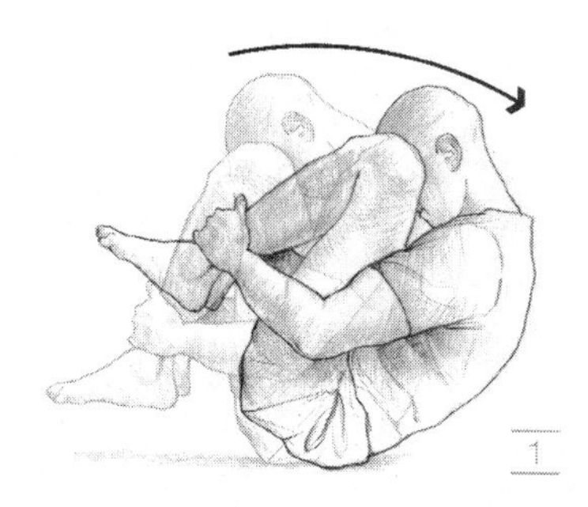

After the single leg circles, roll up to a sitting position. Place your hands on the floor next to your hips. Bring your seat to your feet as you bend your knees. Take hold of your ankles and lift your feet off the floor. Balance on your sit bones. Keep your chin to your chest and try to get your head between your knees. Draw your thighs against your chest. Pull your powerhouse in as you inhale and roll backward.

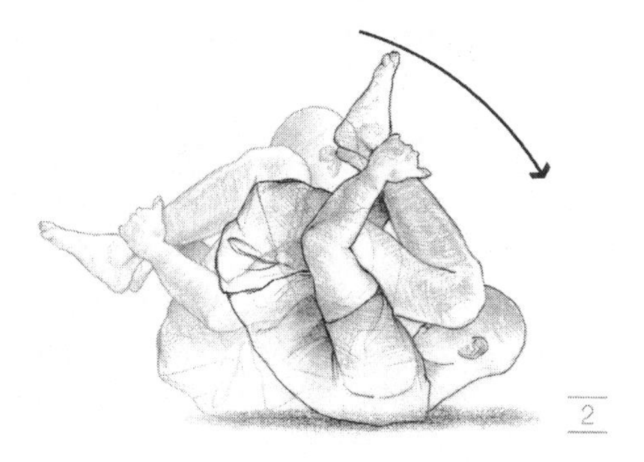

Roll the length of your spine but keep your neck off the floor.

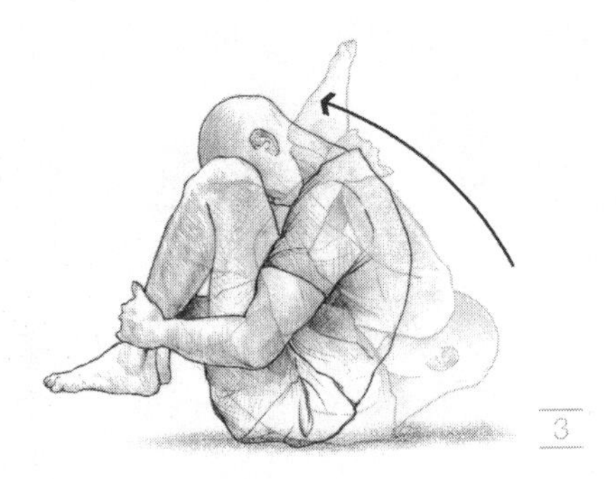

Exhale, keeping your powerhouse pulled in, and roll back up to the original position.

Perform 6 times.

THE BEAST WITHIN

BODY POSITION Try to remain tight like a small package during the entire exercise. Keep your head between your knees and your feet as close to your buttocks as possible. It may take some time before you can assume this ideal position. Think of maintaining a long rounded spine. In Pilates, we sometimes refer to this as your "c-curve."

THE MIND IN MOTION Roll straight back and straight up; don't veer off to the side. Keep your shoulders down and relaxed. Don't throw your head back to initiate the movement or kick your legs for help. Keep your chin to your chest and the powerhouse in. Don't push out the abdominals. If your knee is injured, you have difficulty rounding your back, or your girth makes it difficult to grab hold of your ankles, then hold your hands underneath your legs (on your hamstring muscles) instead. If this exercise is easy for you, then try holding your left ankle with your right hand and grasp your right wrist with your left hand—and roll away!

CAUTIONS If you have neck, shoulder, back, scoliosis, or hip problems, leave this exercise out. If your scoliosis is very slight, you may try it, but concentrate on rolling straight. Don't kick your legs to initiate rolling, as this will result in a precarious movement that lacks powerhouse control.

THE SINGLE LEG STRETCH

BENEFITS: STRENGTHENS THE POWERHOUSE; STRETCHES THE LEGS, HIPS, AND LOWER BACK

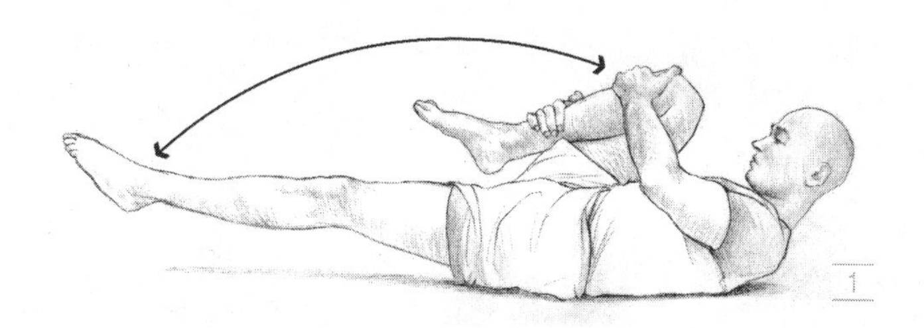

After rolling like a ball, lie on your back with your chin to your chest. Pull your powerhouse in. Bend your right leg into your chest, pulling your right knee (with both hands on your shin) toward your right ear as you inhale. Keep your left leg extended with your toes pointed forward and down.

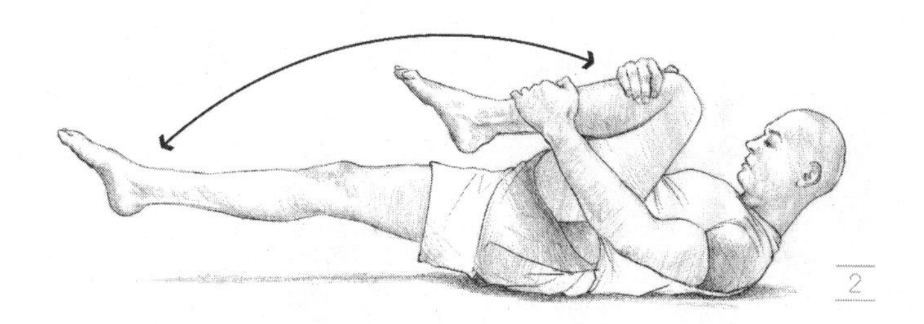

Switch legs as you exhale.

Perform up to 10 times with each leg.

THE BEAST WITHIN

BODY POSITION This is the first exercise in what is commonly referred to as both "the stomach series" and the "series of five." The following four exercises maintain the same body position as this one, and they fully work the powerhouse. From your tailbone to the tips of your shoulder blades, keep your spine on the mat. Where the five exercises vary are in the motions of the arms and legs. Ideally, your extended leg should be level with your eyes or about two inches off the floor. Keep your abdominals in. The buttock of the extended leg should be engaged, with the toes pointed forward and down. Clasp your right ankle with your right hand when you fold your right leg to your chest, and clasp your left ankle with your left hand when you fold your left leg to your chest.

THE MIND IN MOTION If your neck is injured or gets fatigued, you may lower it to the floor. Move through this exercise smoothly. Don't shrug your shoulders up; keep them away from your ears. If your back is injured or sore, you may keep your extended leg at a higher angle off the ground or skip the exercise altogether. If you have knee problems, try pulling your leg in from the back of the thigh (the hamstring muscle). This will allow for less flexion (bend) in your knees. You may also breathe by exhaling as you pull each leg and drawing a short inhalation each time you switch legs.

Once you've mastered this illustrated version, try skimming the floor lightly with your foot when you extend each leg out. For an additional challenge, try keeping your hands behind your head and pull your legs in with only your powerhouse.

CAUTIONS Proceed slowly or leave this exercise out if any of the modifications for the neck, shoulders, back, or knees do not help.

THE DOUBLE LEG STRETCH

BENEFITS: STRENGTHENS THE POWERHOUSE AND BUTTOCKS; STRETCHES THE HIPS, LEGS, AND LOWER BACK; AND OPENS THE SHOULDERS

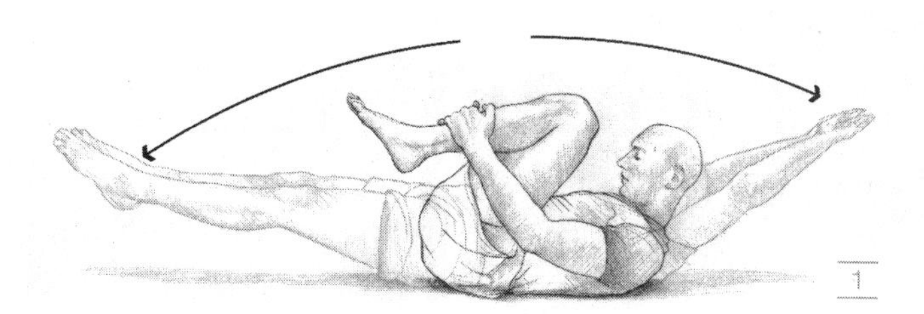

Remain in the same position that you were just in for the Single Leg Stretch, but this time bring *both* knees to your chest and grasp each ankle. Pull your powerhouse in. Inhale as you extend your legs out and reach with your arms straight back behind your head.

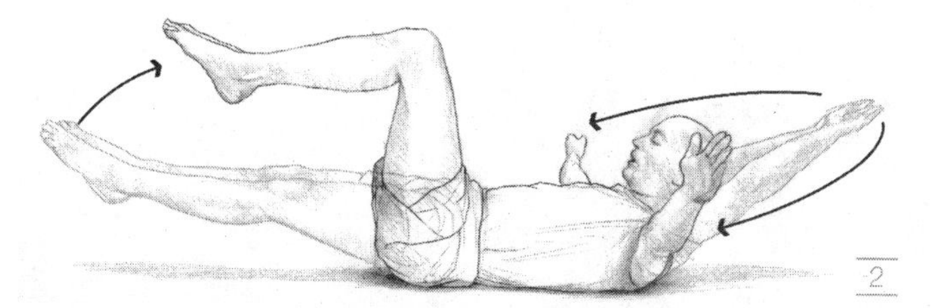

Exhale as you circle your straight arms around and fold your knees back to your chest.

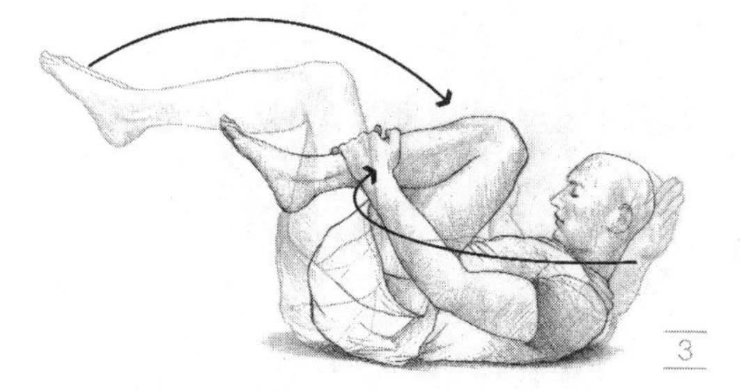

Complete the exhale and hug your ankles or shins with your chin to your chest.

Perform between 5 and 10 times.

THE BEAST WITHIN

BODY POSITION Keep your tailbone pressed down and flat throughout the exercise. Anchor your spine to the mat from your tailbone to the tips of your shoulder blades. Keep your neck long; you should not feel any strain in the front of it.

THE MIND IN MOTION Measure your control of this exercise by three criteria. First, keep your abdomen pulled in and firm; don't let it rise or release when you extend your legs out. Second, do not allow your lower back to arch. If it does, try extending your legs out at a higher angle. Third, your lower back should not hurt. If it does, and lifting your legs higher doesn't relieve the pain, leave this exercise out. Don't thrust your legs out. The movement in this exercise should be smooth like a glider cutting through the air. If you have a neck injury, you may leave this out or try it with your head resting on the floor or on a pillow. If you don't have much neck strength or endurance, lower your head to the mat before it fatigues and then continue the exercise. If you have knee problems or are overweight, hug underneath your thighs on the hamstring muscles, instead of your ankles, when you draw your legs in.

To make this exercise more challenging, progressively lower your legs until you can do the exercise with them extended 2 inches off the mat or at eye level. You may also try placing your hands along the outside of your thighs when your legs are extended. This position resembles standing at attention.

CAUTIONS Men tend to lose the powerhouse connection by using only arm, shoulder, and leg strength when the arms and legs extend. To prevent this, make certain you extend the legs out to a height that you can control, with the powerhouse engaged throughout the movement. Proceed slowly or leave this exercise out if the above modifications don't alleviate pain in your neck, shoulder, back, hip, or knee problems.

THE SINGLE STRAIGHT LEG STRETCH

BENEFITS: STRENGTHENS THE POWERHOUSE AND LENGTHENS THE LEGS

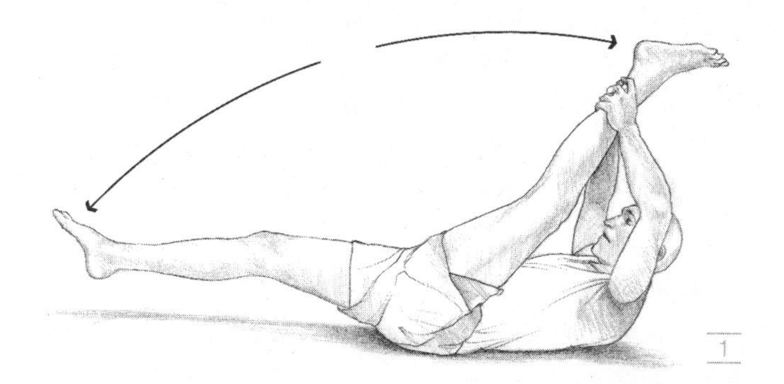

Upon finishing the Double Leg Stretch, you should be hugging both ankles. Now take hold of your left leg with both hands, and straighten your left leg to the ceiling. Keep your right leg straight and suspended off the floor. Pull your powerhouse in and inhale.

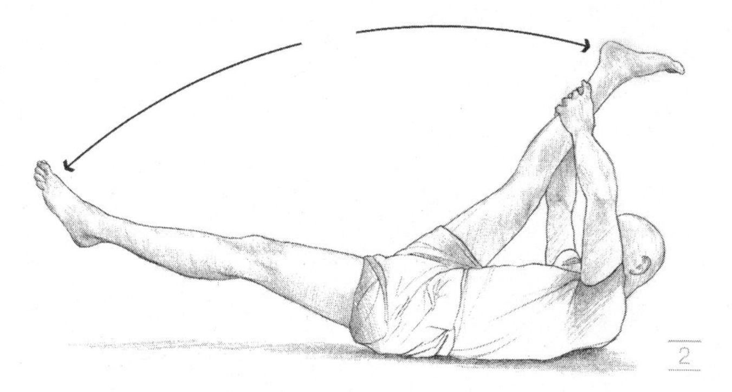

Switch legs in a scissor-like fashion and pull your right leg as you exhale. Keep your abdomen pulled in and firm.

Perform 5 to 10 times.

THE BEAST WITHIN

BODY POSITION From your tailbone to the tips of your shoulder blades, keep your spine flat on the mat throughout the exercise. Hold your hands anywhere on your leg that allows you to maintain a straight leg and an anchored torso.

THE MIND IN MOTION If your neck becomes tired, lower your head. If this exercise aggravates your back, then keep your extended leg either higher in the air or bent at the knee with your foot on the floor when you pull your other leg up. If your knees are problematic, try performing the exercise by pulling on the hamstring muscle.

If you're more advanced, work your powerhouse harder by placing your hands alongside your body or beneath your bottom with palms facedown on the mat, and rapidly kick your legs one at a time. It will look as if you are trying to kick your ears with a single straight leg, and then the other, and so on. If you try this more difficult variation, don't let your lower back arch.

CAUTIONS Men tend to have tight hamstring muscles and tight backs, which makes this a challenging exercise. Do not pull your leg so hard that your upper back peels off the floor. If the above modifications do not help, then leave this exercise out for any neck, shoulder, back, hip, or knee problems.

THE DOUBLE STRAIGHT LEG STRETCH

BENEFITS: STRENGTHENS THE POWERHOUSE

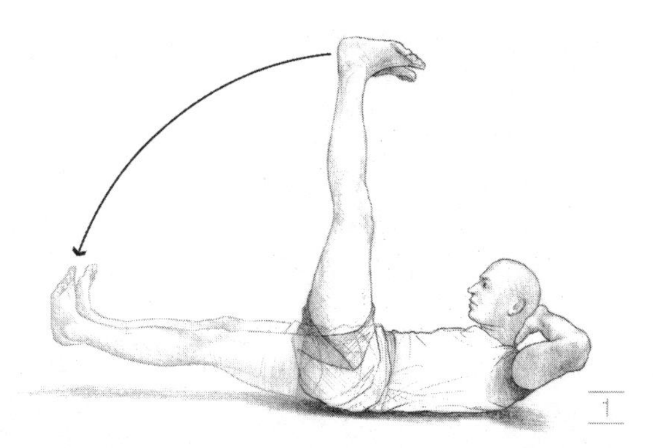

After you finish the Single Straight Leg Stretch, extend both legs up and together toward the ceiling. Your spine should remain touching the floor from your tailbone to the tips of your shoulder blades. Keep your hands behind your head with tightly interlaced fingers, or hand over hand. Pull your powerhouse in. Lower both legs in a controlled descent while inhaling.

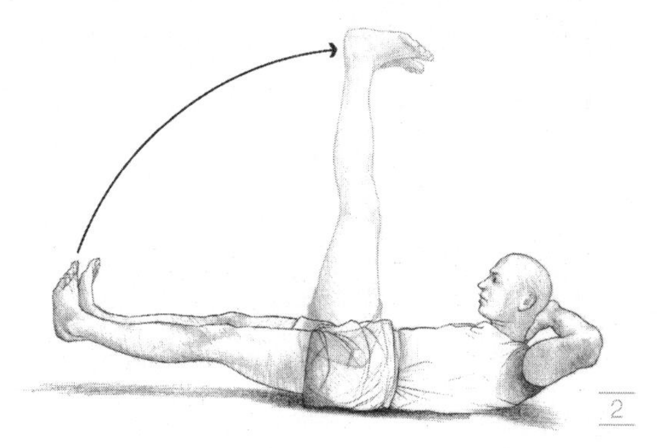

Exhale as you lift both legs back up toward the ceiling, until your thighs are vertical to the floor.

Perform 5 to 10 times.

THE BEAST WITHIN

BODY POSITION Anchor your body to the floor. The illustrations show the chin jutting forward; the chin position is slightly exagerated to convey the importance of not pulling your head up with your hands. Rather, lift your upper body with your upper abdominals while keeping your elbows wide. Keep your toes either pointed or flexed (as illustrated). I turn out my legs a bit to avoid fatiguing my hip flexors on the front tops of the thighs. It is fine to have the knees slightly bent, if you can not yet straighten your legs. Make sure to start and finish with your thighs perpendicular to the floor.

THE MIND IN MOTION When you first begin, play it safe and perform this exercise with a small range of motion by lowering your legs a few inches at most and then return to the starting position. As you lift your legs, it helps to think of lengthening your hamstrings through your calves, all the way to your feet. Control the Double Leg Stretch by keeping your stomach pulled in and firm. Your lower back shouldn't arch or hurt. If it does hurt, or if you have neck and shoulder problems, try placing your hands under the buttocks, head on the floor, and lower your legs with a small range of motion. Keeping a small range of motion also helps if you have heavy legs, until you strengthen the powerhouse.

CAUTIONS Men tend to have tight legs and backs. If you have tight legs, your knees may naturally stay slightly bent, which is fine. But if you have a weak powerhouse and/or a tight back, be careful not to arch your lower back. Leave this exercise out if the modifications for your neck, shoulder, back, or hip problems don't help.

THE CRISSCROSS

BENEFITS: STRENGTHENS THE POWERHOUSE AND WORKS THE WAIST

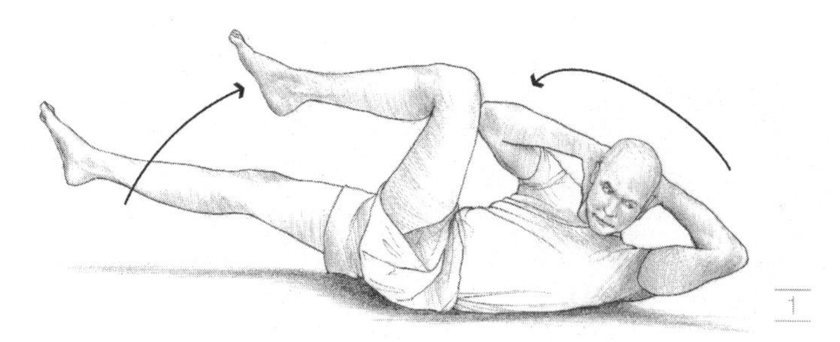

From the Double Straight Leg Stretch, bend your knees and then extend your right leg out at an angle between 30 and 45 degrees. Your left leg should create a 90-degree angle at the knee, with a vertical thigh and a horizontal shin. Hold your hands centered behind your head, with your fingers tightly interlaced, or hand over hand. Keep your shoulders lifted off the mat, and pull the powerhouse in. Twist your torso to the left, touching your right elbow to your left knee and inhale. Hold your breath while in this position for two full seconds (i.e., one Mississippi, two Mississippi).

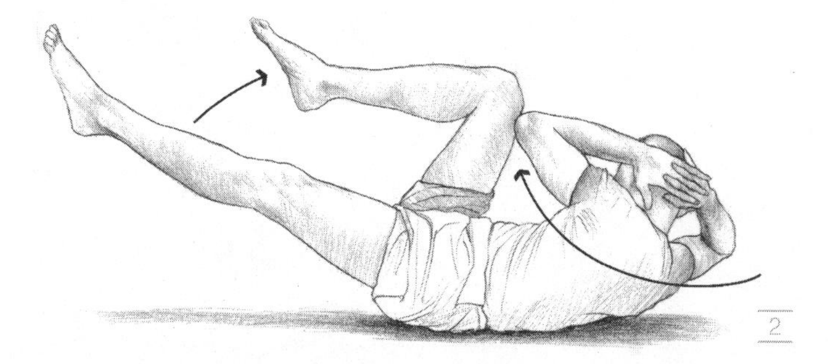

Switch legs as you twist your torso to the right, touching your left elbow to your right knee and exhale, releasing the exhalation in this position for two full seconds.

Perform 5 times for each side.

THE BEAST WITHIN

BODY POSITION It is easy to cheat in this exercise. That said, don't cheat. Keep the thigh of your bent leg vertical, as opposed to drawing the knee in farther. This will make you use your powerhouse to lift your torso high enough to reach the bent knee. Keep your fingers tightly interlaced so you're not tempted to let your hands slide apart when you're reaching your elbow toward your knee. Keep both shoulders lifted off of the mat.

THE MIND IN MOTION If you want to be a bit more dynamic, you may also perform the Crisscross without the two count pause in each position. Without the pause, you will resemble a boxer in training as you move smoothly from knee to knee. Keep your powerhouse tight, tight, tight; don't release your stomach muscles. Here's another variation which engages a different area of the powerhouse. Instead of touching the elbow to the opposite knee, bring the elbow all the way over your body, as if to touch the floor on the opposite side with it.

CAUTIONS Proceed slowly or leave this exercise out if you have neck, shoulder, rib, or back problems.

THE SPINE STRETCH FORWARD

BENEFITS: LENGTHENS THE SPINE AND LEGS AND STRENGTHENS THE POWERHOUSE

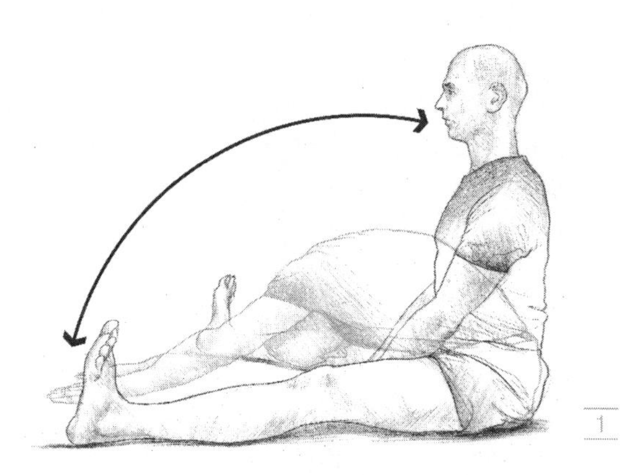

After the Crisscross, sit up tall with your legs straight and more than shoulder width apart. Keep your feet flexed at the ankles, with your knees rotated toward the ceiling. Rest your hands lightly on the floor in front of you. Bring your chin to your chest and, as you exhale, slide your hands and body in front of you as far as you can go. Then inhale as you stack your vertebra up one at a time until you are sitting up tall again.

Perform 3 to 5 times.

THE BEAST WITHIN

BODY POSITION Nowadays this exercise is often done with the arms extended out and parallel to the floor. This "hands on the floor" variation structures the movement of the spine nicely. You may do either version.

THE MIND IN MOTION Keep your powerhouse pulled in and up at all times. Keep your neck long throughout the exercise. If you have difficulty sitting up tall, try bending your knees as much as is necessary to allow for a tall spine. Pull your shoulders down as you return to the starting position. If keeping your ankles flexed and your legs straight makes your hip flexors cramp, then stop the exercise, lie back, and rotate your legs left and right at the hip sockets to release the cramp. In future workouts, try pointing your feet and/or turning them out so you don't experience the same cramp.

CAUTIONS The tightness in many men's bodies inhibit the range of motion. That's okay. This exercise will work to loosen your tight legs and back. If you are overweight, your girth may also hinder the range of motion—but your commitment to get fit will take care of that in just a matter of time! Leave this exercise out if it aggravates your neck, shoulders, or back.

THE OPEN LEG ROCKER

BENEFITS: STRENGTHENS THE POWERHOUSE; LENGTHENS THE SPINE AND LEGS; WORKS THE LUNGS; MASSAGES THE BACK

You've just finished the Spine Stretch Forward. Exhale as you lean back and pull your powerhouse in as if preparing to absorb the impact of a cannonball hitting your stomach. Bend your knees and take hold of your ankles.

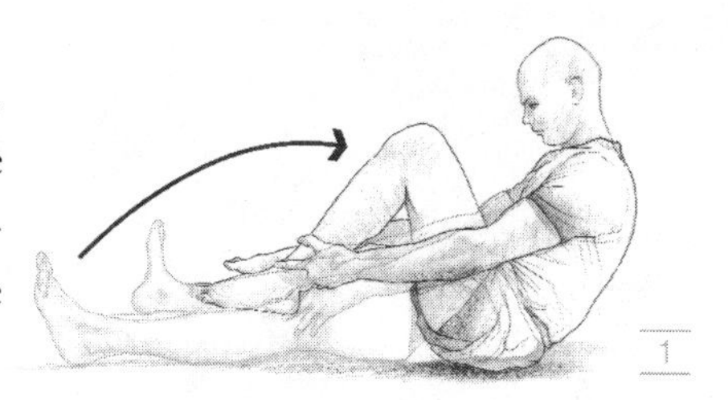

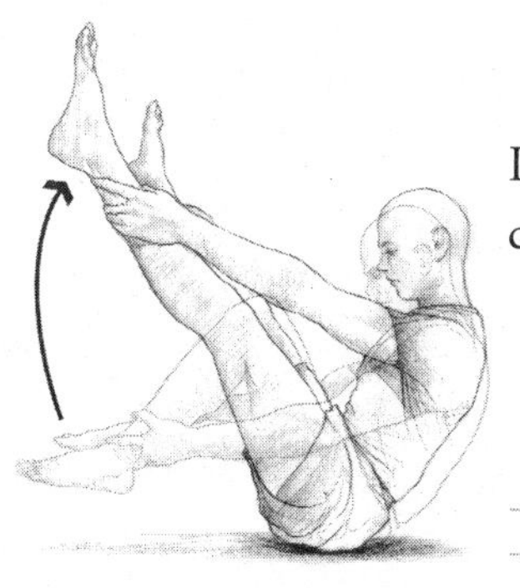

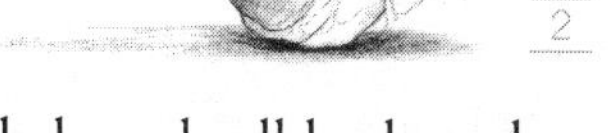

Inhale and straighten your arms and legs. Bring your chin to your chest. Balance yourself on your sit bones.

Exhale and roll backward one vertebra at a time onto your upper back.

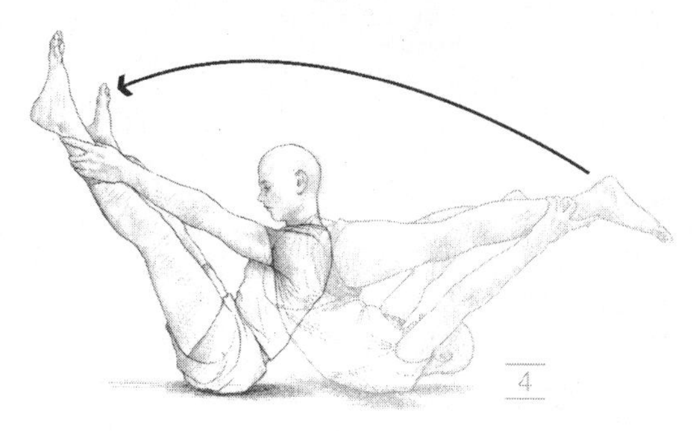

Pull your powerhouse in. Inhale as you roll back up and balance upon your sit bones.

Perform 6 times.

THE BEAST WITHIN

BODY POSITION Adjust your leg spread to allow yourself to balance before rolling back. The closer your legs are together, the harder it will be to balance. Try six inches outside of shoulder width to shoulder width as your starting position. Keep your arms and legs straight. This exercise will reveal any disparity there might be between your flexibility and strength. If you're flexible enough to hold your ankles with straight arms and legs while maintaining a tall back, but unable to roll back up from the floor and balance in the sitting position, your powerhouse probably isn't strong enough yet.

THE MIND IN MOTION If you have trouble rolling up on the first repetition, try opening your legs wider. Or, instead of holding your ankles, try holding your shin, calves, or even your hamstrings—wherever you can maintain straight arms and legs to roll up into a balanced position. Hold your powerhouse in firmly. Don't arch your lower spine when balancing. Don't roll onto the top of your neck. If you find rolling is too difficult, try balancing in the first position (see illustration 1). Then progress to balancing in the second position (see illustration 2).

For a fun challenge, try to touch your toes on the floor behind you when you roll backward. For an even greater challenge, bring your legs together and hold onto your toes as you perform the exercise." Good luck!

CAUTIONS Men tend to have some difficulty straightening their legs. Grasp anywhere along your legs that allows you to keep them straight throughout the exercise. Use your powerhouse to motor the roll, not the momentum of dropping your head or kicking your legs. Leave this exercise out if you have neck, shoulder, hip, or back problems. Leave this out if you have scoliosis. If your scoliosis is very slight, you may try it, but be certain to roll straight.

THE CORKSCREW

BENEFITS: STRENGTHENS YOUR POWERHOUSE, SHOULDERS, BUTTOCKS, AND ARMS; STRENGTHENS AND LENGTHENS YOUR WAIST AND SIDES

After the Open Leg Rocker, lie down on the floor from your head to your toes. Press your arms into the floor along your sides with your shoulders drawn down and away from your ears. Pull your powerhouse in. Exhale and bring your straight legs up perpendicular to the floor. Your entire spine should be flat on the floor.

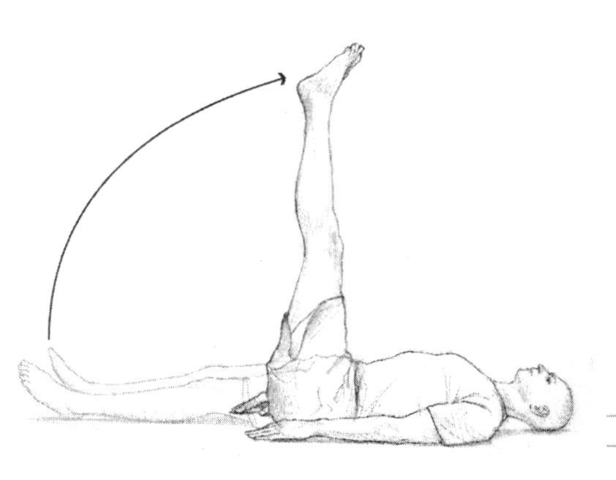

1

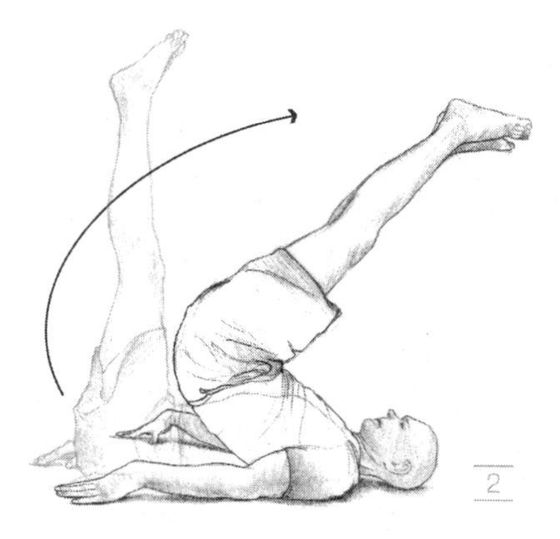

2

Inhale as you press your hands and arms into the floor. Using your powerhouse, peel your hips and then your spine up one vertebra at a time off the mat—until your knees are suspended over the lower region of your face. This will require you to be perched on your mid to upper back.

Drive your hips forward as you continue to press your arms into the floor, and squeeze your buttocks as your straight legs reach up to the ceiling. Keep your stomach pulled in.

3

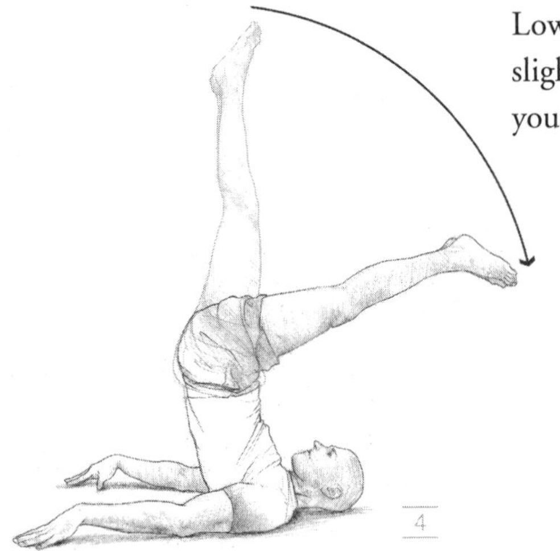

Lower both legs together to an angle that's slightly above parallel to the floor, while keeping your spine and hips lifted.

4

Exhale and lower the right side of your body to the floor as you begin to circle your legs around in a clockwise direction.

5

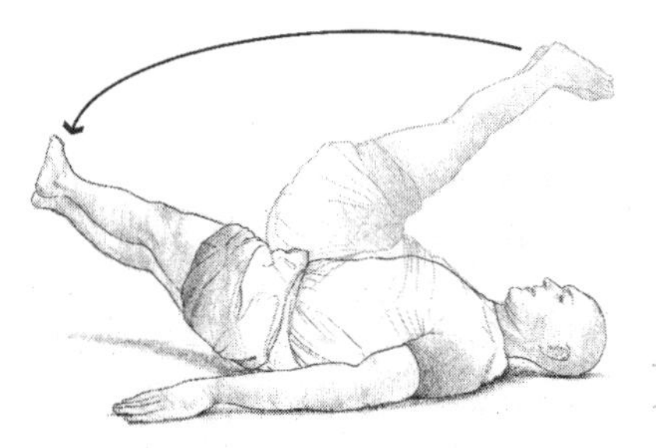

Once the entire right side of your torso is down, continue to circle your legs around clockwise.

6

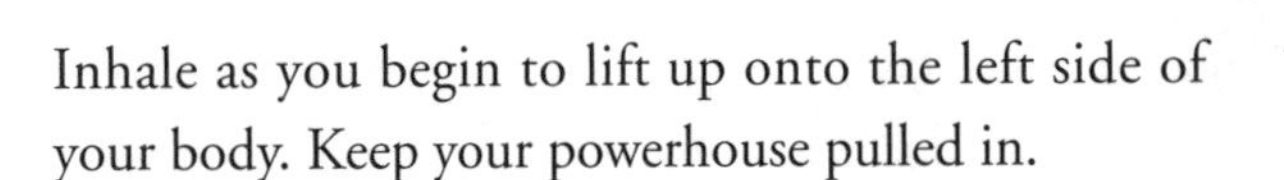

Inhale as you begin to lift up onto the left side of your body. Keep your powerhouse pulled in.

7

Continue up the left side of your body.

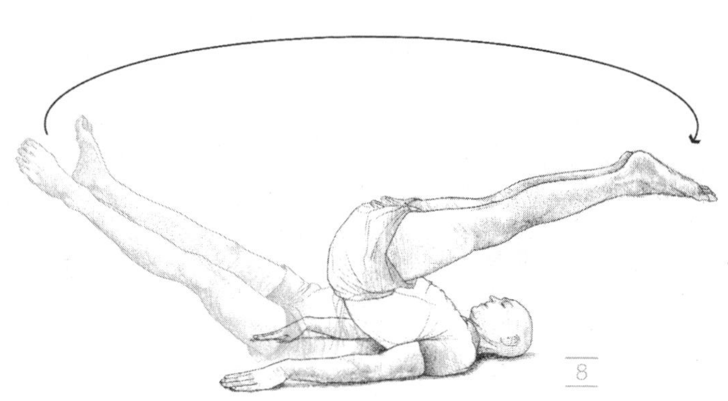

Your legs arrive overhead at an angle just above parallel to the floor with your weight evenly distributed across your upper back, shoulders, and arms.

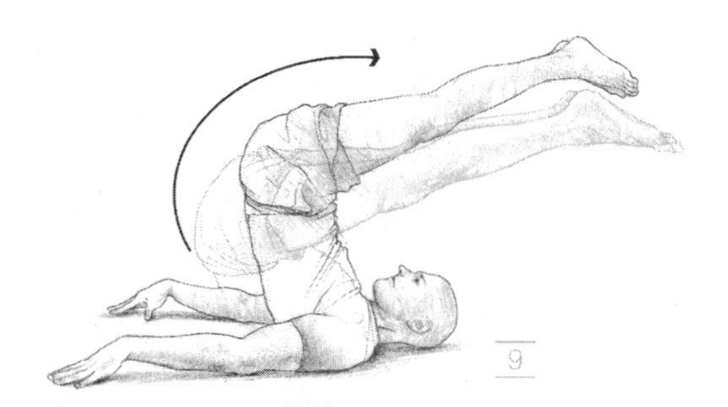

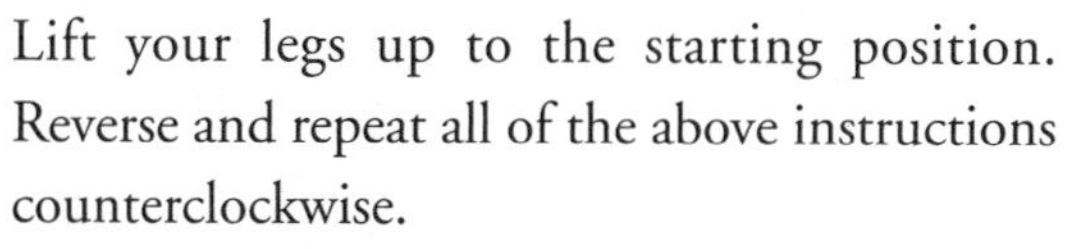

Lift your legs up to the starting position. Reverse and repeat all of the above instructions counterclockwise.

Perform 3 times in each direction.

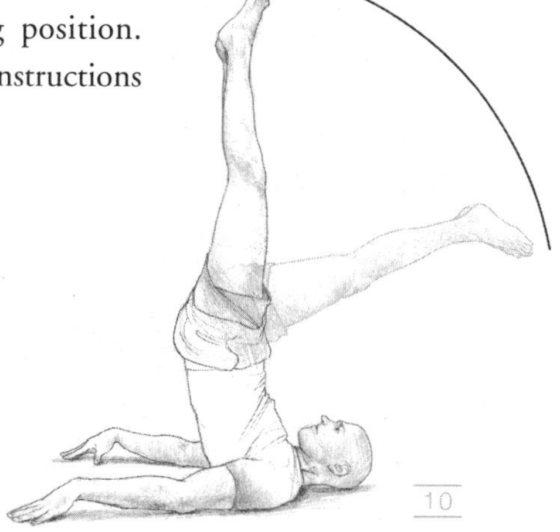

THE BEAST WITHIN

BODY POSITION The illustrations depict the advanced variation of the Corkscrew. It requires a bit of practice to do it this way. Reach your arms long toward your feet, and anchor your shoulders and arms down onto the mat. At all times keep your shoulders away from your ears. Keep your knees and elbows locked so that all four limbs remain straight throughout the exercise.

THE MIND IN MOTION The easiest way to learn the Corkscrew is to begin by lying on your back with only your legs in the air, as demonstrated in the first illustration. Do not lift your bottom in the air at this point. Circle your legs around clockwise, then circle them counterclockwise. Exhale during the first half of each circle and inhale during the second half of each circle. Control the entire movement. Don't allow momentum to take away your control. If a tight back or tight legs makes it difficult, try the exercise with bent knees. If you have a vulnerable lower back, keep your hands under your buttocks when circling without lifting your hips and spine. You mustn't allow your lower back to arch up off the mat when your buttocks, spine, and torso are on the floor. When you have mastered this "spine down" version, you may then progress to lifting your hips slightly at the end of each circle (see the hip lift in illustration 2, but do not lift as high off the ground). Finally, you may attempt the complete Corkscrew sequence as illustrated.

For more of a challenge, lower your feet as low as possible (see illustration 5), with your hips lifted up as you begin to circle your legs around. Keep your powerhouse pulled in throughout the movement.

CAUTIONS Proceed slowly, according to the suggested modifications, or leave this exercise out if you have neck, shoulder, elbow, back, or hip problems.

THE SAW

BENEFITS: STRENGTHENS THE WAIST AND POWERHOUSE; WORKS THE LUNGS; LENGTHENS THE LEGS AND SPINE; OPENS THE CHEST

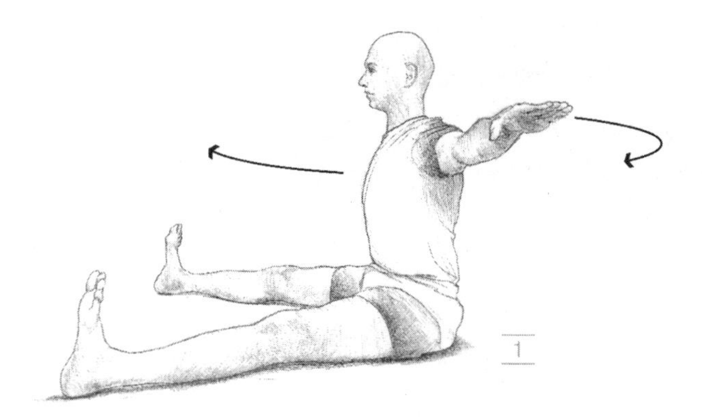

Sitting up tall after the Corkscrew, flex your ankles and open your legs a few inches more than shoulder width apart. Hold your arms up and outstretched to the sides. Pull your powerhouse in. Lock your shoulder blades back and inhale.

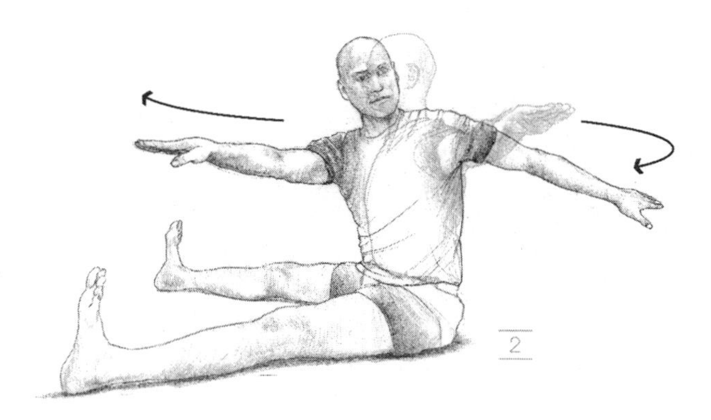

Twist your torso to the left.

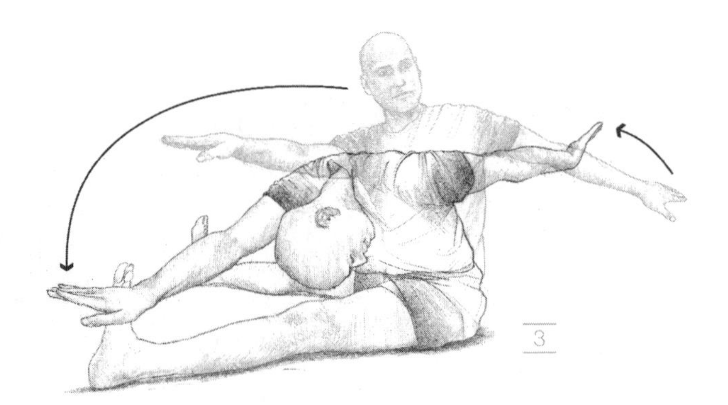

Bend forward and "slice" the outside of your left foot with your forward-reaching right hand. Simultaneously, reach back with your left hand palm up, and exhale. Sit up tall and untwist to the starting position, (see illustration 1). Repeat on the opposite side.

Perform 3 times on each side.

THE BEAST WITHIN

BODY POSITION Keep your powerhouse in. Your legs should be anywhere from shoulder width to slightly wider than shoulder-width apart. Your arms should be straight and long, stretching out in opposite directions at all times.

THE MIND IN MOTION If you find that your lower back is rounded and you cannot sit up tall, bend your knees as much as necessary to sit upright. (*Note:* Bent knees may inhibit your ability to stretch forward.)

To get the most out of this exercise, focus on keeping the hip down as you reach toward the opposing foot. Also focus on reaching your hands in opposite directions to maximize the opening and twisting of your chest.

CAUTIONS Men commonly have a limited range of motion due to tight shoulders, backs, and hamstring muscles. The exercise functions to open these tight areas. Proceed slowly if you have neck or shoulder problems. Skip this exercise if you have rib or back problems.

THE SWAN DIVE

BENEFITS: LENGTHENS THE SPINE; STRENGTHENS THE BACK, ARMS, AND BUTTOCKS

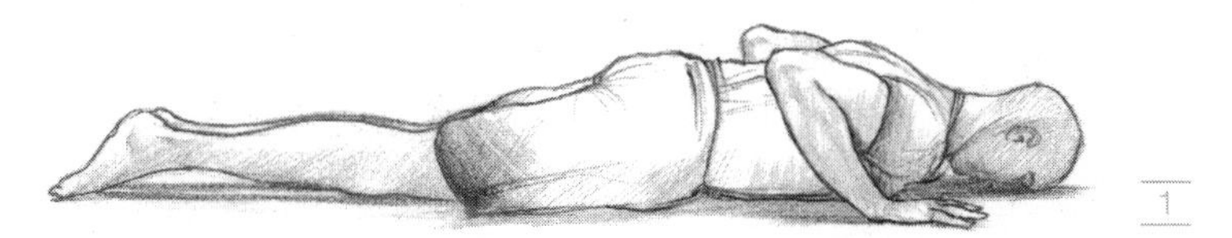

After the Saw, turn over onto your stomach. Touch your forehead to the floor and place the palms of your hands down under your shoulders.

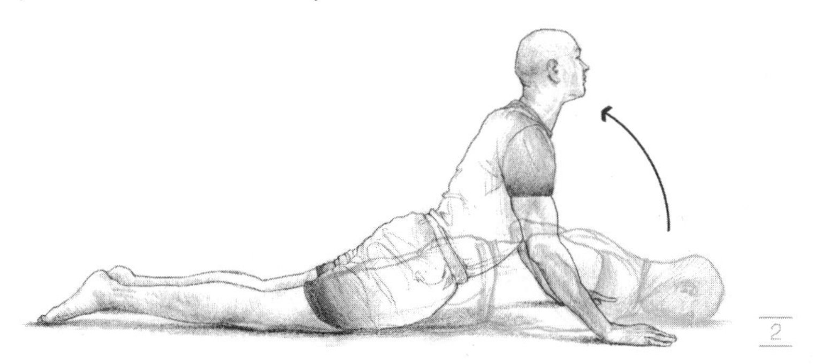

Inhale as you draw your powerhouse in, while lifting your chest high into the air. Keep your shoulders down and back.

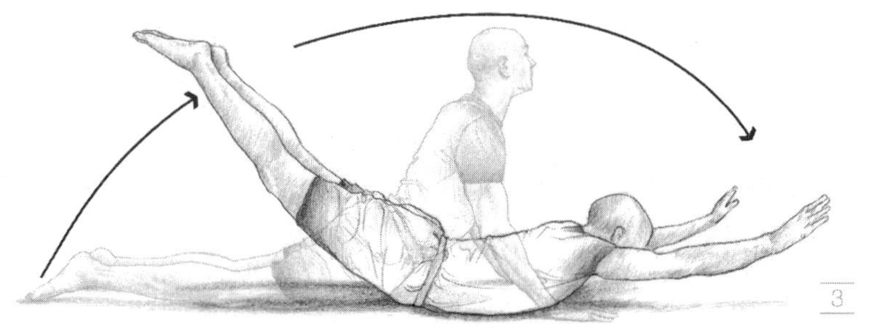

Shoot your hands forward and up off the floor as you rock forward and exhale.

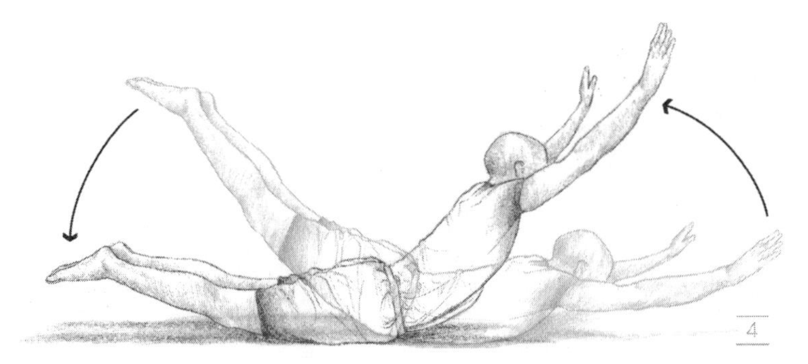

Inhale as you lift your chest (with your hands still elevated off the floor) and rock backward.

Rock up and down 6 times.

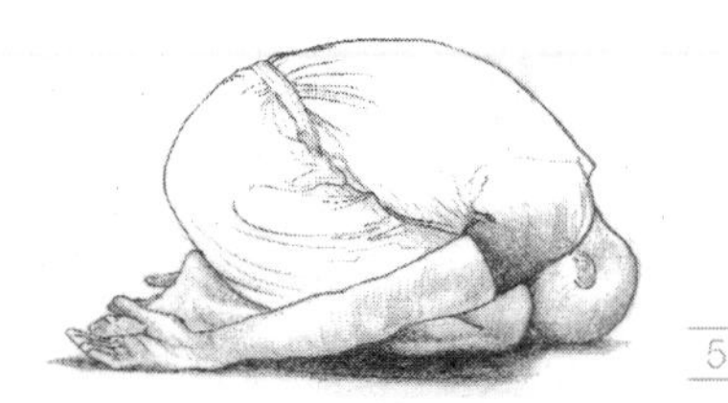

Sit back on you heels with your forehead on your knees. Breathe in this position for up to 5 breaths to release your back muscles.

THE BEAST WITHIN

BODY POSITION To begin, lift your upper body as high off the mat as you can. Think of your entire spine and body lengthening upward. It helps to imagine someone pulling your legs out of your hips.

THE MIND IN MOTION If necessary, try holding just the first position for many workouts to let your body open up and strengthen before attempting to rock back and forth. If this is too difficult, try lifting your upper body with your forearms anchored (instead of your hands) on the floor.

While rocking, you may extend your hands palm up as if you just dunked a basketball and are hanging backward from the rim. You may also rock with your arms out to the sides instead of forward. If you do it with your arms out to the sides, try rotating your palms up and back when your chest is lifted, and rotate your palms forward and down when your legs are in the air. If sitting back on your heels hurts your knees (see illustration 5), then turn onto your back and hug your legs to your chest by holding the backs of your thighs (your hamstrings).

CAUTIONS Since the Swan Dive is not particularly friendly to the male anatomy, adjust yourself accordingly before rocking! Due to tight backs, hip flexors, and shoulders, men typically find these back-bending exercises difficult, especially in the beginning. Leave this exercise out if you have neck, shoulder, rib, back, hip, or knee problems.

THE SINGLE LEG KICK

BENEFITS: STRENGTHENS THE LEGS, BUTTOCKS, POWERHOUSE, BACK, SHOULDERS, AND ARMS

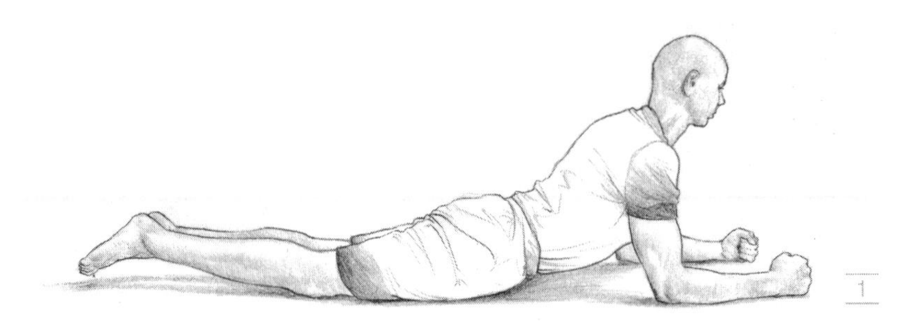

From sitting back on your heels at the end of the Swan Dive, bring yourself forward onto parallel forearms with tight fists. Pull your powerhouse in and lift your spine. Draw the shoulders down and back. Lift your feet slightly off the mat with your toes pointed. Keep your stomach lifted off the floor.

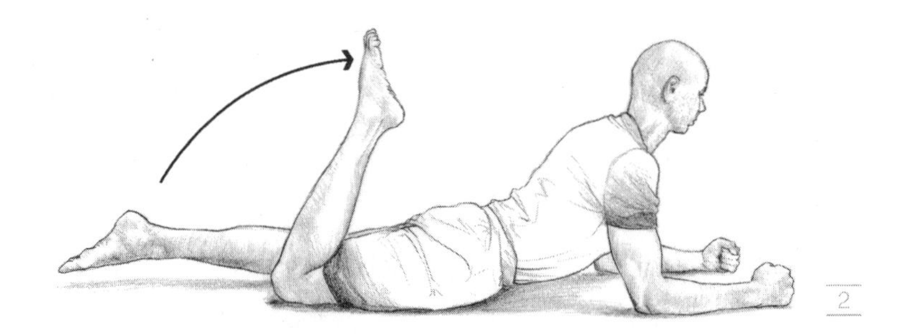

Inhale and kick your right heel twice toward your right buttock.

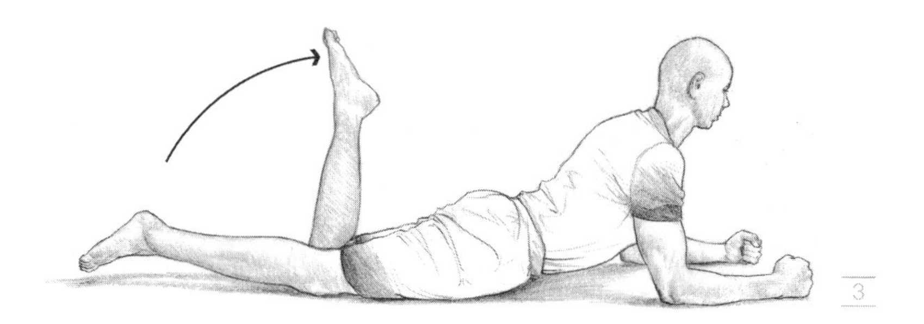

Exhale and kick your left heel twice toward your left buttock.

Perform 6 times with each leg.

THE BEAST WITHIN

BODY POSITION Keep your spine lifted and long with your forearms pressing firmly into the mat. Your nonkicking foot should remain lifted off the mat while you kick with the other one. When your legs are lifting off the floor, you should be able to feel it in the backs of the legs and buttocks. Keep your powerhouse pulled in and up at all times and your shoulders down and back. Don't let your neck and head collapse into your shoulders.

THE MIND IN MOTION If you have a tight back, you might not be able to lift your spine that much (see illustration 1). Just do your best and don't let your spine or stomach sink. Instead of double kicking toward your bottom, try a single kick.

CAUTIONS Proceed slowly or leave this exercise out if you have any neck or shoulder problems. Leave this exercise out if you have any elbow, rib, back, or knee problems.

THE DOUBLE LEG KICKS

BENEFITS: STRENGTHENS THE BACK, BUTTOCKS, ARMS, LEGS, AND POWERHOUSE; OPENS THE CHEST AND SHOULDERS

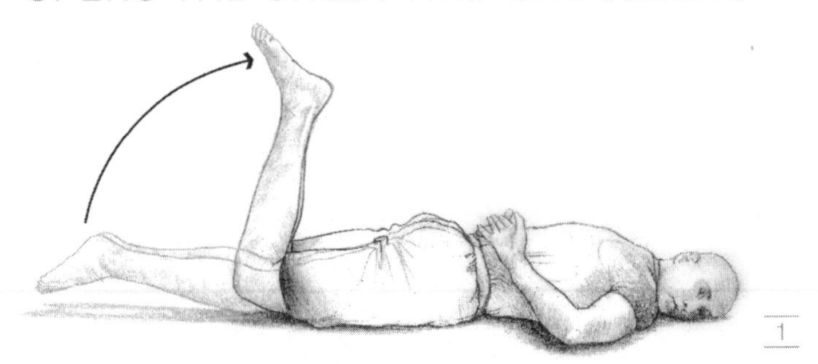

Lie down on your chest and stomach with your left cheek on the mat and your hands on top of each other placed on your lower back. Your elbows should be down at your sides. Pull your powerhouse in. Exhale as you bend your knees to 90 degrees, lift them both off the floor, and drive your hips into the mat.

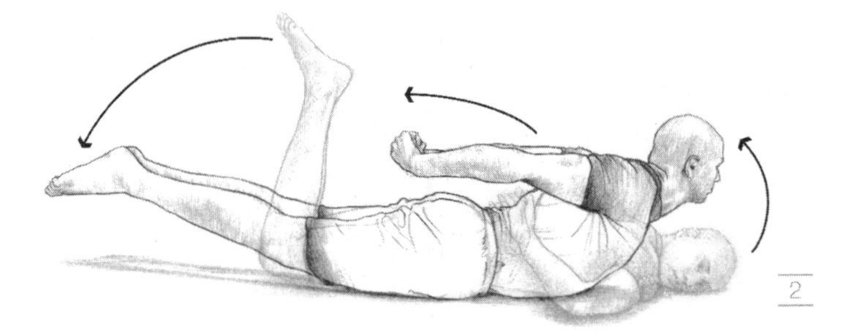

Inhale as you lift your head, look forward, and lift your chest off the floor. Simultaneously straighten your legs and arms and lift them as high as you can. Keep your head lifted as far as comfortably possible. Lift your entire spine by engaging your buttocks while firmly holding in your powerhouse. Lower yourself back down to the starting position (see illustration 1) but with your right cheek on the mat.

Repeat 6 times, starting alternately on the right cheek 3 times, and then the left cheek 3 times.

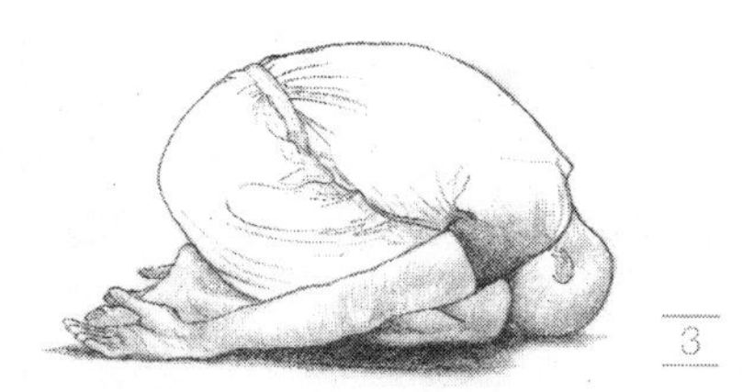
3

As performed at the end of the Swan Dive, sit back on your heels at the end of this exercise to release your back muscles. You may get into this position at any time during the exercise, whenever you need to release pressure or tightness in your back.

THE BEAST WITHIN

BODY POSITION Simply follow the key points that accompany the first illustration.

THE MIND IN MOTION As in the Swan Dive and Single Leg Kicks, protect your private area before you begin. Keep your powerhouse in. Move smoothly and keep your legs tightly together throughout the exercise. Don't throw your body up haphazardly. When you lift your body, hold your arms as straight and as high off your bottom as possible, and lengthen your entire spine. If your upper back is too tight to clasp your hands together, you may keep them apart while reaching your palms up toward the ceiling and your fingers extended toward your feet. You may also clasp a face towel with your hands about four inches apart. When you lift off the floor, try to tear the towel in half. Your chest and shoulders will feel more open. If you are able to clasp your hands together, on the very last repetition you may separate them and press the backs of your hands into the floor to maximize the extension of your spine.

CAUTIONS Leave this one out if you have neck, shoulder, rib, back, hip, or knee problems.

THE NECK PULL

BENEFITS: STRENGTHENS YOUR POWERHOUSE WHILE LENGTHENING YOUR SPINE AND LEGS

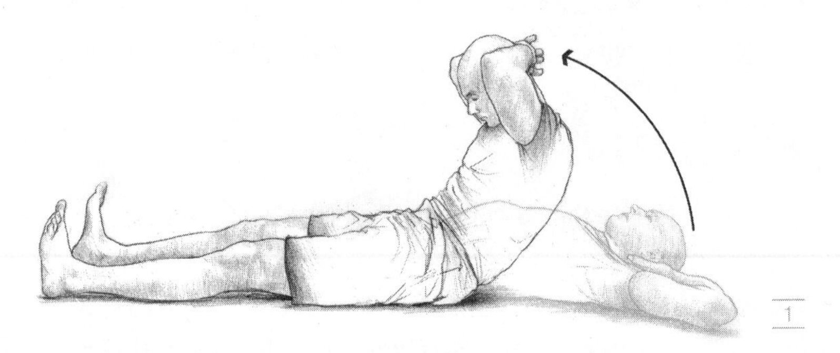

After the Double Leg Kicks, turn over onto your back. Interlace your fingers tightly behind your head and flex your ankles, with your feet hip-width apart. Lock your knees and align them with the ceiling. Inhale and bring your chin to your chest as you begin to round your spine off the floor one vertebra at a time. Keep your stomach in.

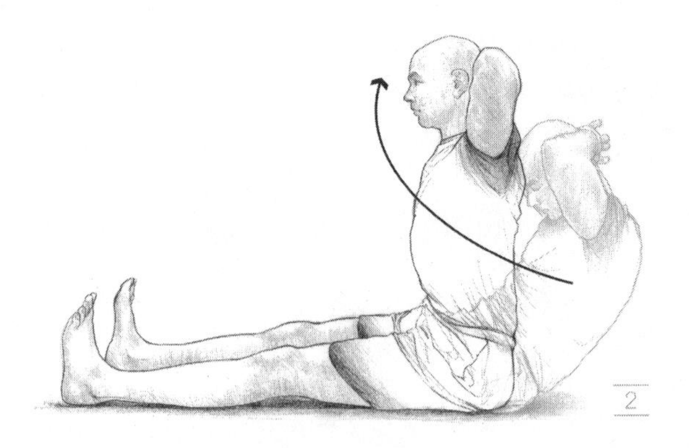

Exhale as you continue to round your torso up, then sit up tall with your elbows wide. Keep your stomach firmly in.

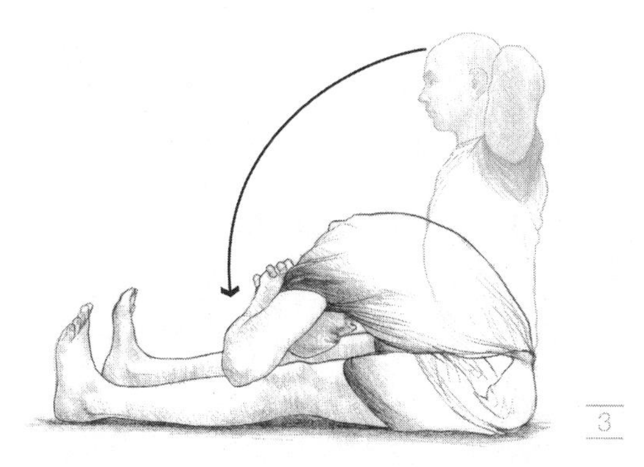

Lengthen your body forward, bringing your forehead between your legs. Keep your powerhouse pulled in and up.

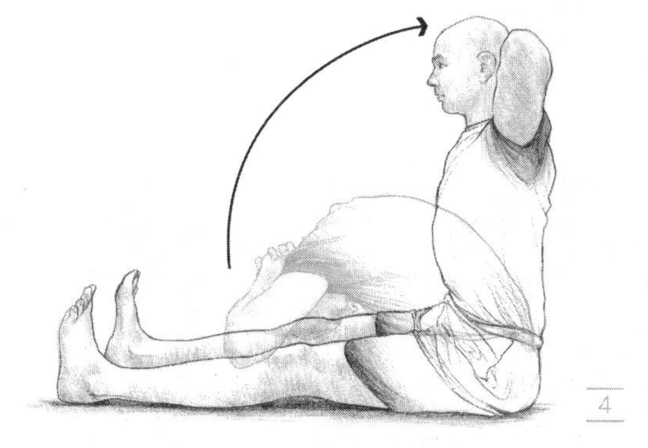

Inhale and sit up tall with your powerhouse pulled in and up.

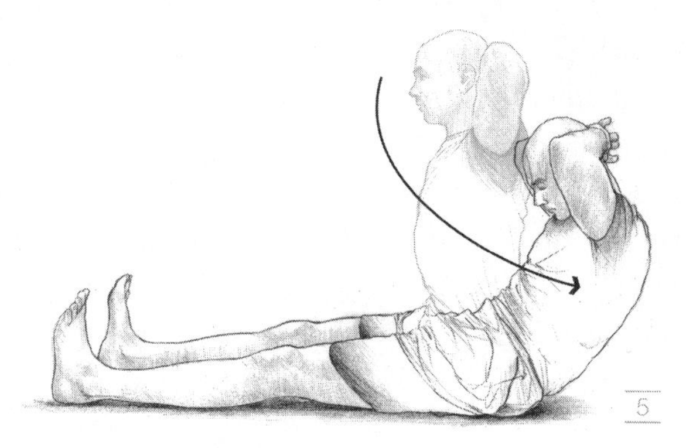

Begin exhaling as you roll your vertebra down one at a time. Hold your powerhouse in firmly.

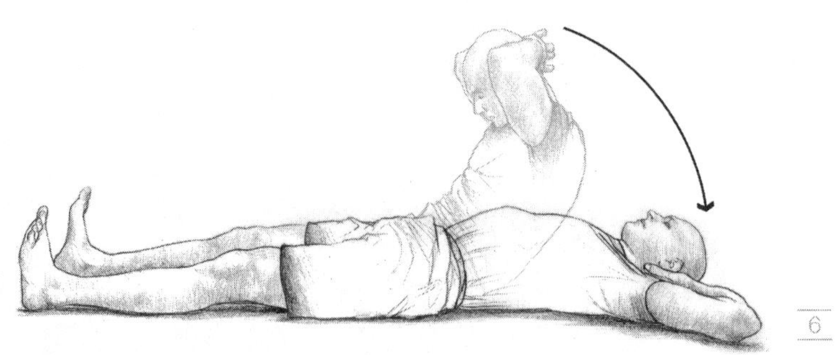

Complete the exhalation and finish in the starting position.

Perform 5 times.

THE BEAST WITHIN

BODY POSITION Keep your ankles flexed throughout the exercise. Don't let your fingers slide apart. You may also try the hand over hand position behind your head or neck instead of interlacing your fingers. Hold your stomach in firmly; keep your neck long throughout the movement. If you focus on pressing your legs down into the floor, everything will work properly. Fundamentally speaking, this is an old-fashioned straight leg sit-up.

THE MIND IN MOTION If getting up is difficult at first, try doing it with bent legs anchored with a strap over the tops of your ankles, or with your feet under a safe, comfortable piece of furniture. This way, you can also walk your hands underneath your thighs as you round your back up off the floor for additional assistance; but don't try this last modification if you have ankle problems. Don't throw yourself with momentum.

To make this exercise more challenging, from the upright position on your sit bones (see illustration 4) lower your torso to the mat with a straight spine instead of a rounded one. You won't be able to maintain this straight spine all the way to the floor; eventually you will have to roll. To make this even harder, come back up for another repetition when the tips of your shoulder blades touch the floor, instead of lowering your shoulders and head all the way down.

CAUTIONS Leave this one out if you have neck, shoulder, or back problems.

THE SCISSORS

BENEFITS: STRENGTHENS THE POWERHOUSE AND LEGS WHILE OPENING THE HIPS

After the Neck Pull, place your arms alongside your body. Pull in your powerhouse and lift your legs to the ceiling as you exhale.

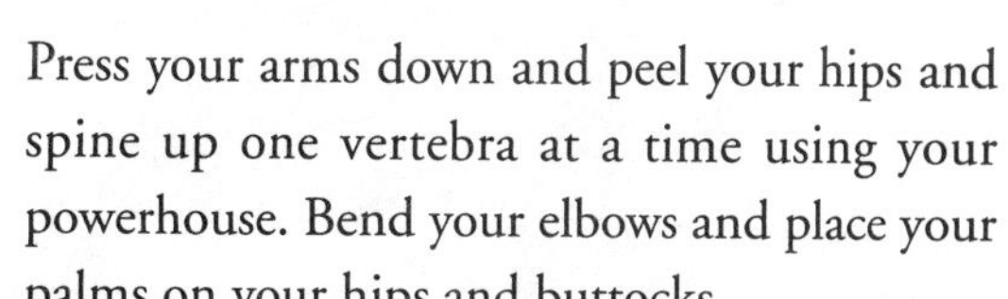

Press your arms down and peel your hips and spine up one vertebra at a time using your powerhouse. Bend your elbows and place your palms on your hips and buttocks.

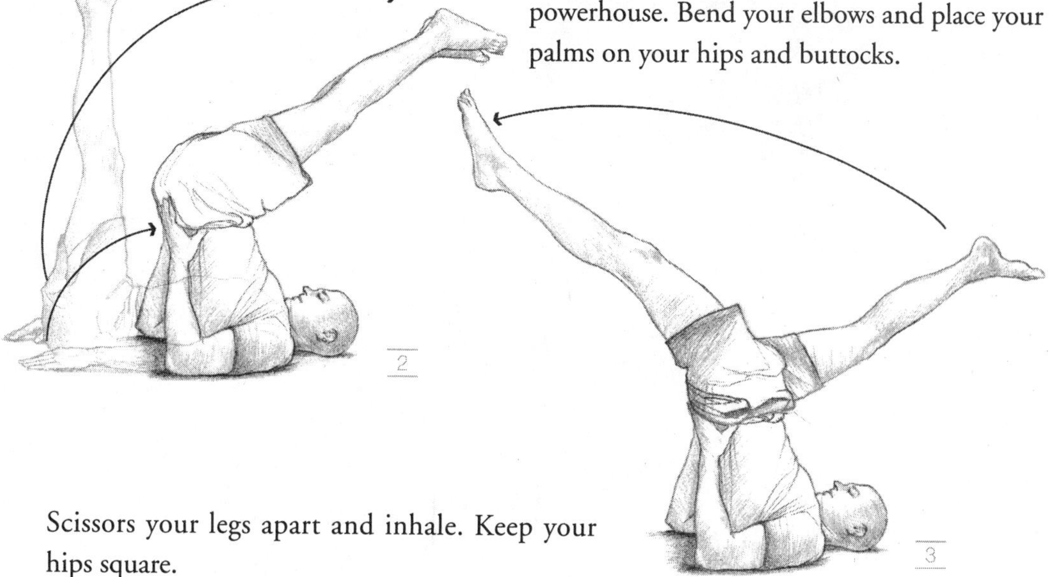

Scissors your legs apart and inhale. Keep your hips square.

Switch legs and exhale. Keep your hips square.

Perform 5 times. The count should be: "1 and 1, 2 and 2, etc," with your legs switching and passing each other back and forth on each beat. (See illustrations 3 and 4).

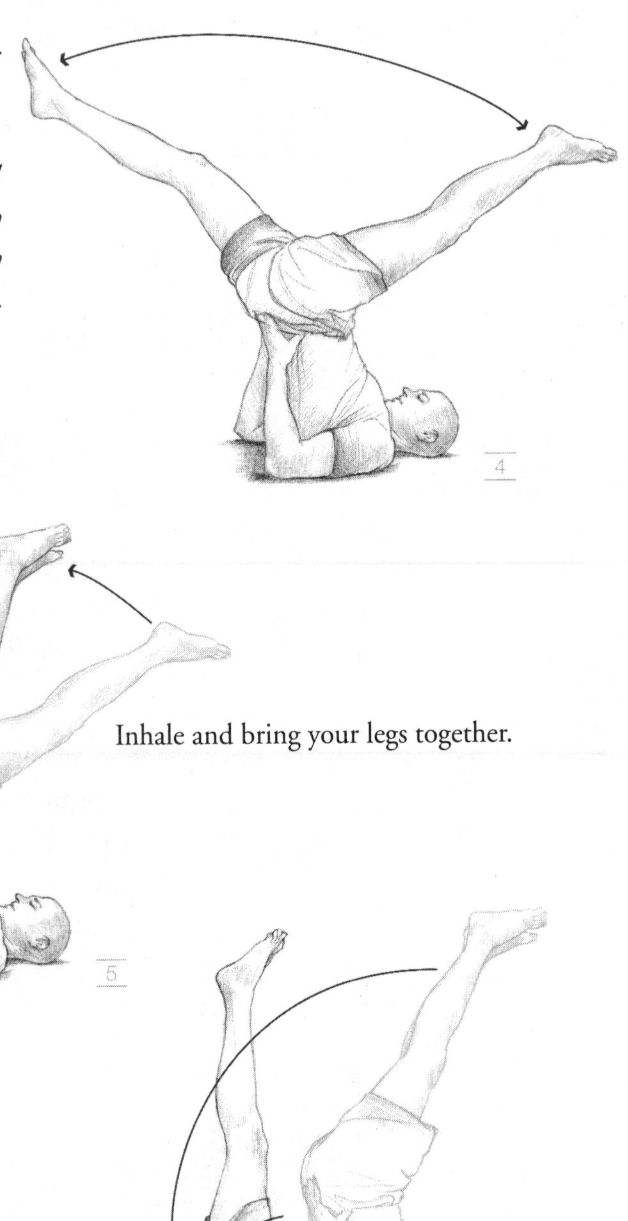

Inhale and bring your legs together.

Bring your arms down alongside the body. Roll your spine down with control.

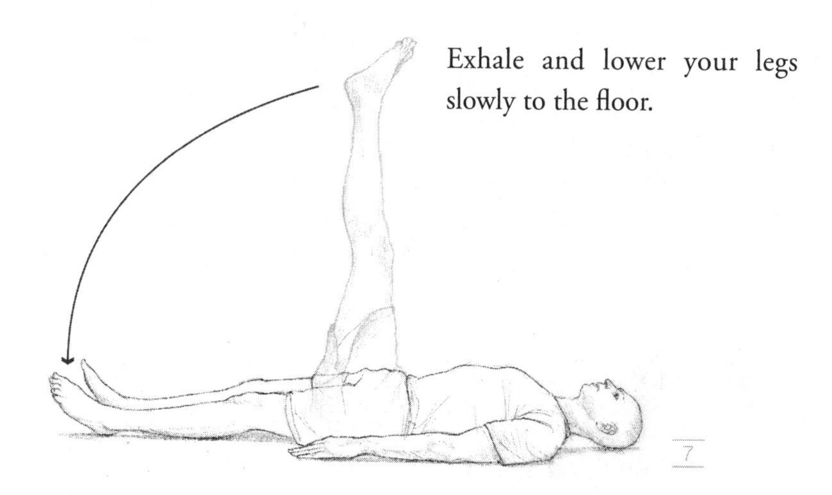

Exhale and lower your legs slowly to the floor.

THE BEAST WITHIN

BODY POSITION Hold your body firmly in the upright position with an engaged powerhouse. Be careful not to strain your neck when you first bring your legs up and over. When your legs are in the air, the weight of your body should be distributed in your arms and upper back.

THE MIND IN MOTION When you scissor your legs apart, keep your hips square. Keep your knees locked and legs straight throughout the movement. When you descend to the floor, focus on keeping your toes over your body in a range from the sternum (most difficult) to the top of the head (least difficult) until your tailbone touches the floor. If you allow your toes and feet to fall over or past your head as you descend, you won't be working your powerhouse nearly as much as you should. To feel the difference: First, bring your toes over the sternum when your legs are together in the air, and try to lower your body from here. Then bring your toes over the top of your head, and try lowering your body from there. It makes a world of difference.

CAUTIONS Leave this one out if you have neck, shoulder, wrist, elbow, back, hip, or knee problems.

THE BICYCLE

BENEFITS: WORKS THE POWERHOUSE AND LEGS; OPENS THE HIPS AND CHEST

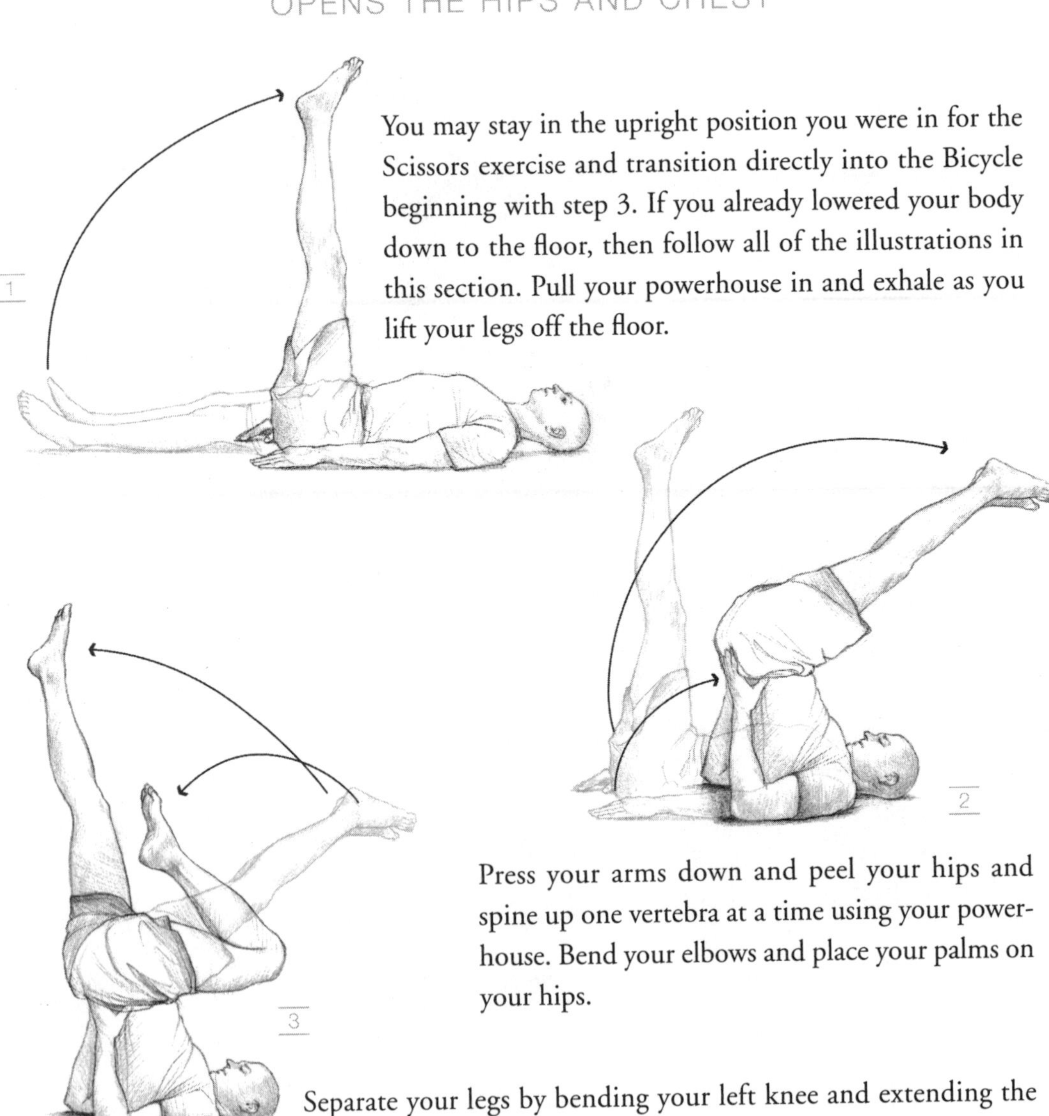

You may stay in the upright position you were in for the Scissors exercise and transition directly into the Bicycle beginning with step 3. If you already lowered your body down to the floor, then follow all of the illustrations in this section. Pull your powerhouse in and exhale as you lift your legs off the floor.

Press your arms down and peel your hips and spine up one vertebra at a time using your powerhouse. Bend your elbows and place your palms on your hips.

Separate your legs by bending your left knee and extending the straight locked right leg away from your bent leg. Inhale.

Bend your right knee and straighten your left leg, moving both legs in opposite directions. Exhale.

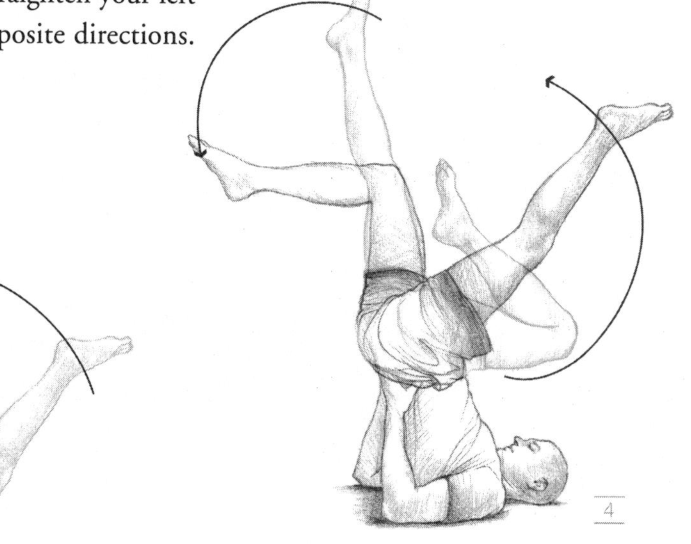

Continue the motions of bending one knee and straightening the other leg while they move in a fluid alternating motion, as if you were riding a bicycle. Alternate your inhalations and exhalations.

Perform 5 times with each leg in one direction and then reverse the cycling for 5 repetitions with each leg in the opposite cyclical direction—as if you were pedding backward.

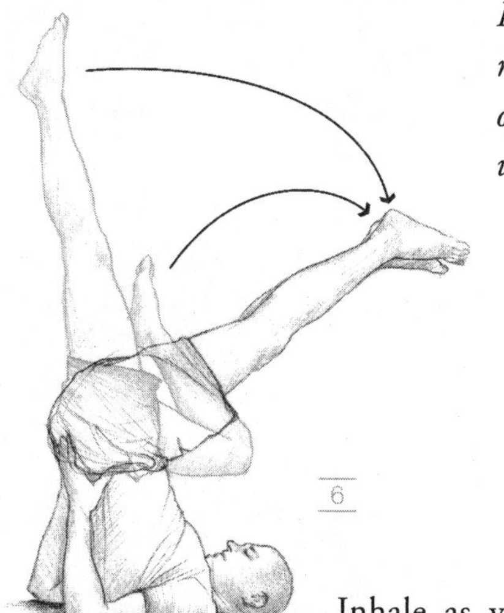

Inhale as you bring your legs together and hold them at a 45-degree angle above your head.

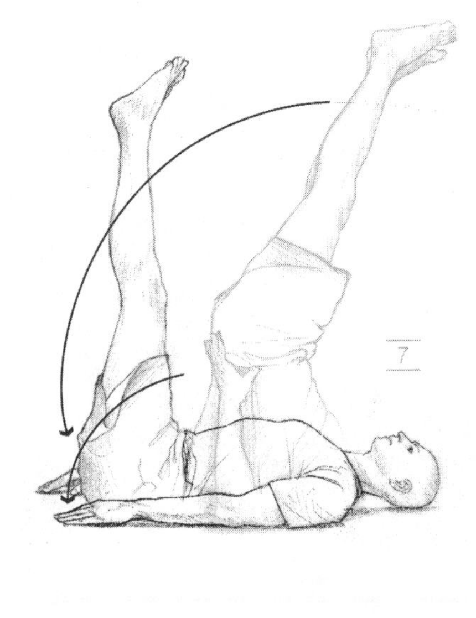

Now lift your legs up, bringing your toes level with your eyes. Lower your arms to the floor. Pull your powerhouse in and lower your spine down to the floor one vertebra at a time.

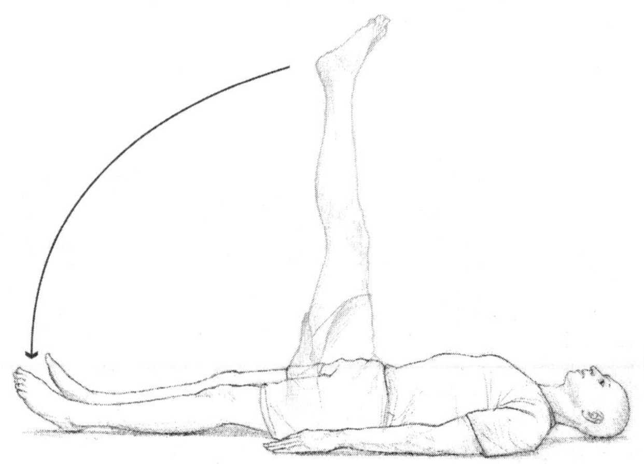

Exhale and slowly lower your legs to the floor.

THE BEAST WITHIN

BODY POSITION Again, as in the Scissors exercise, stabilize your body by firmly holding in the powerhouse. Keep your hips square and stable. Do not let your hips wiggle or twist from side to side. Feel that your weight is evenly distributed from your elbows to your shoulders and across your upper back. Be careful not to strain your neck when you bring your legs up.

THE MIND IN MOTION When you straighten a leg, try to keep the knee locked and the leg straight to achieve your full range of motion, before you bend it to switch legs (see illustrations 3 to 5).

CAUTIONS Men typically have trouble straightening their legs, keeping their hips square, and bringing their body up with control. The tendency is to muscle the body up with the arms and momentum, instead of using the powerhouse, which can result in pushing the back of the head into the mat. This is not good for the neck. Leave this one out if you have neck, shoulder, wrist, elbow, back, hip, or knee problems.

THE SHOULDER BRIDGE

BENEFITS: STRENGTHENS THE LEGS, HIPS, BUTTOCKS, AND BACK WHILE OPENING THE CHEST AND HIP FLEXORS

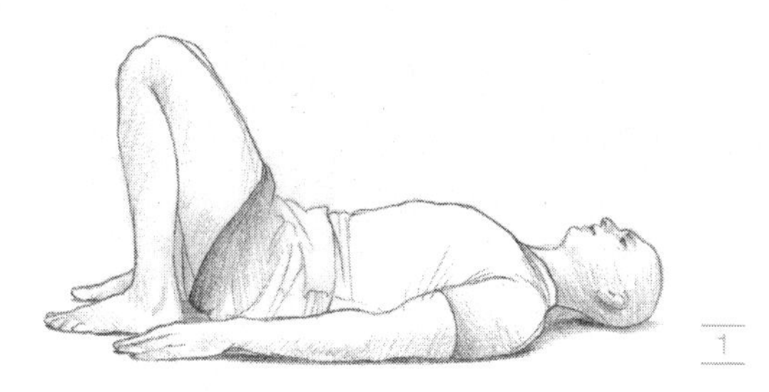

1

After the Bicycle exercise, stay lying on your back but bend your knees and keep your feet flat near your bottom. Keep your arms extended alongside your body with your shoulders down and away from your ears.

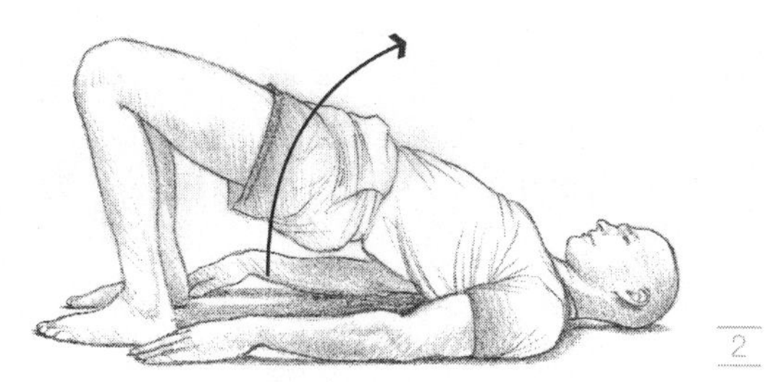

2

Exhale as you drive your hips up toward the ceiling.

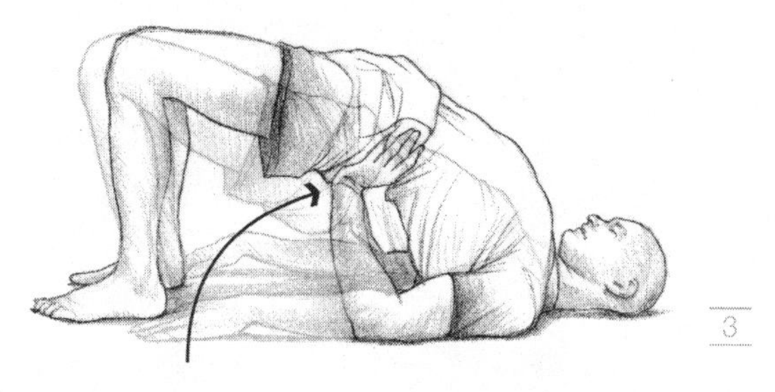

3

Bend your elbows and take hold of your waist. Keep your elbows underneath your hands.

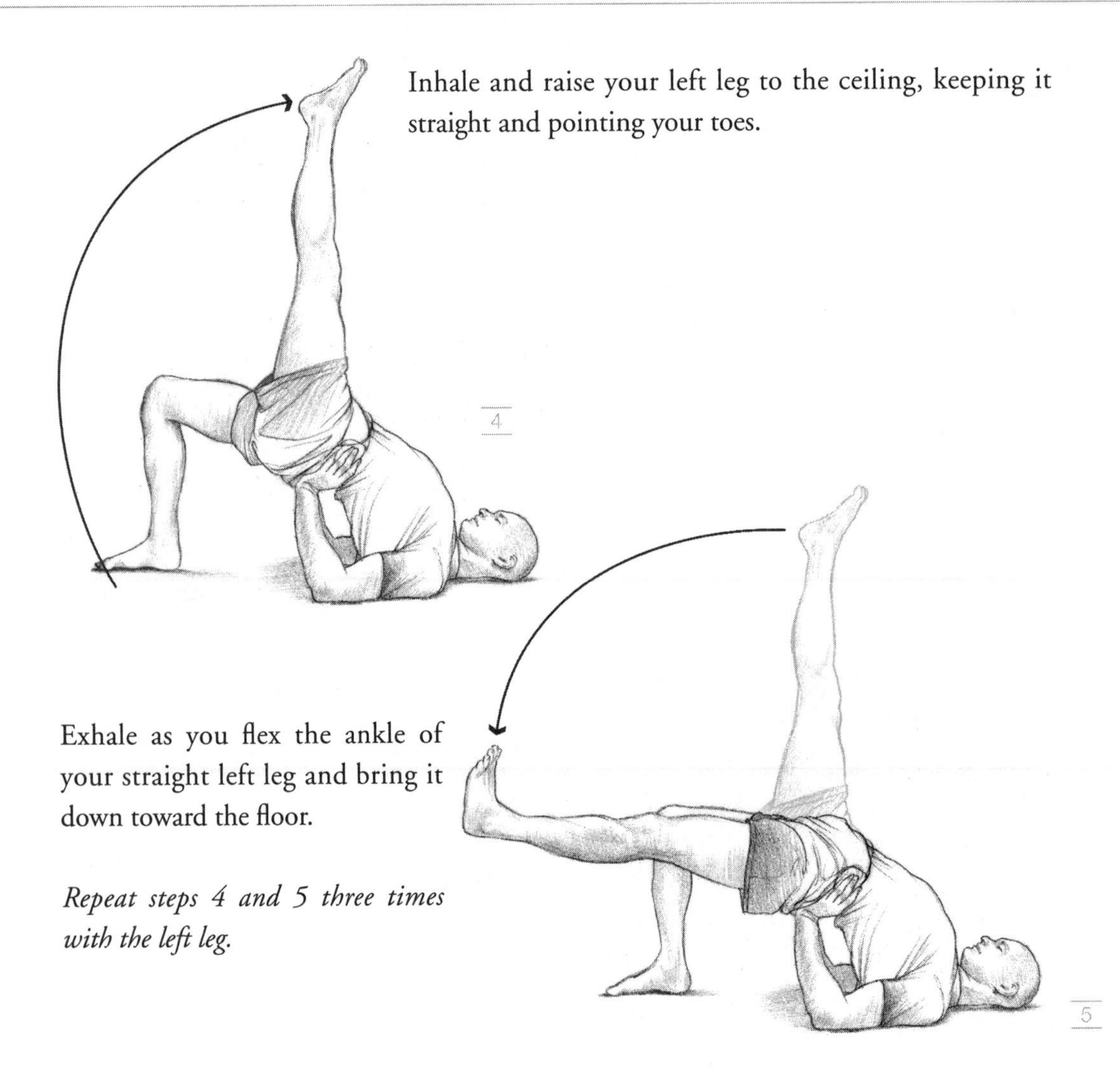

Inhale and raise your left leg to the ceiling, keeping it straight and pointing your toes.

Exhale as you flex the ankle of your straight left leg and bring it down toward the floor.

Repeat steps 4 and 5 three times with the left leg.

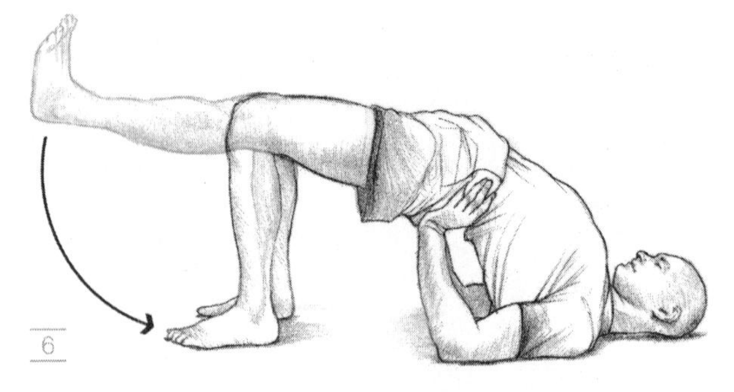

Bend your left knee and place your left foot flat on the floor.

Perform steps 4 and 5 another 3 times, but with the right leg.

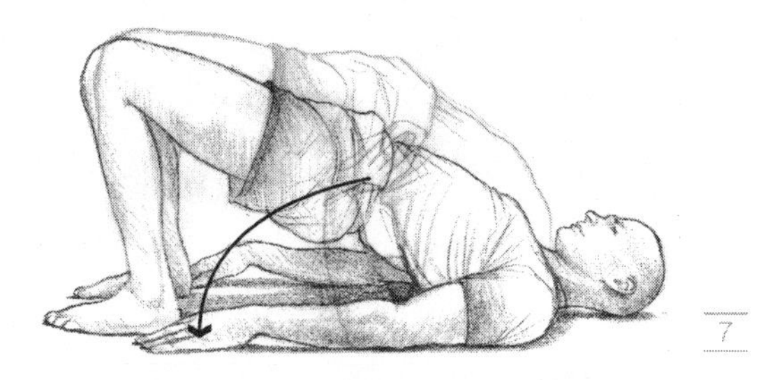

After a total of 6 repetitions (3 times with each leg) inhale and lower your arms.

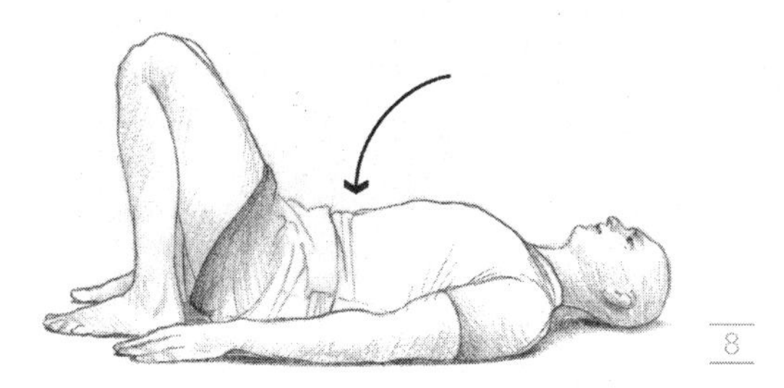

Exhale as you lower your spine and hips to the floor.

THE BEAST WITHIN

BODY POSITION The shoulder bridge distributes the body weight onto the shoulders, arms, and feet. Squeeze your buttocks hard. Keep your hips lifted, even, and stable. Keep your chest lifted and open.

THE MIND IN MOTION This exercise may be hard on your wrists. If so, play with your hand position to alleviate any pain or discomfort. If you cannot find a comfortable position for your hands, then keep your arms straight on the mat with your fingers reaching long toward your feet (see illustration 2). Keep the knee of your kicking leg locked. If you have tight hip flexors and/or a tight back and need help acclimating to this exercise, just practice lifting your hips into the air and lowering them back down onto the floor.

CAUTIONS Men tend to have tight hip flexors and backs, which make back bending difficult. Leave this exercise out if you have neck, shoulder, wrist, elbow, back, hip, or knee problems.

THE SPINE TWIST

BENEFITS: STRENGTHENS THE WAIST AND POWERHOUSE

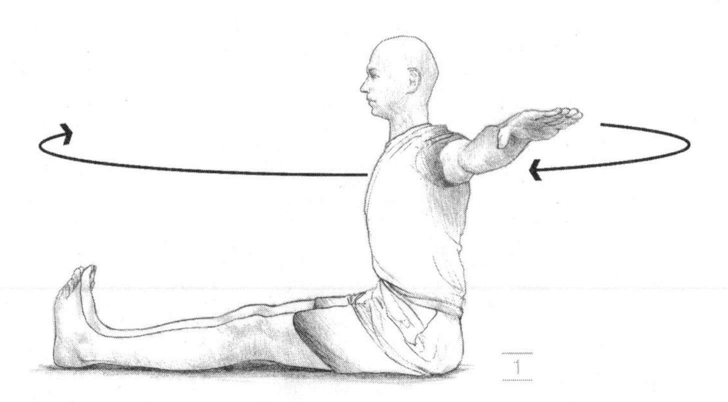

After the Shoulder Bridge, roll up with control—one vertebra at a time—until you are sitting up tall. Squeeze your buttocks together. Flex your ankles and lock both of your knees. Spread your arms straight out to the sides as you engage your shoulder blades, thus opening your chest and drawing your arms back. Keep your powerhouse firmly in.

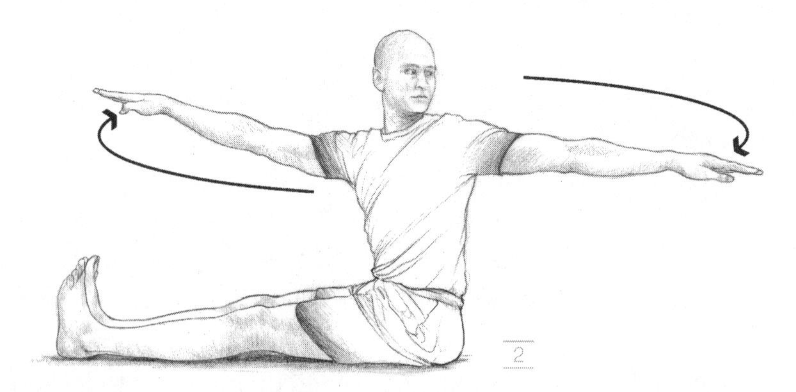

Exhale as you twist your torso to your left. Inhale and return to the starting position. Keep your powerhouse pulled in.

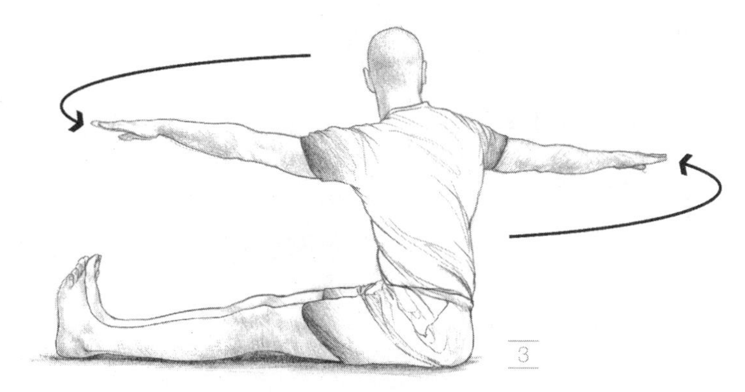

Exhale as you twist to your right. Inhale and return to the starting position.

Perform 3 to 5 times in each direction.

THE BEAST WITHIN

BODY POSITION Sit up tall on your sit bones. If you find it too difficult to sit up tall without rounding your lower back, then bend your knees as much as necessary to acheive this position. Keep your hips square and stable. Your neck should be straight and long; be careful not to bend it to one side as you twist. Keep your arms and legs long and locked (unless you need to bend your knees up per the above modification). Keep your shoulders down and away from your ears.

THE MIND IN MOTION Think of yourself spiraling upward as you rotate your spine. Make sure your feet stay glued together. If they shimmy or slide when you twist, this means your hips are not remaining stable. If your hip flexors cramp, try pointing your toes and turning them out slightly, or lie down on your back and rotate your legs inwardly and outwardly to relax the cramp. It also helps to lightly massage your hip flexors with your thumbs.

CAUTIONS Tight backs tend to cause men to slouch in this exercise. Just remember to bend your knees to help you sit up tall, if necessary. Proceed slowly if you have neck or shoulder problems. Leave this exercise out if you have rib, back, or hip problems.

THE JACKKNIFE

BENEFITS: STRENGTHENS THE POWERHOUSE, BUTTOCKS, ARMS, UPPER BODY, AND HIPS

After the Spine Twist, lie down on the floor on your back from your head to your toes. Your entire spine should be on the floor. Place your arms along your sides with your shoulders down and away from your ears. Your feet are in Pilates stance. Pull the powerhouse in, and exhale as you bring your legs up so that they are straight and vertical to the floor. Your entire spine should *still* be on the floor at this point.

1

Inhale as you press your hands and arms into the floor. Using the powerhouse, roll your hips and spine one vertebra at a time off the mat, until your knees are approximately over the lower region of your face.

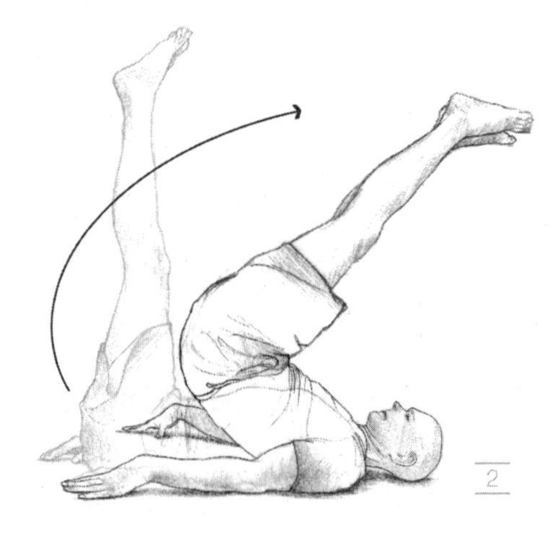

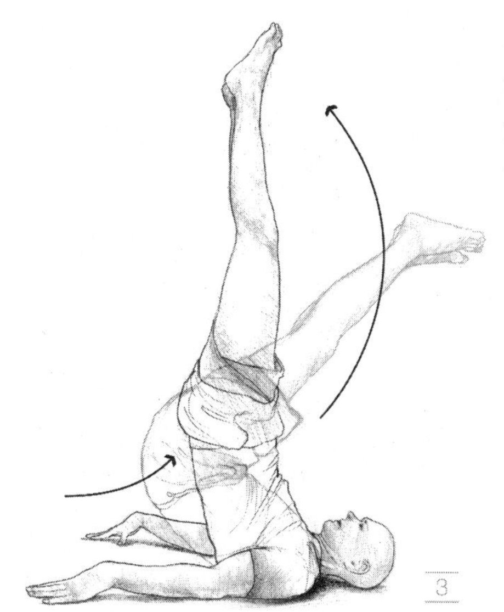

Drive your hips forward and squeeze your buttocks as you reach up toward the ceiling with your legs. Hold this upright position for a controlled moment, keeping your stomach pulled in.

Exhale and slowly lower your spine down one vertebra at a time onto the mat. When your mid to lower spine touches the floor, begin inhaling. Keep your powerhouse firmly in.

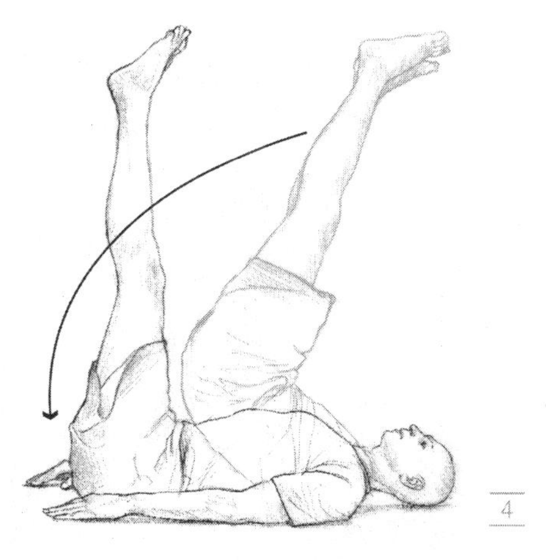

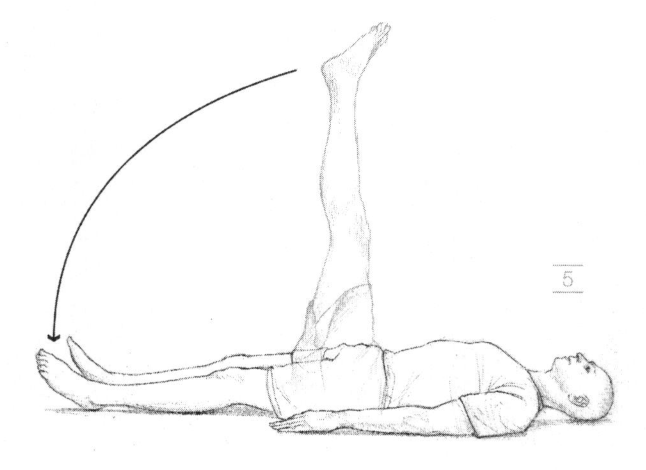

Lower your feet to the floor or, if you can, to an ideal height of 2 inches off the floor. Again, keep your stomach drawn in. Your spine should be completely flat on the floor.

Perform 3 or 4 times

THE BEAST WITHIN

BODY POSITION Maintain a long body. Be sure not to arch your lower spine in this starting position.

THE MIND IN MOTION Don't haphazardly throw yourself up into the air. Focus on using your powerhouse to help control the movement. When your legs are in the air, your bodyweight is distributed throughout your upper back, shoulders, and arms. When you hold the upright position (see illustration 3) keep your toes hovering over the region between your eyes and sternum so that you feel your powerhouse working to control your descent to the floor (as in the Scissors and Bicycle exercises). If you bring your feet too far over your head, you will do two things: First, you will potentially transfer your weight to your neck, which can be dangerous. Second, and equally important, you drastically reduce the work in your powerhouse. Be sure to keep your knees locked throughout the movement. Also try to keep your arms long and straight on the floor, although a lack of flexibility and/or anatomical make up may hinder your elbows or wrists from remaining straight. Keep your shoulders down, even though they may want to roll up off the mat when you lower your legs. To make the movement easier to control, until your powerhouse becomes stronger, try ending each repetition with your spine down and your legs pointed toward the ceiling (see illustration 1).

To make this exercise even more challenging than it already is, try a few repetitions with your palms facing up as you lower your body toward the floor. Hold your powerhouse firmly in throughout the exercise; don't let it release.

CAUTIONS Men tend to lift themselves with upper body strength and momentum rather than the powerhouse. Straightening the legs is also tough for men. If you are overweight or have heavy legs, you will find this exercise difficult to perform. Leave it out if you have neck, shoulder, elbow, hip, or back problems.

THE SIDEKICKS

BENEFITS: STRENGTHENS THE POWERHOUSE, LEGS, AND HIPS; STRETCHES THE HIPS AND LEGS

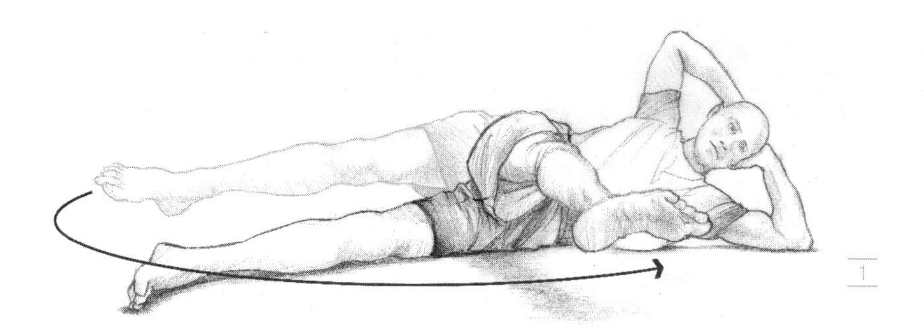

After you finish the Jackknife, turn onto your left side and grasp the back of your head with both hands. Bring both legs forward about 30 to 45 degrees from the line of your spine, keeping your tailbone back and your spine long. Keep your powerhouse in. Lift your top leg about 2 to 3 inches and point your toes. Inhale and, with a controlled kick, bring your leg forward.

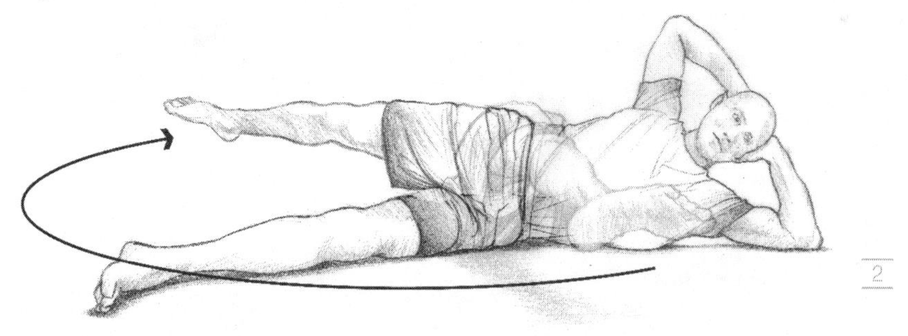

Reverse the direction and bring your leg back, past the starting position and reaching behind you in a controlled fashion as you exhale. Keep your stomach firmly in.

Perform 5 to 10 times on each side. (You should kick forward and backward, forward and backward, etc., in a steady and continuous motion until you're ready to switch sides.)

THE BEAST WITHIN

BODY POSITION Your shoulders should remain stable and your body anchored to the mat. Don't let your top shoulder and hip roll forward or back; they should be in line with your spine, which should remain in the starting position at all times. Use your powerhouse to stabilize your hips, your nonkicking leg, and torso. Maintain your balance and move only your kicking leg, which you may turn out from your hip (as illustrated on page 89) or not. Keep your top shoulder down and away from your ear. Hold your abdominals firmly in place.

THE MIND IN MOTION This is a good example of "range serving the ego and control serving the soul." Kick your leg only as far as you can while controlling the rest of your body. If this hurts your neck or you have neck or shoulder problems, then simply straighten your lower arm onto the floor and try the exercise with your head lying on your bicep. To help stabilize yourself, you may place your top hand palm down on the mat in front of you.

CAUTIONS Men tend to have a limited range of motion in this exercise. Leave it out if you have back or hip problems.

TEASER I

BENEFITS: STRENGTHENS THE POWERHOUSE AND LEGS; IMPROVES BALANCE AND COORDINATION

After the Sidekicks, lie on your back with your feet in Pilates stance. Pull your stomach in, exhale, and lift your legs together about 30 to 45 degrees off the floor. Your entire spine should be flat on the floor.

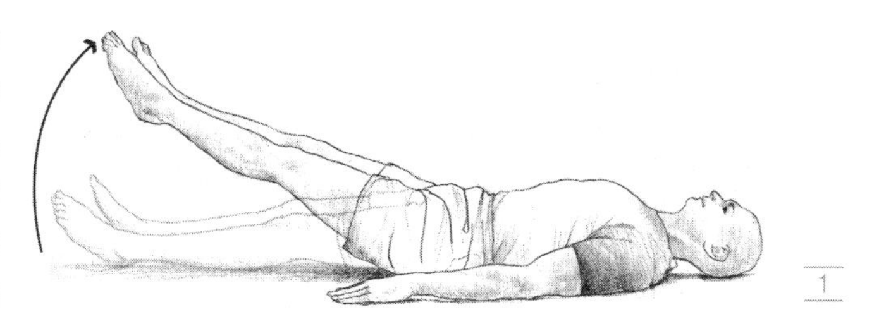

Reach your arms together over your head.

2

Inhale and bring your arms straight up, keeping your shoulders down and away from your ears.

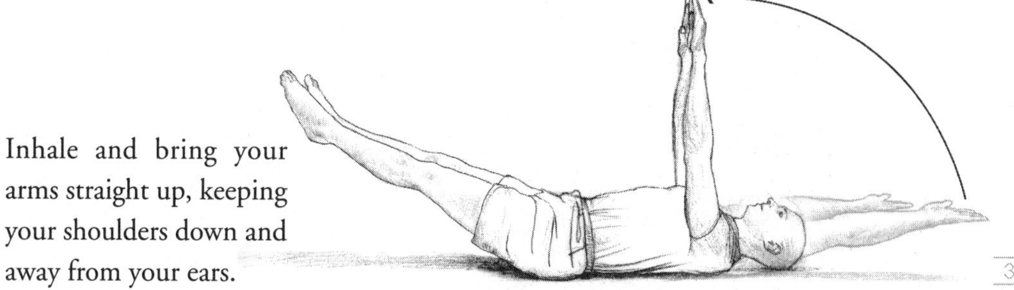

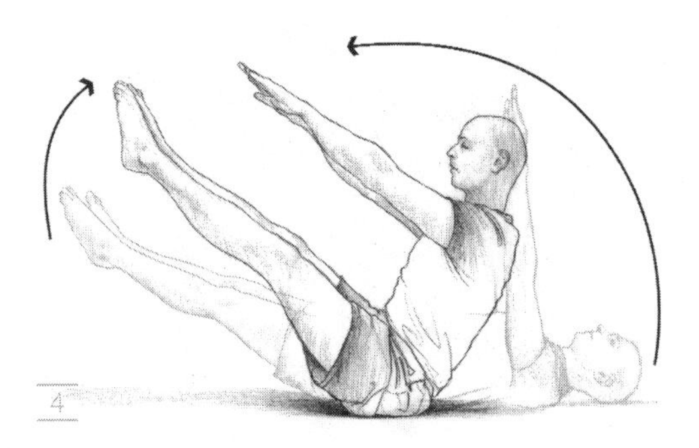

Lift your head and roll up—off the floor one vertebra at a time up—as you begin to exhale. Think of reaching past your toes. If necessary, adjust the height of your legs so that your thighs and torso create the letter "V." (Ideally, your toes should be in line with your eyes.) Bring your arms and thighs parallel to each other.

Inhale and lift your arms straight up toward the ceiling.

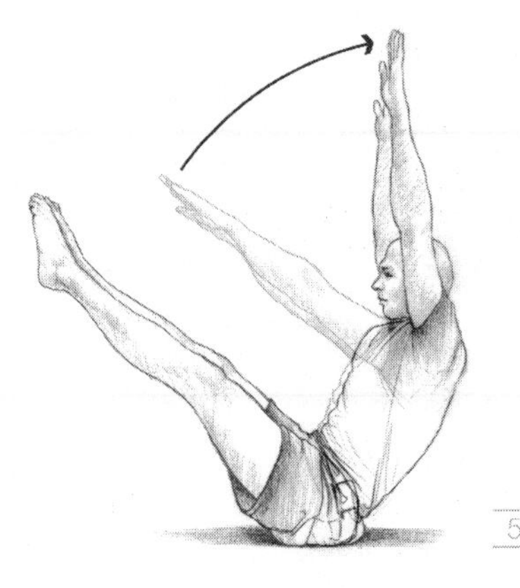

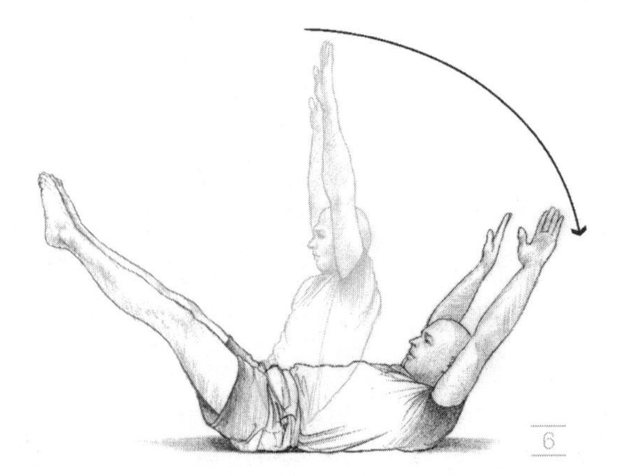

Keep your powerhouse in as you begin to exhale and lower your spine down—one vertebra at a time—to the floor.

Finish exhaling and lower your head and arms. Keep your legs lifted for the next repetition.

Perform 3 times.

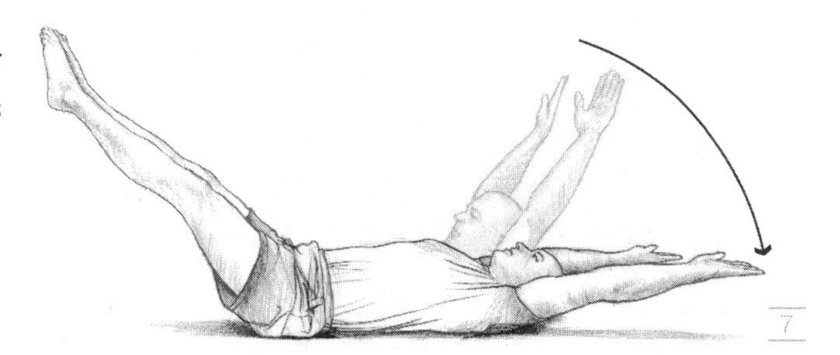

THE BEAST WITHIN

BODY POSITION If you find your lower back arching or straining while in the starting position, then start with bent knees.

THE MIND IN MOTION Do not throw yourself up into the Teaser. Roll up with control. If necessary, bring your knees to your chest and then straighten them out to assume the starting position with your legs in the air. You may also perform this exercise with bent knees throughout, if you find it too difficult to control the movement with straight legs. It is more important to have a lifted lower back throughout steps 4 and 5 than to have straight legs with a sagging lower back. Eventually, you'll be able to straighten your legs as your powerhouse becomes stronger. Don't arch your back. Keep your abdominals in. Keep your feet turned out so your hip flexors stay relaxed. (You may perform the exercise without turning your feet out.) If your lower back hurts, lower yourself to the mat and hug your shins to relieve the pressure. If you cannot roll up into the Teaser, try placing the heels or soles of your feet against a wall at Teaser leg height and let your knees bend or remain straight as you roll up. You may also try placing your heels on a low chair so that your legs form the same 30- to 45-degree angle. If your feet are too high, you will not be able to roll up.

CAUTIONS If you are among a small minority of men who experience discomfort in the tailbone during this exercise, place a small rubber pad underneath your tailbone or leave the exercise out entirely. If none of the modifications help and you simply find this exercise too difficult, practice the Roll Up (see page 33) as an alternative. Leave the Teaser out if you have neck, shoulder, hip, or back problems.

TEASER II

BENEFITS: STRENGTHENS THE POWERHOUSE AND LEGS; IMPROVES BALANCE AND COORDINATION

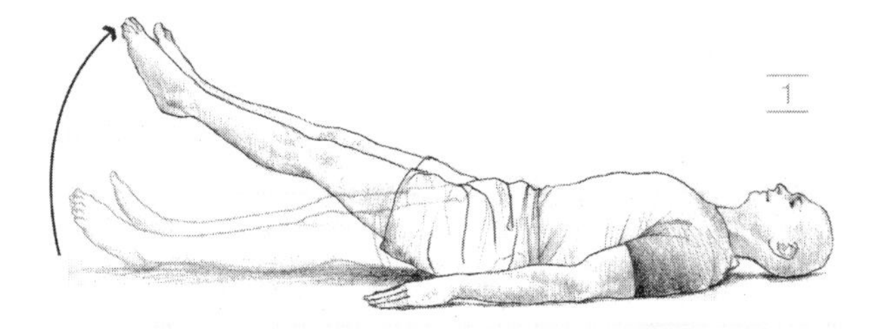

1

Pull your stomach in, exhale, and lift your legs about 30 to 45 degrees off the floor. Your entire spine should be on the floor, and your feet should be in Pilates stance.

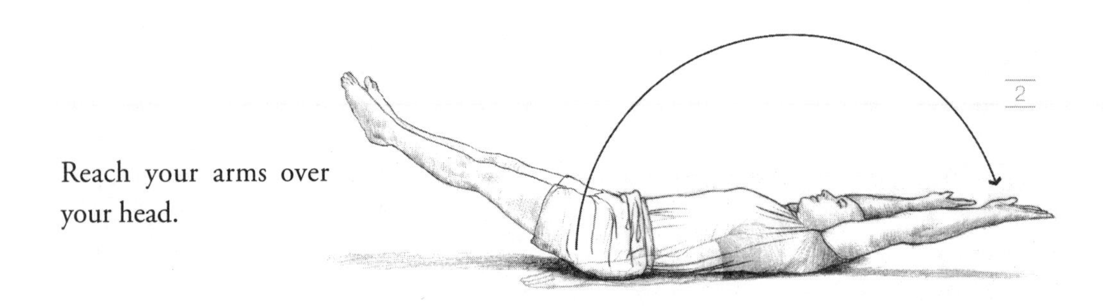

2

Reach your arms over your head.

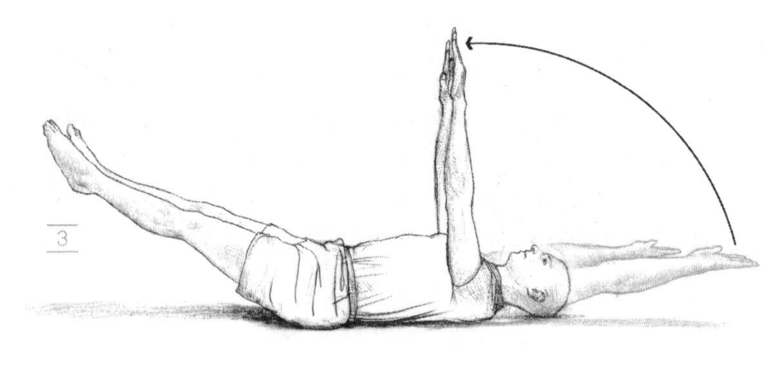

3

Inhale and bring your arms up, keeping your shoulders down and away from your ears.

Lift your head and roll up—one vertebra at a time—off the floor as you begin to exhale. Adjust the height of your legs so that your thighs and torso create the letter "V." Bring your arms and thighs parallel to each other.

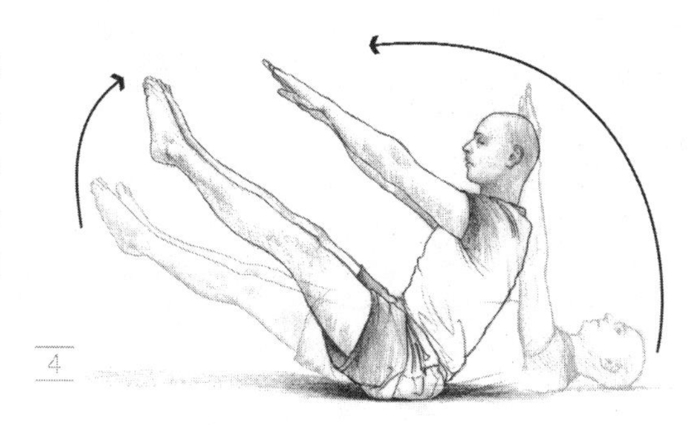

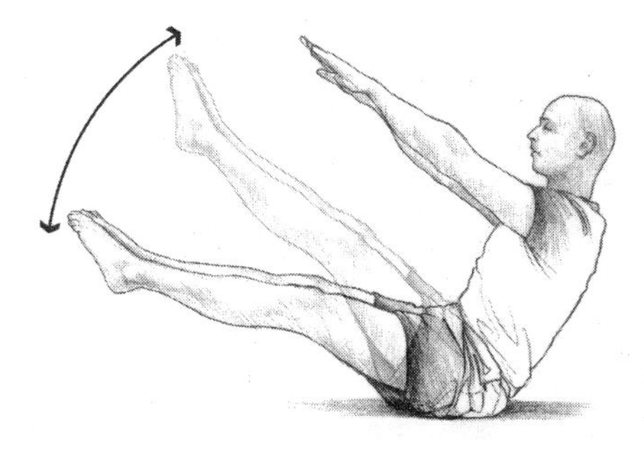

Inhale as you lower your legs and exhale as you lift your legs. Keep your powerhouse in.

Perform these leg raises 3 times.

Keep your powerhouse in and inhale. Then, exhale and lower your spine down—one vertebra at a time—to the floor.

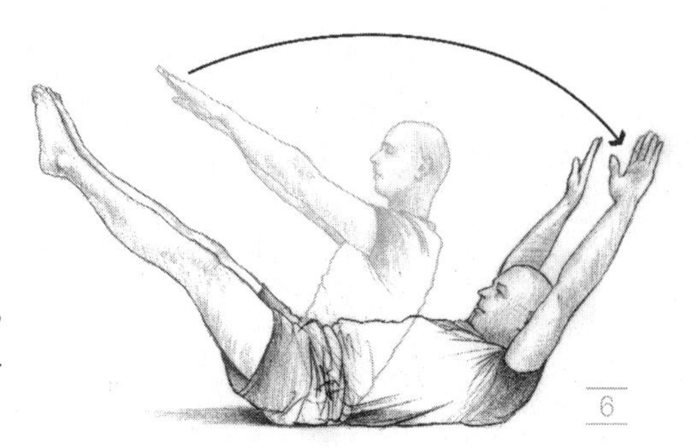

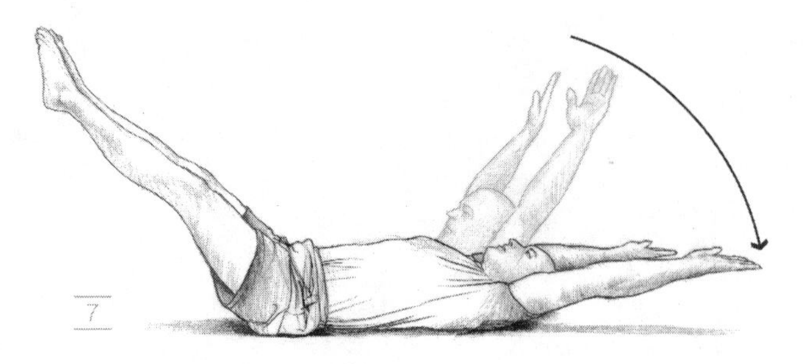

Finish exhaling and lower your head and arms.

Perform this exercise 1 time with the 3 leg lifts.

THE BEAST WITHIN

All of the information from Teaser I applies here. Lower your legs only as much as you can while maintaining abdominal control. Your back should not hurt. If your lower spine starts to hurt or arch, cease this exercise, lie on your back, and hug your shins to your chest. Practice Teaser I for a while before trying Teaser II again.

TEASER III

BENEFITS: STRENGTHENS THE POWERHOUSE AND LEGS; IMPROVES BALANCE AND COORDINATION

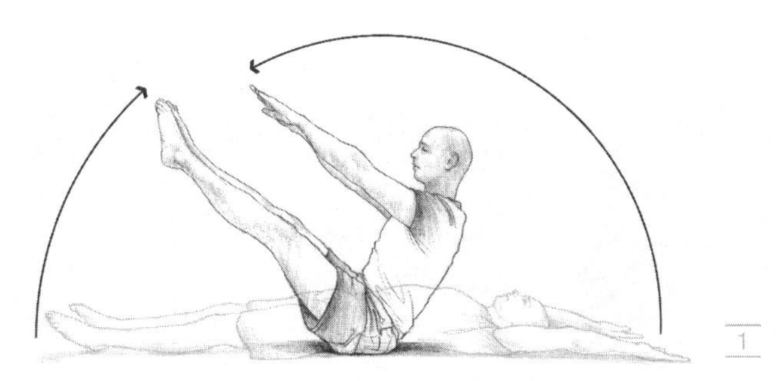

1

Lie down on your back in the same starting position as in Teaser I and II. Inhale and pull your powerhouse in. Exhale and fold your body into the Teaser position.

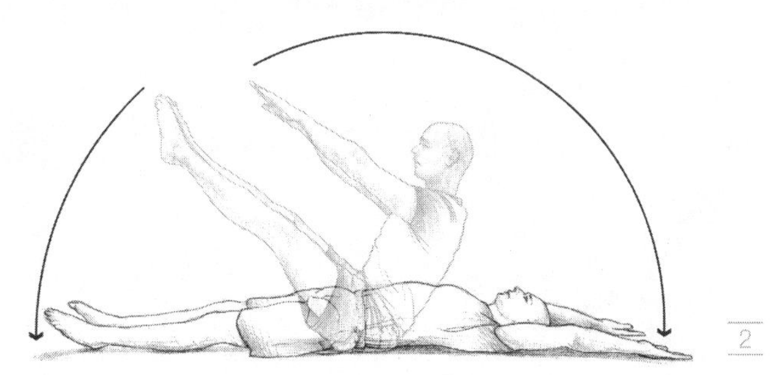

2

Inhale when you reach the top of the Teaser position and exhale as you lower your legs and upper body to the floor simultaneously.

Perform 3 times.

THE BEAST WITHIN

All the information from Teaser I and II applies here. Control your movement as you fold your body up. Don't throw your body around recklessly.

TEASER IV

BENEFITS: STRENGTHENS THE POWERHOUSE; IMPROVES BALANCE AND COORDINATION

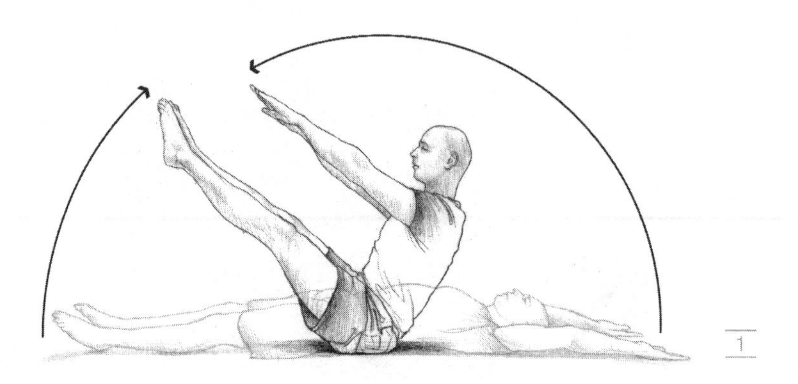

Again, start by lying on your back with your arms reaching above your head. Inhale. Exhale and fold your body up into the Teaser position.

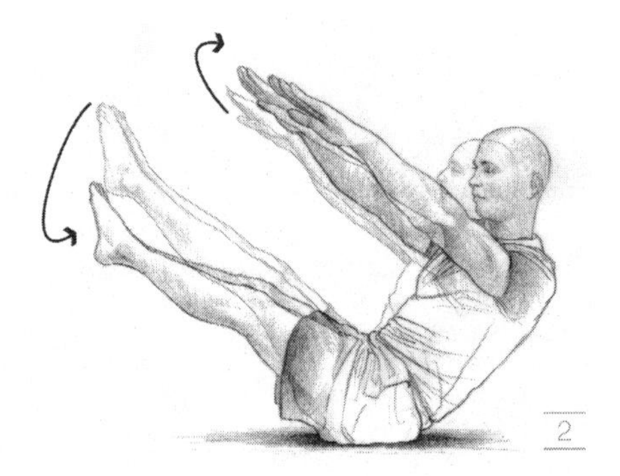

Inhale and pull your powerhouse in. Twisting from your waist, circle your upper body and arms counterclockwise (to the left). Simultaneously circle your legs and lower body clockwise (to the right).

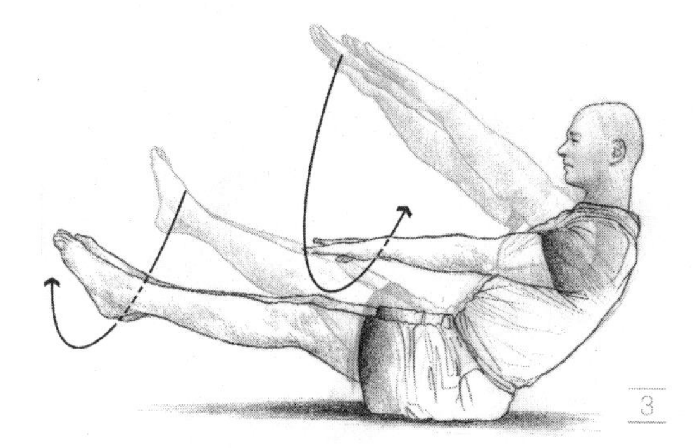

Start to exhale as your arms and legs begin the second halves of their respective circles.

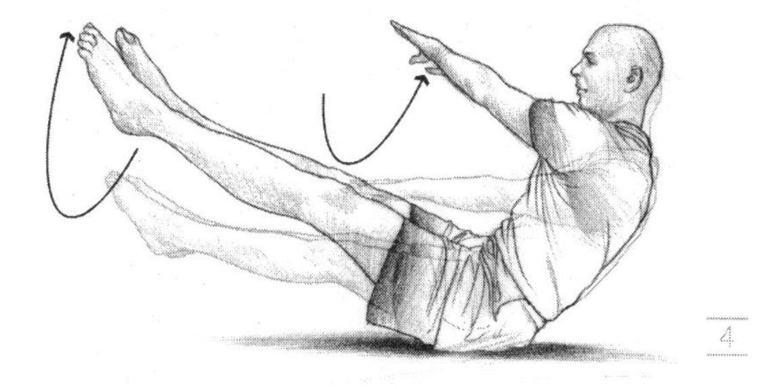

Continue to exhale as you complete the circle.

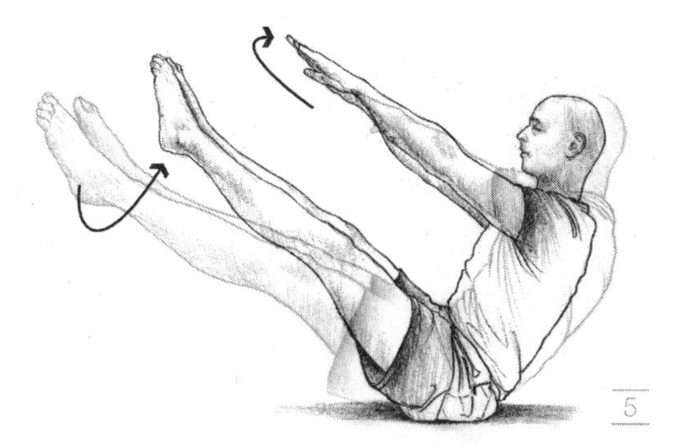

Finally, arrive back to the Teaser position. Reverse the directions, with your arms now circling clockwise and your legs circling counterclockwise. This represents 1 repetition.

Perform for a total of 3 repetitions.

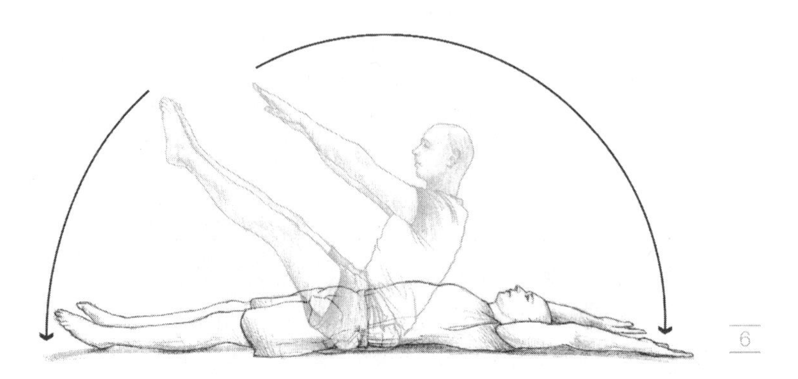

Inhale upon completing the reverse circles. Exhale and lower your entire body down to the floor.

THE BEAST WITHIN

THE MIND IN MOTION All of the information for Teasers I to III also applies here. Do not attempt the Teaser IV until you can execute the other Teasers quite perfectly. The leg lifting, coordination, and balancing aspects of this Teaser are what make it difficult. Remember, don't sag or arch your lower back! Keep your abdominals firmly in place. If anything hurts, leave this exercise out, heal your body, and master the other Teasers. This is a difficult Teaser, as it's basically a combination of the Hip Circles (coming up next on page 99) and Teaser III. A strategic approach would be to master those two exercises first, and then return here to Teaser IV.

People are frequently confused by the coordination that this exercise requires. Simply put, there are four variations of this Teaser IV: (1) Circle both your arms and your legs upward, but in opposite rotational directions—clockwise and counterclockwise. (2) Circle both your arms and your legs downward, but in opposite rotational directions. (3) Circle your arms upward as you circle your legs downward, in opposite rotational directions. (4) Circle your arms downward as you circle your legs upward, in opposite rotational directions.

CAUTIONS Leave out the Teaser IV if you have neck, shoulder, hip, or back problems.

THE HIP CIRCLES

BENEFITS: STRENGTHENS THE POWERHOUSE, HIPS, AND LEGS; STRETCHES THE CHEST AND SHOULDERS

After the Teaser exercises, sit up tall. Slide your hands back as you firmly pull your powerhouse in.

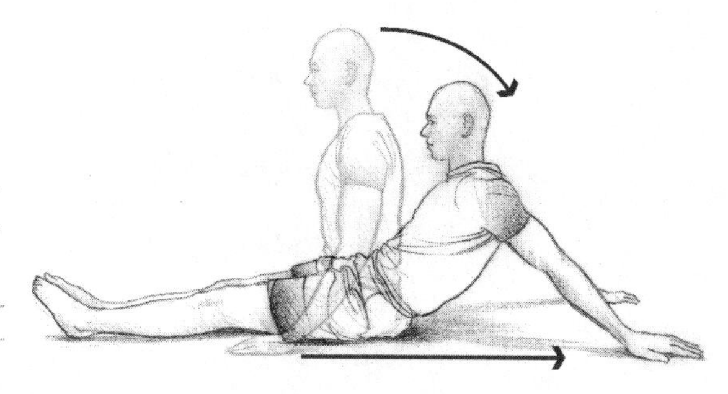
1

Inhale and lift your straight legs up while keeping your powerhouse in.

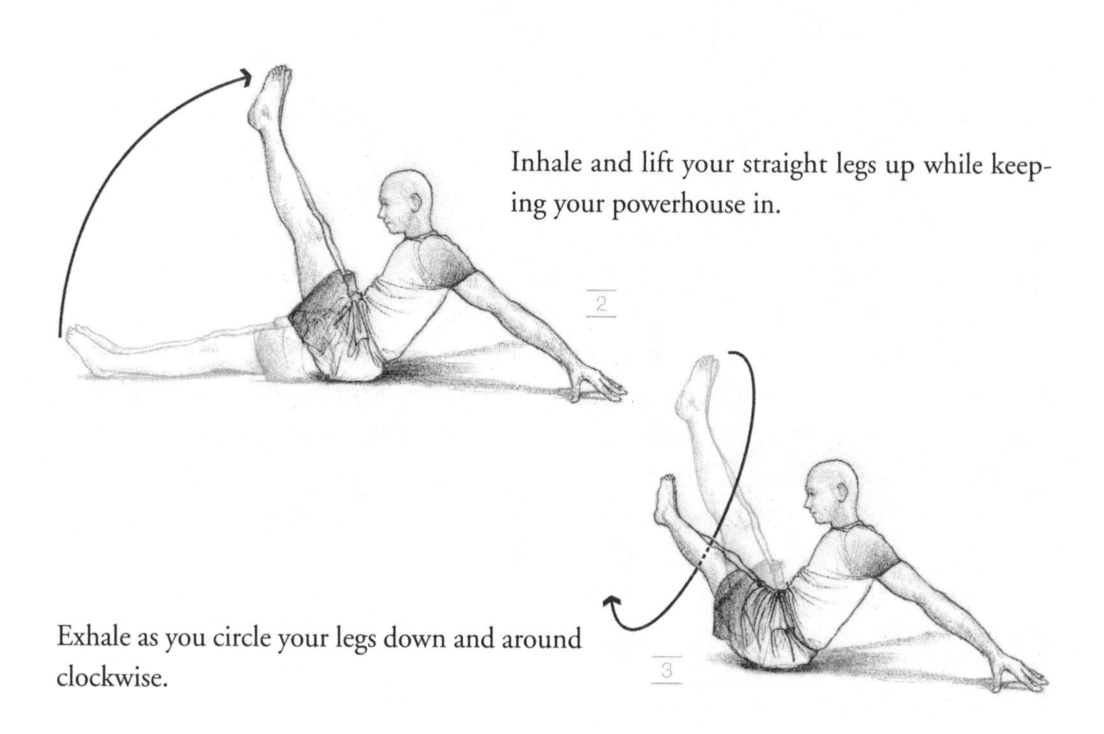
2

3

Exhale as you circle your legs down and around clockwise.

Inhale as you begin to circle your legs up. Keep your powerhouse pulled in and up.

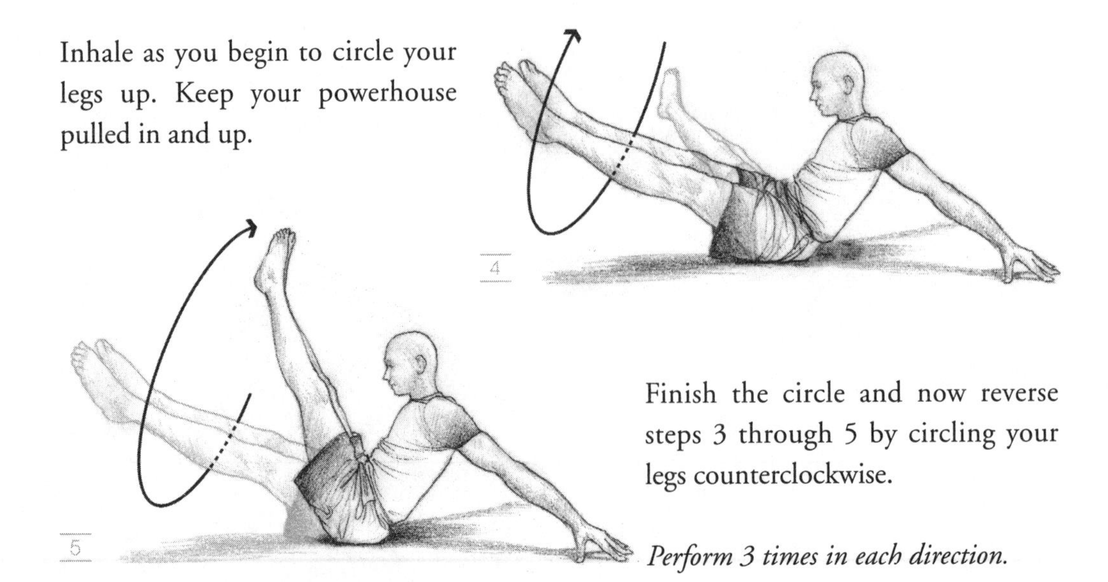

Finish the circle and now reverse steps 3 through 5 by circling your legs counterclockwise.

Perform 3 times in each direction.

THE BEAST WITHIN

BODY POSITION Keep your chest either lifted or inward. Try each variation and see which one works better for you. I prefer to keep my chest inward because it simply feels better for my body. Keep your legs straight with your knees locked. Keep your neck long and your shoulders down and away from the ears.

THE MIND IN MOTION When you first try this exercise, you may keep your elbows bent and your forearms on the floor with your palms down. If you have tight leg and back muscles as many men do, you may bend your knees slightly to avoid straining your lower back. As you get stronger with this easier variation, try it with straight arms and/or straight legs as illustrated. If your hip flexors cramp, then lie on the floor and rotate your legs inward and outward to release the cramp. You may also rub your hip flexors with your thumbs.

For an extra challenge, simply keep your legs straight and try to touch your knees to your nose at the completion of each circle (see illustration 5).

CAUTIONS Don't throw your legs around. Don't allow your lower back to arch. Leave this exercise out if you have neck, shoulder, wrist, back, or hip problems.

SWIMMING

BENEFITS: STRENGTHENS THE ARMS, SHOULDERS, BACK, BUTTOCKS, AND LEGS; LENGTHENS THE SPINE

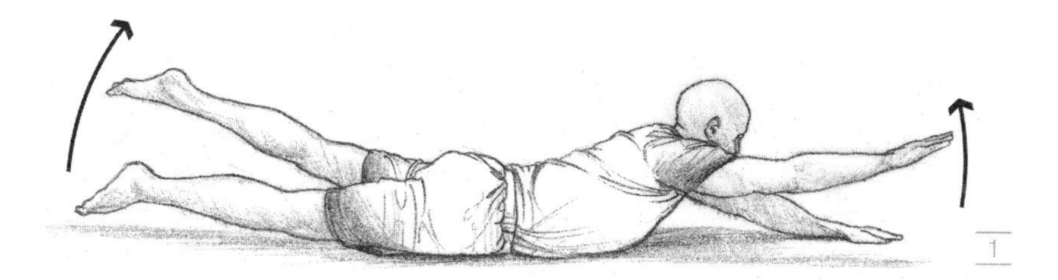

After you complete the Hip Circles, turn over onto your stomach. Exhale and pull your powerhouse in. Lift your right arm and left leg into the air. This is 1 stroke.

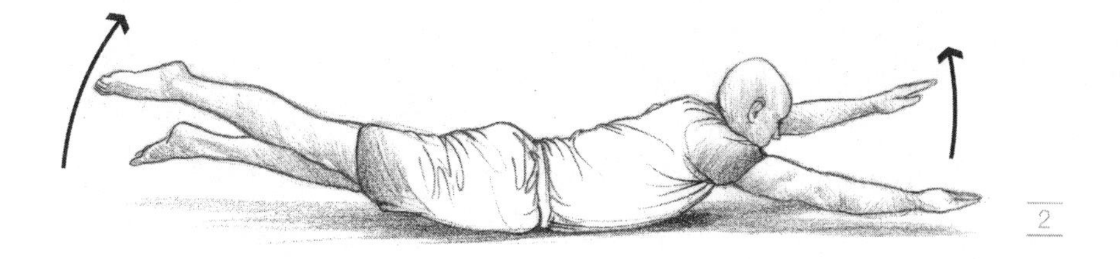

Then lift your left arm and right leg while lowering your alternate limbs to slightly off the floor. Continue alternately raising your right arm and left leg, then your left arm and right leg, while keeping all four limbs off the floor at all times. Sustain continuous movement as if you're swimming, inhaling for 5 "strokes" and exhaling for 5 "strokes." This is counted as 1 set.

Perform 3 to 4 sets.

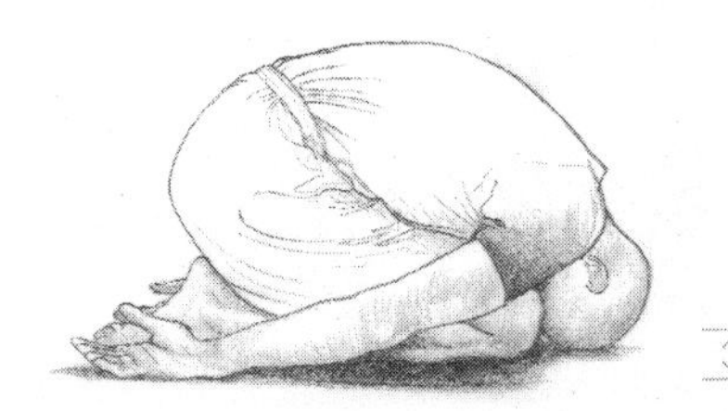

Sit back on your heels with your forehead touching your knees and/or the floor as at the end of the Swan Dive (see page 63).

THE BEAST WITHIN

BODY POSITION Keep your body lifted as high off the floor as possible. Keep your elbows and knees locked and straight. Don't let your arms or legs touch the floor. Keep your shoulders down and away from your ears.

THE MIND IN MOTION A stroke is defined as the single lifting motion of an arm and its opposite leg. Lift the entire length of your body as you feel your spine lengthen. Squeeze your bottom, hold your powerhouse in, and keep your sternum lifted off the floor. If you can not completely straighten your elbows and knees, then just keep them as straight as possible, allowing them to bend only slightly. If you begin to feel discomfort in your lower back, stop the exercise and sit back on your heels (see illustration 3). If you are overweight, leave this exercise not until you slim down a bit.

CAUTIONS Men tend to have tightness in the back, which can make it difficult to lift and lengthen the spine in this exercise. Leave this one out if you have neck, shoulder, rib, back, or knee problems.

THE LEG PULL DOWN

BENEFITS: STRENGTHENS THE ARMS, CHEST, BACK, POWERHOUSE, BUTTOCKS, AND LEGS WHILE STRETCHING THE BACKS OF THE LOWER LEGS

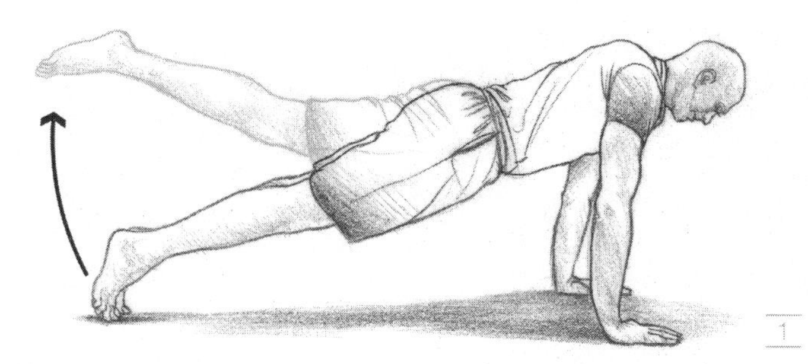

1

After the Swimming exercise, pull your powerhouse in, exhale, and lift your body into a push-up position. Inhale and lift your right leg up with your foot pointed long.

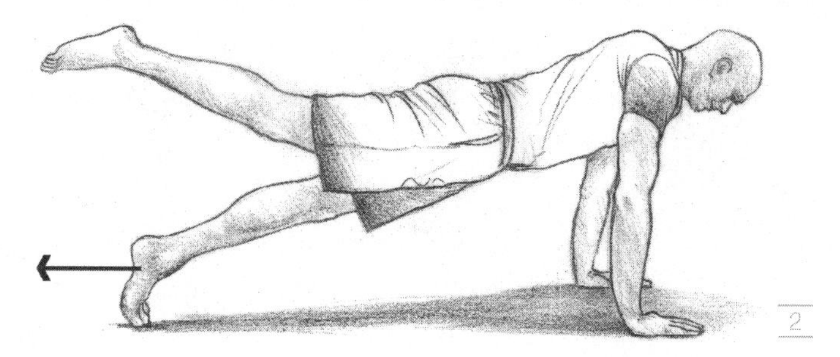

2

Lower your left heel back.

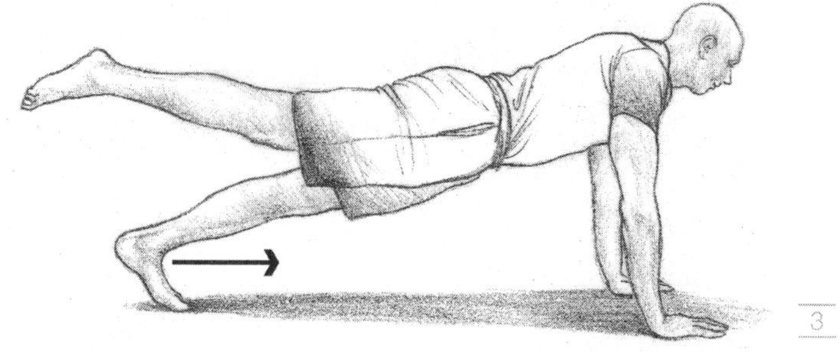

3

Start to exhale as you pull your powerhouse in and bring your left heel back over the toes.

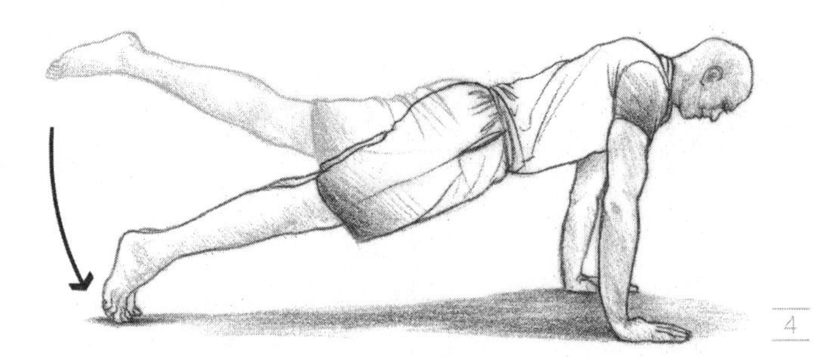

Finish exhaling and lower your right leg back down to the floor. Repeat the exercise, lifting your left leg and engaging your right ankle.

Perform 3 times on each leg.

THE BEAST WITHIN

BODY POSITION When you assume the initial Push-up position, keep your fingers splayed out, your wrists directly under your shoulders, your elbows locked, and your shoulders pulled down and away from your ears. Also keep your legs together with your knees locked. Tuck your tailbone and squeeze your bottom before lifting your leg. If tucking your tailbone is uncomfortable, try a slight tuck. Keep your body firm and rigid throughout the exercise.

THE MIND IN MOTION Don't release your powerhouse; keep it drawn firmly in, especially when you lift your leg and hold it in the air. Your hips must remain square. Focus on tightening your whole body. Since this exercise is an all around strength builder, men acclimate well to it, but sometimes have difficulty keeping the hips stable throughout the movement. If your wrists hurt, try propping yourself up on the first two knuckles of your fists, or simply leave it out. You may also perform this exercise with an arched, extended, spine when your leg is in the air. In other words, when your leg is in the air, lift it as high as you can and look up toward the ceiling. This will arch your back. Keep your powerhouse pulled in.

CAUTIONS Leave this exercise out if you have neck, shoulder, back, wrist, elbow, or ankle problems. If you are overweight and the weight of your stomach strains your lower back, leave this exercise out.

THE LEG PULL UP

BENEFITS: STRENGTHENS THE ENTIRE BODY—THE LEGS, BUTTOCKS, ARMS, SHOULDERS, BACK, AND POWERHOUSE; OPENS UP THE CHEST

After completing the Leg Pull Down, turn over. Pull your powerhouse in. Place your hands flat onto the mat, straighten your arms and legs, and lift your bottom into the air as you exhale. Keep your buttocks engaged. Inhale and lift your left leg as much as you can toward your face with a controlled kick.

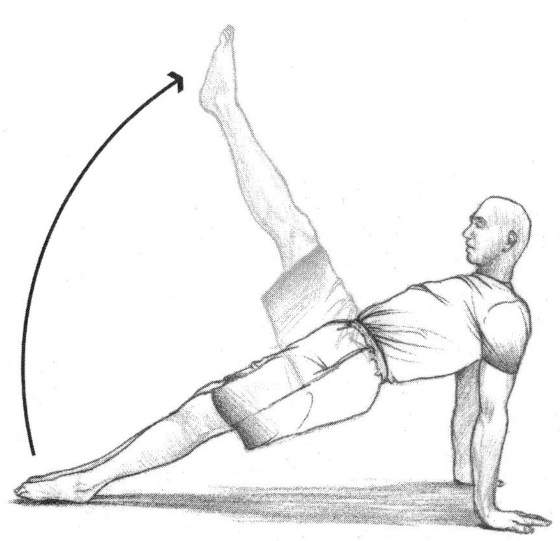

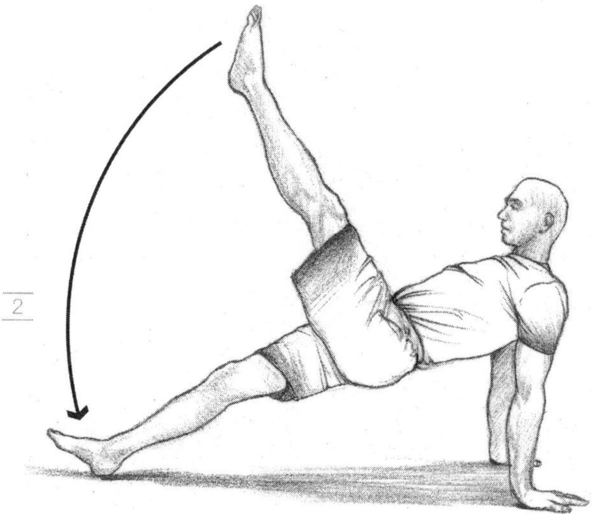

Exhale as you lower your leg back down to the floor. Lift and lower your right leg in the same manner.

Perform 3 times, alternating legs within each repetition.

THE BEAST WITHIN

BODY POSITION Remember to keep your shoulders down and away from your ears. Keep your neck long and upright, or you may hold it in a straight line with the rest of your spine as you look up to the ceiling. You must keep your hips square and lifted. Don't drop your buttocks to the floor. Keep your knees and elbows locked.

THE MIND IN MOTION If you find it too difficult to lift your legs when you start out, simply hold the first position and breathe in and out a few times. Perform the exercise like this until you gain the strength to hold yourself without struggle. Keep your bottom up when you lift one of your legs. It's okay to turn your leg out when you lift it, but always raise it with control. Don't throw it haphazardly. Don't "turtle" your head down into your shoulders. You may turn your fingers in any direction that doesn't hurt your wrists.

CAUTIONS Men tend to have a small range of motion when lifting their legs. As always, control is more important than range. Leave this exercise out if you have neck, shoulder, wrist, elbow, back, hip, knee, or ankle problems.

THE KNEELING SIDEKICKS

BENEFITS: STRENGTHENS THE ARMS, LEGS, AND POWERHOUSE; LENGTHENS THE LEGS, AND WAIST

After the Leg Pull Up, kneel on your right knee. Place your right hand with a straight arm on the floor and position your left hand on the left side of your head. Look forward or down at your right hand. Bring your left leg up in line with your body. Pull your powerhouse in. Inhale and kick your leg forward.

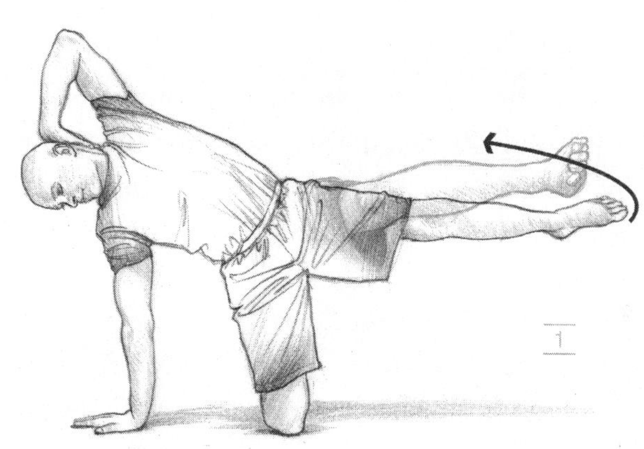

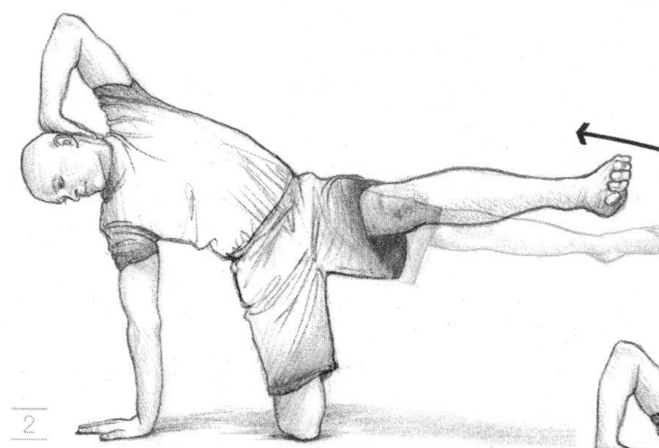

Begin to exhale as you kick your leg backward.

Finish exhaling as you reach your kicking leg all the way behind you.

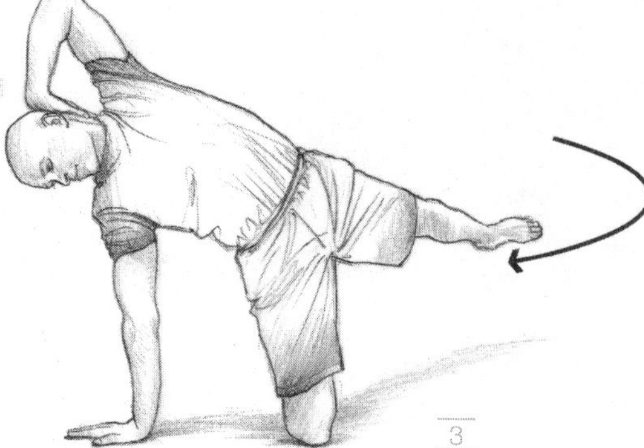

Perform 3 to 4 times with your left leg, then switch sides and perform 3 to 4 times with your right leg.

THE BEAST WITHIN

BODY POSITION Many men typically have tight hips, and they often have difficulty keeping their leg raised throughout this exercise. Keep the shoulder of your supporting arm pulled down and away from your ear; do not let yourself sink into the supporting shoulder. Keep your neck long and your chest open. Engage your powerhouse throughout the exercise. Keep the knee of your extended leg locked.

THE MIND IN MOTION Don't contract the hip flexors of your supporting hip when your kicking leg travels forward. You'll know if you do, because your buttocks will push back and most likely sink down a bit. If you keep your hips stabilized and forward during the movement, you will have few to no problems with the hip flexors of your supporting leg. If you find it difficult to keep your leg up or you experience a cramp, try holding the first position with your extended leg not lifted but straight in line with your body with only your foot placed on the floor. If you have no trouble doing this, then try holding the first position (as illustrated) for a few breaths. Finally, once you've strengthened your hips and legs in this manner over the course of a few work-outs, try the complete exercise. Instead of kicking, you may also circle your leg as you hold the body position (as in illustration 1). Think of circling your leg as if the foot were scraping the inside of a medium-sized jar. Your kicking range is secondary to maintaining control. Control your body throughout the exercise.

CAUTIONS Leave this exercise out if you have neck, shoulder, wrist, back, hip, or knee problems.

THE SIDE BEND

BENEFITS: STRENGTHENS THE UPPER BODY, WAIST, LEGS, ARMS, AND POWERHOUSE; OPENS THE SIDES OF THE BODY; IMPROVES BALANCE AND COORDINATION

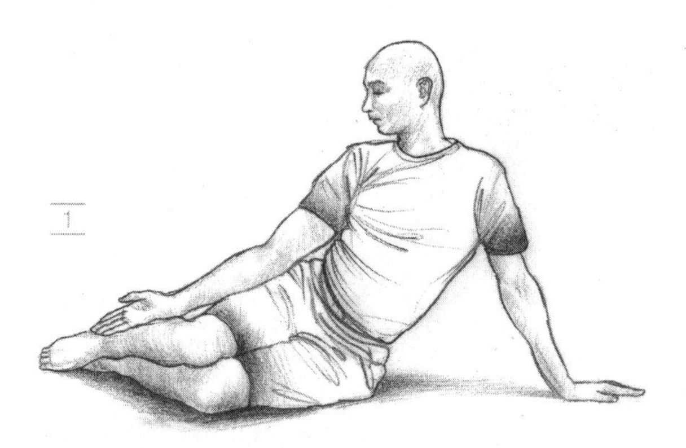

Sit down on your left hip, bend your knees slightly, and place your left hand flat on the floor a short distance away from your seated hip, keeping your left arm straight. Reach your right hand, palm up, toward your toes. Stack your feet on top of one another. Look down to your right hand.

Inhale and pull your powerhouse in and up. Simultaneously lift your hips and body into a straight line with straight legs as you reach your right arm overhead and look either forward or to your left hand.

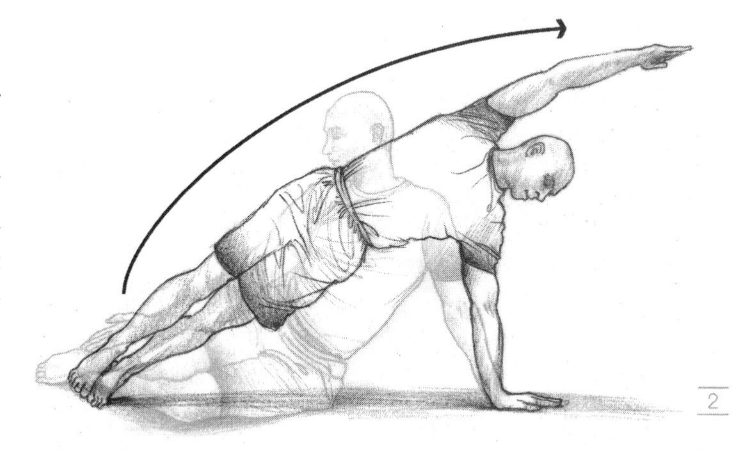

Exhale and lower your hips to the ground as you arc your right hand back toward your toes, and again look at your right hand. Keep your legs straight and lower your hips until your left knee is lightly touching the floor.

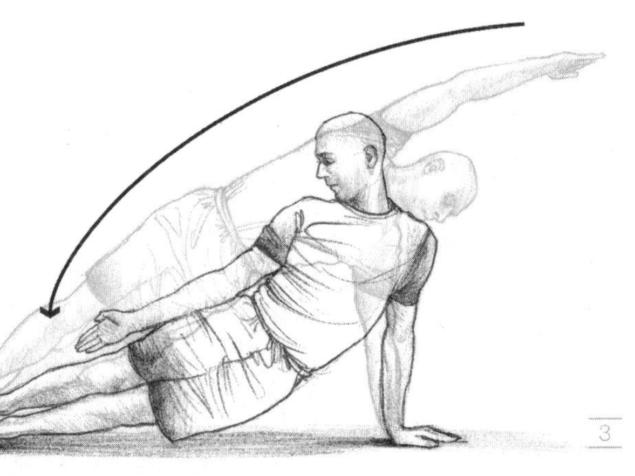

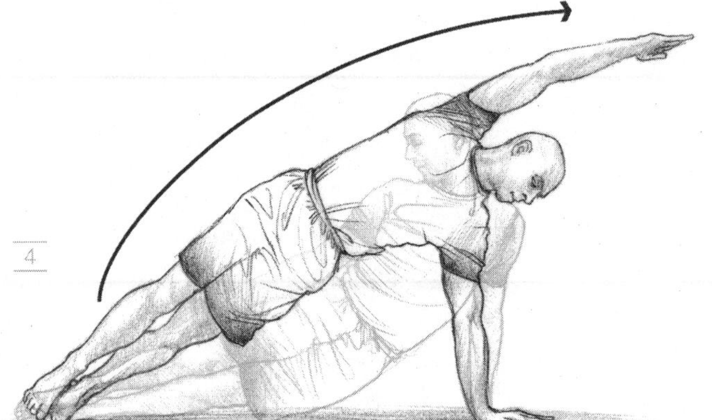

Inhale and lift your hips and body up into a straight line with straight legs as you reach your right arm overhead again.

Lower and lift your hips for a total of 5 repetitions.

Lower your body down to the starting position as you exhale.

Repeat this exercise in its entirety on your opposite side.

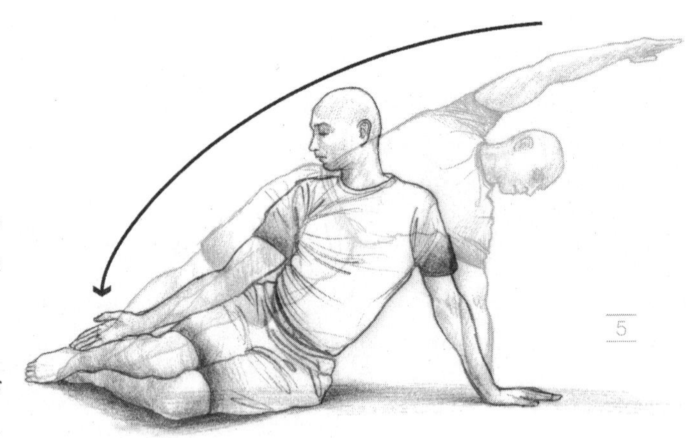

THE BEAST WITHIN

BODY POSITION The illustrations demonstrate a more difficult version of the Side Bend, with your feet stacked on top of each other. When you first try this exercise, for better balance, place your top foot on the floor in front of the other foot so that they are heel-to-toe. Keep your supporting shoulder down and squarely in its socket. Do not sink into your supporting shoulder. It helps to tighten the armpit of your supporting arm and think of pushing your body away from the floor.

THE MIND IN MOTION Lower yourself down until the knee of your lower leg lightly touches the floor. Don't lower yourself all the way and sit on your hip until you need to switch sides or have completed the exercise. Don't let your top hip roll forward or backward. Keep your hips squarely aligned. When your body is lifted, you may look forward or at your supporting hand (as illustrated). Keep your powerhouse firmly in and your spine long.

CAUTIONS Leave this exercise out if you have neck, shoulder, wrist, back, hip, foot, or ankle problems.

THE BOOMERANG

BENEFITS: LENGTHENS THE LEGS AND SPINE; OPENS THE CHEST, SHOULDERS, AND HIPS; STRENGTHENS THE POWERHOUSE; MASSAGES THE SPINE; DEVELOPS BALANCE; WORKS THE LUNGS

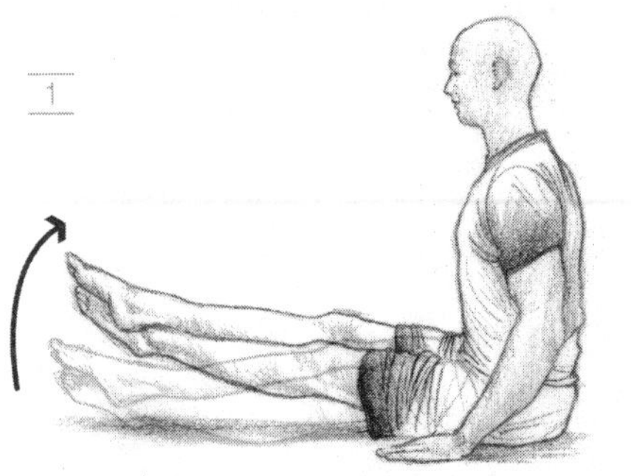

Pull your powerhouse in and up as you sit up tall with your hands palm down on the floor beside your hips. Cross your right ankle over your left ankle. Inhale. Lift your legs using your powerhouse as you begin to roll backward.

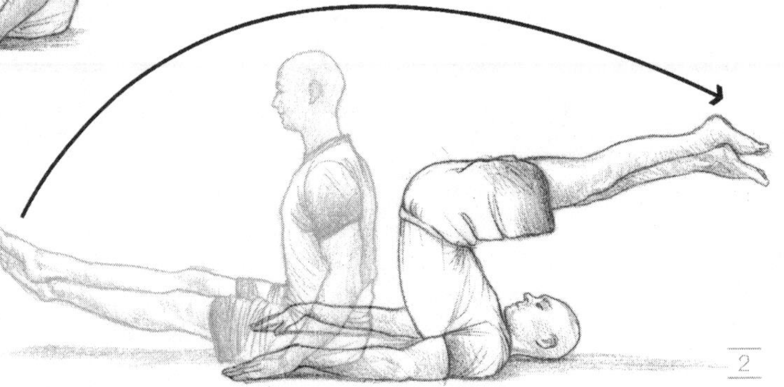

Exhale and roll onto your upper back, keeping your spine and hips lifted. Your arms should now be long with palms facing down on the mat, helping to support you.

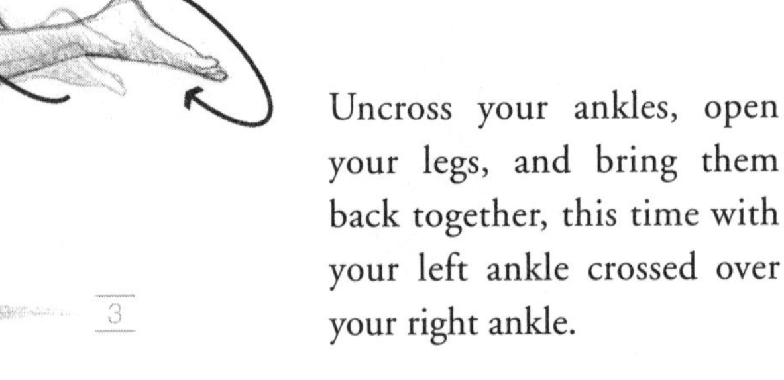

Uncross your ankles, open your legs, and bring them back together, this time with your left ankle crossed over your right ankle.

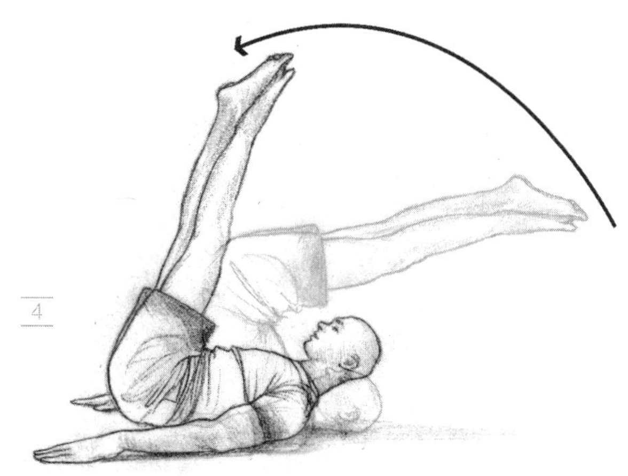

Inhale and roll forward, keeping your powerhouse in.

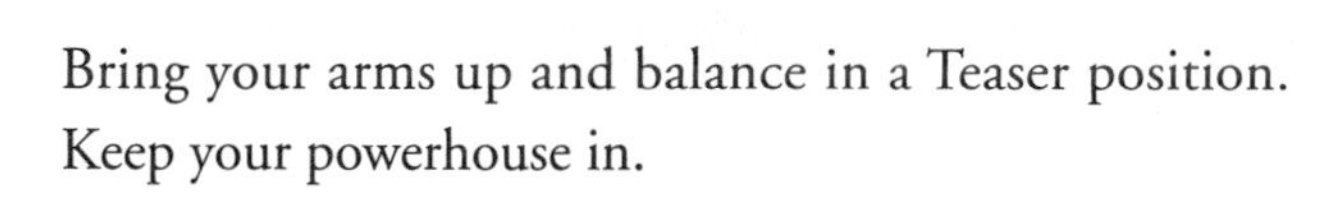

Bring your arms up and balance in a Teaser position. Keep your powerhouse in.

5

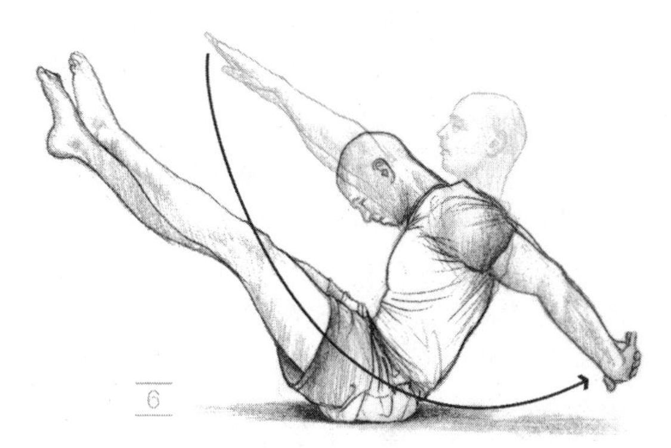

Bring your arms behind you and clasp your hands together. Reach your arms and legs up and lengthen them away from each other as you pull your powerhouse in.

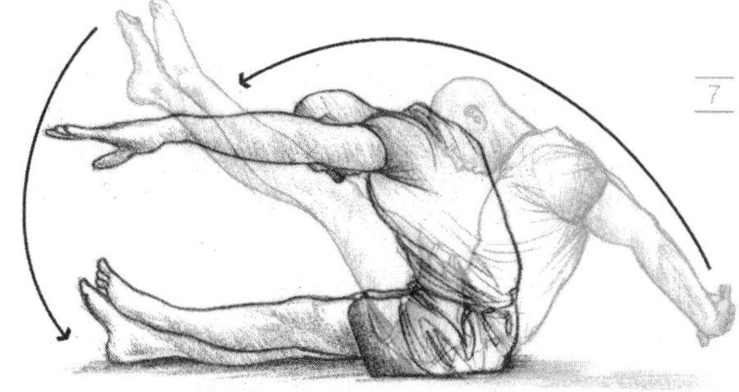

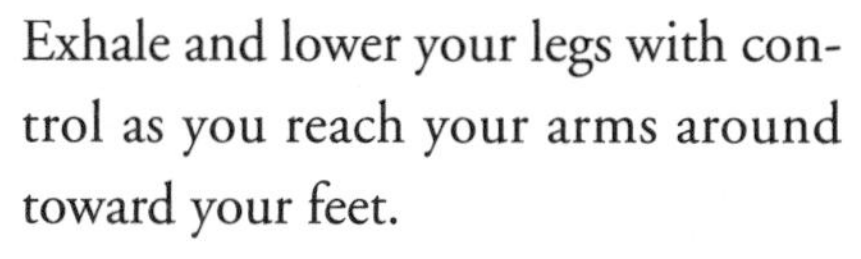

Exhale and lower your legs with control as you reach your arms around toward your feet.

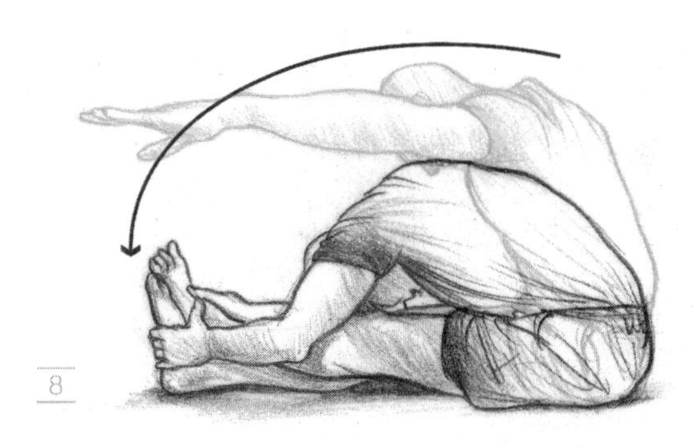

Bring your forehead to your legs as you complete the exhale. Stretch like this momentarily.

Perform 6 times.

THE BEAST WITHIN

BODY POSITION The Boomerang engages your entire body. Lengthen your legs through your toes as you pull your powerhouse in. Your hands should be anchored on the floor as you begin to roll back.

THE MIND IN MOTION Be sure to have mastered Teaser I before attempting this exercise. Your legs should rise at the same time as (or just before) you roll on your spine. To accomplish this, you must keep your powerhouse firmly drawn in as you roll backward. If you leave your legs on the ground as you roll backward and *then* lift them as a subsequent movement you are not using your powerhouse and you risk hurting your lower back. As in the Roll Over, don't allow your hips to collapse and your legs to fall down onto your face when your bottom is in the air and you're switching the ankle cross (see illustration 3). This is especially important to keep in mind if you have notably heavy legs. Keep your spine and hips lifted. If you can't clasp your hands together in steps 6 and 7 because of a tight back and/or tight shoulders, then reach your hands behind you, palms up and with your arms straight.

CAUTIONS Leave this exercise out if you have neck, shoulder, hip, or back problems, or scoliosis. If your scoliosis is very slight, you may try it, but focus on rolling straight. To avoid injury, it's very important to remember to engage your powerhouse throughout this exercise.

THE SEAL

BENEFITS: MASSAGES AND STRETCHES THE BACK; STRENGTHENS THE POWERHOUSE; OPENS THE HIPS; WORKS THE LUNGS

Sit on your bottom with your knees bent. Feed your hands inside your legs and take hold of the tops of your feet. Bring your chin to your chest. Pull your powerhouse in and balance on your buttocks with your feet in the air. Clap the soles of your feet together 3 times. Inhale and roll backward.

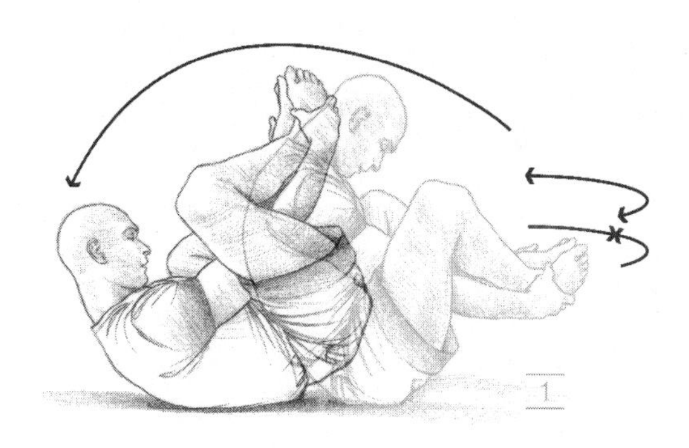

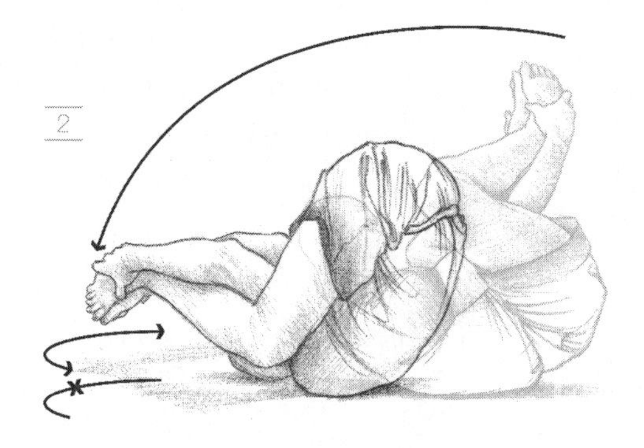

Roll onto your upper back. Clap the soles of your feet together 3 times while in this position.

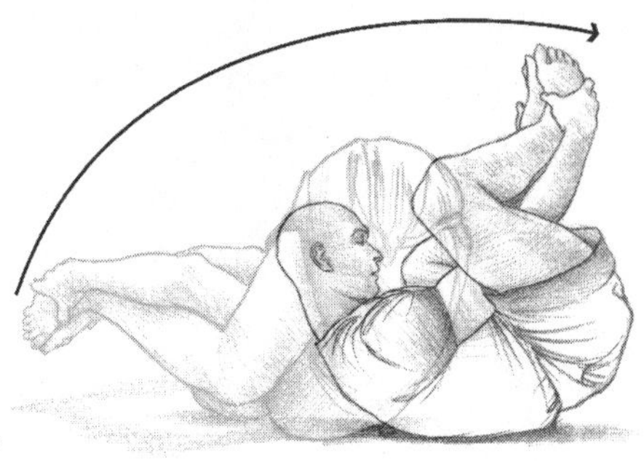

Exhale, pull your powerhouse in, and roll up.

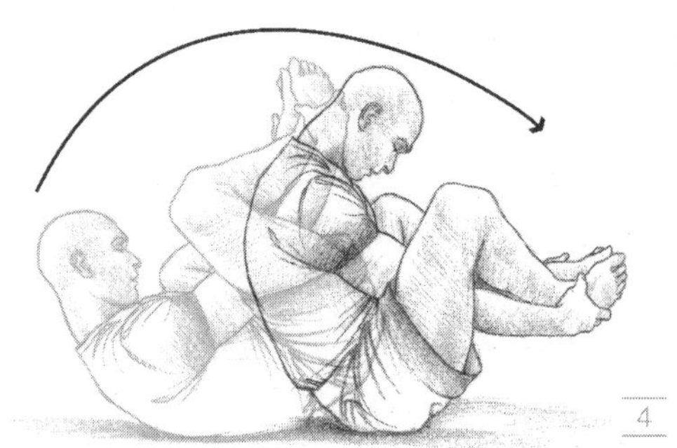

Finish exhaling and balance on your buttocks.

Perform 6 times.

THE BEAST WITHIN

BODY POSITION The Seal opens your hips more than the other rolling exercises. This does not mean, however, that you can relax when performing the Seal. You must hold your powerhouse firmly throughout the motion.

THE MIND IN MOTION Don't throw your head back to initiate the backward roll. Use your powerhouse to control the roll back and the roll up. Holding your powerhouse will also help you maintain the rounded shape of your spine. Roll the full length of your spine, keeping your shoulders down and away from your ears. Men typically find it difficult at first to contort themselves into a small, little package. Being overweight will only make it more difficult. If you have trouble with this position, hold your calves, shins, or ankles. The illustrations demonstrate an easier version of the Seal by touching only the inside edges of the feet together during the clap and roll. To get the most out of this exercise, keep the entire soles of the feet together when you roll. You'll find your knees higher with your hips, and your lower back opened up even more.

CAUTIONS Leave this exercise out if you have neck, shoulder, back, hip, knee problems, or scoliosis. If your scoliosis is very slight, you may try it but focus on rolling straight.

THE CRAB

BENEFITS: STRENGTHENS THE POWERHOUSE; MASSAGES THE SPINE; DEVELOPS FLEXIBILITY IN THE HIPS; WORKS THE LUNGS

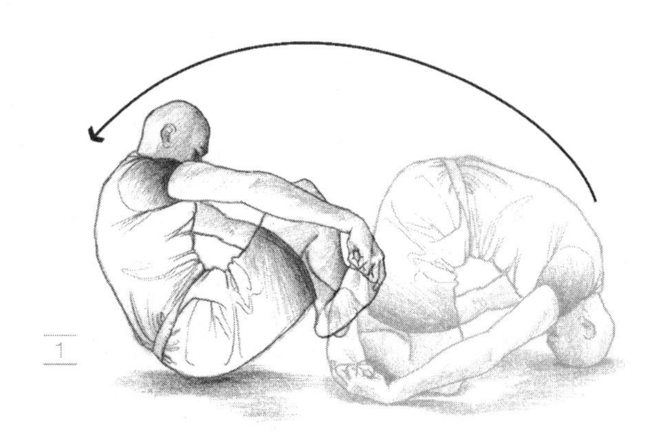

1

Sitting down after the Seal, cross your legs with the calf of your right leg across the shin of your left leg and take hold of your feet. Pull your powerhouse in and up. Bring your chin to your chest. Slowly roll forward onto your knees, bringing your head to the mat as you exhale. This is the starting position. Inhale and roll backward, keeping your powerhouse lifted.

Roll onto your upper back while finishing the inhalation. Keep your powerhouse in.

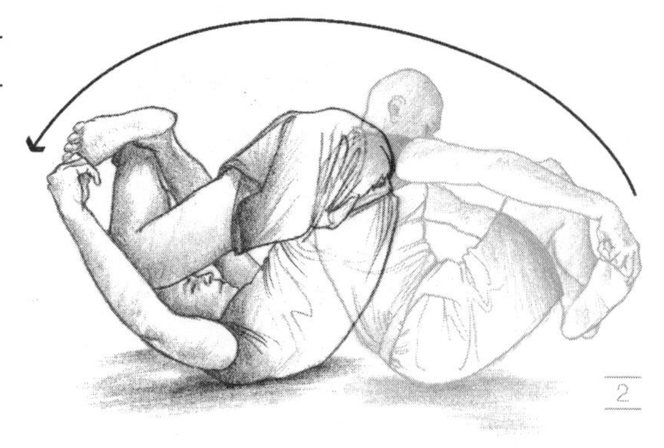

2

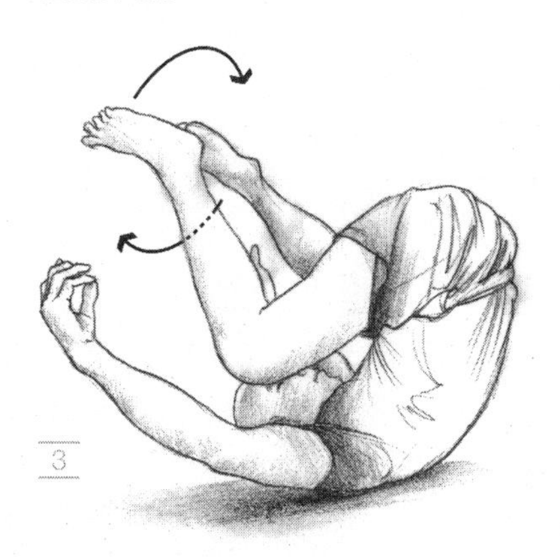

3

Release your feet, open and uncross your legs, but keep them bent.

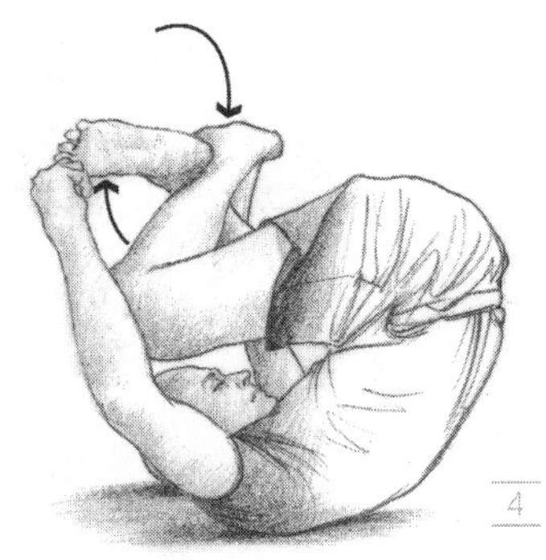

Switch your legs so that the calf of your left leg now crosses over the shin of your right leg. Take hold of your feet.

Exhale and roll up. Pull your powerhouse in and up.

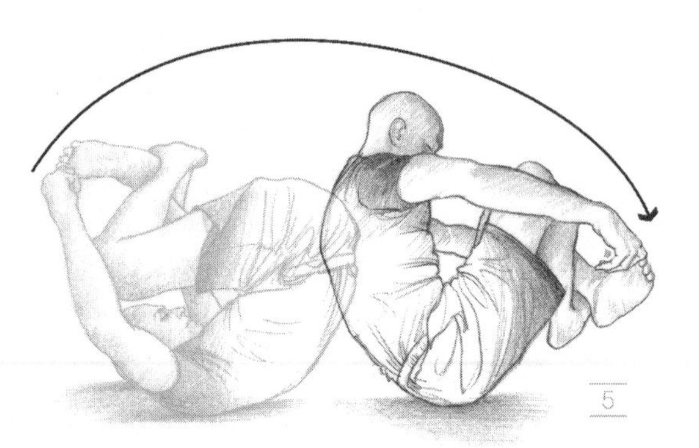

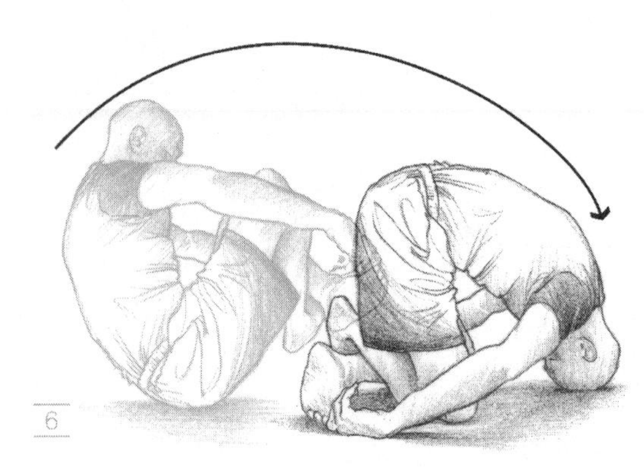

Finish exhaling and roll back onto your knees and head. Keep your powerhouse in and up.

Perform 6 times.

THE BEAST WITHIN

BODY POSITION When your head rests upon the mat, do *not* let your neck (cervical spine) collapse. In other words, don't arch or hyperflex your neck. Keep your neck long. Keep your powerhouse lifted in and up.

THE MIND IN MOTION The Crab is rarely taught, but it's a blast—as long as you keep a few things in mind. When lowering your head to the mat, do it slowly. Do not transfer your body weight to your head as it approaches the mat. Keep your powerhouse in and up when your head is on the floor. Keep your shoulders down and away from your ears.

CAUTIONS Leave this exercise out if you have neck, shoulder, back, hip, knee, or foot problems, or if you have scoliosis. If your scoliosis is very slight, you may try it but focus on rolling straight. Most of all, remember to *protect your neck.*

ROCKING

BENEFITS: STRETCHES THE HIP FLEXORS AND THIGHS; OPENS THE CHEST; STRENGTHENS THE BACK, LEGS, BUTTOCKS, AND POWERHOUSE

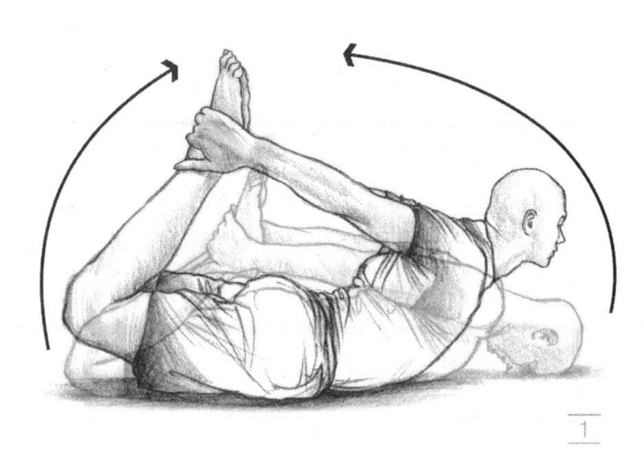
1

After the Crab, lie down on your stomach with your forehead on the mat. Bend your knees and take hold of the tops of your feet with your hands. Keep your legs close together. (If you wish to stretch the front of your legs, you may pull your heels to your buttocks 3 times before proceeding.) Inhale, pull your powerhouse in, and squeeze your buttocks. Simultaneously lift your chest and knees off the mat. Hold for an exhalation.

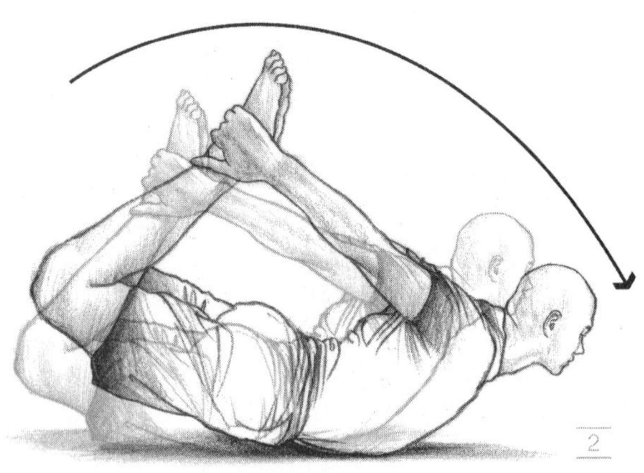
2

Inhale and rock your body forward.

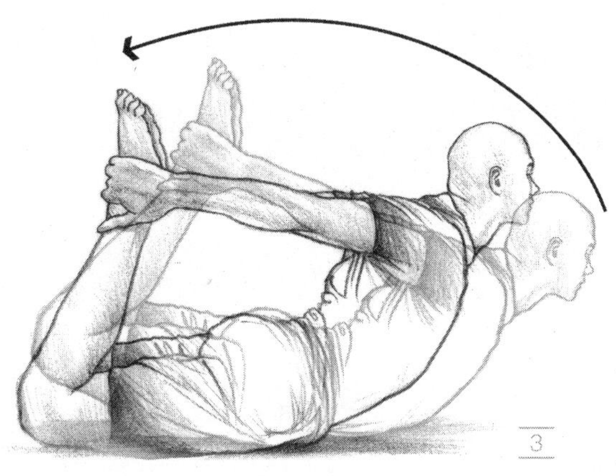

Exhale and rock your body backward.

Perform 5 times.

THE BEAST WITHIN

BODY POSITION When you are lifted in the starting position, keep your chest and knees off the mat. Keep your back lifted and your neck long. Attempt to maintain straight arms.

THE MIND IN MOTION This can be an uncomfortable position for men, so adjust accordingly beforehand! Squeeze your buttocks while you rock. Use your abdominal muscles to rock back and forth. Don't rock with your head; keep your head lifted up and back as far as comfortably possible. You may touch your chin lightly to the floor on the forward rock.

CAUTIONS Tight backs, shoulders, and hip flexors often make it difficult for men to lift off the floor or even reach their feet at all. Lengthen your whole body upward instead of straining your lower back when you lift off the floor. Leave this exercise out if you have neck, shoulder, rib, back, hip, ankle, or knee problems.

THE CONTROL BALANCE

BENEFITS: DEVELOPS FLEXIBILITY, BALANCE, COORDINATION, AND POWERHOUSE STRENGTH

After Rocking, turn over onto your back. Place your arms straight alongside your body with your palms down, and keep your shoulders down and away from your ears. Start with your spine on the floor. Pull your powerhouse in. Exhale and lift your legs up.

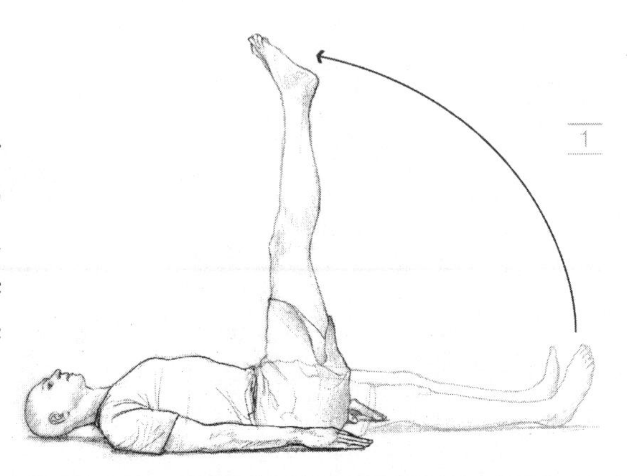

Roll up your hips and then your spine one vertebra at a time until your toes rest on the floor behind your head; your ankles should be flexed. Take hold of your ankles with your hands.

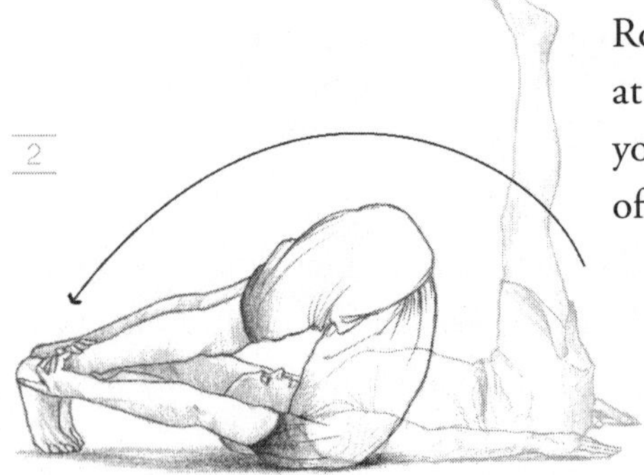

3

Release your left leg and clasp your right ankle with both hands. Inhale and extend your left leg to the ceiling with your foot pointed.

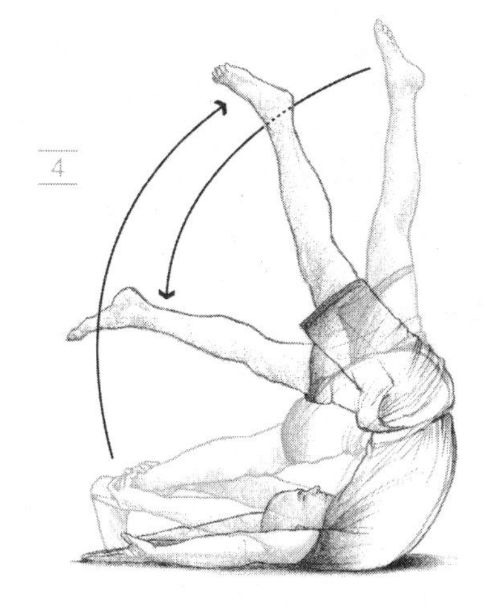

Release your right ankle. Exhale and switch your legs.

Clasp your left ankle with both hands. Extend your right leg to the ceiling as you finish exhaling.

Perform the leg switch (steps 3 to 5) 6 times.

5

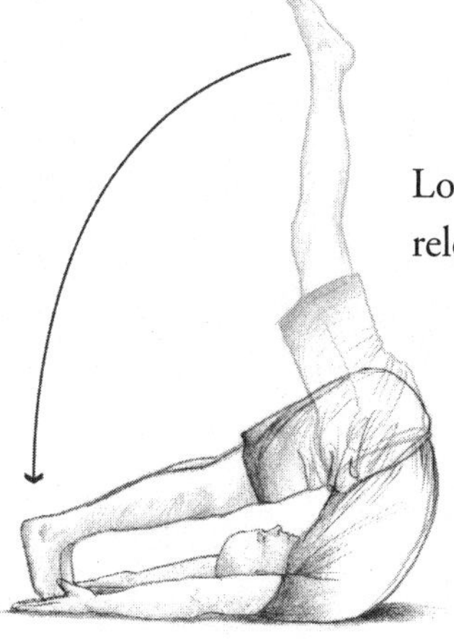

Lower your right leg to the floor and release your hands as you inhale.

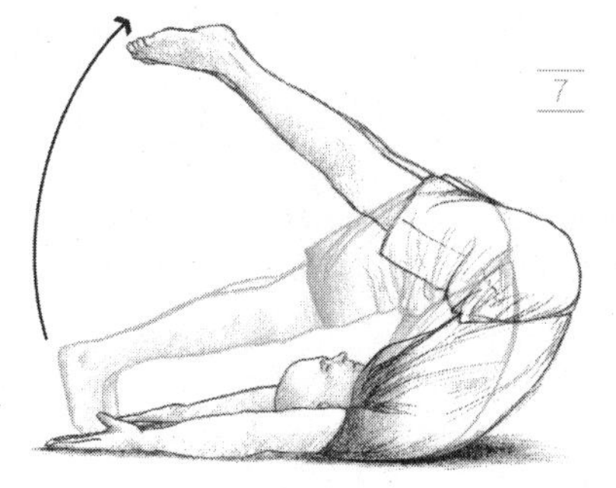

Keep your powerhouse pulled in. Roll your spine down to the mat one vertebra at a time.

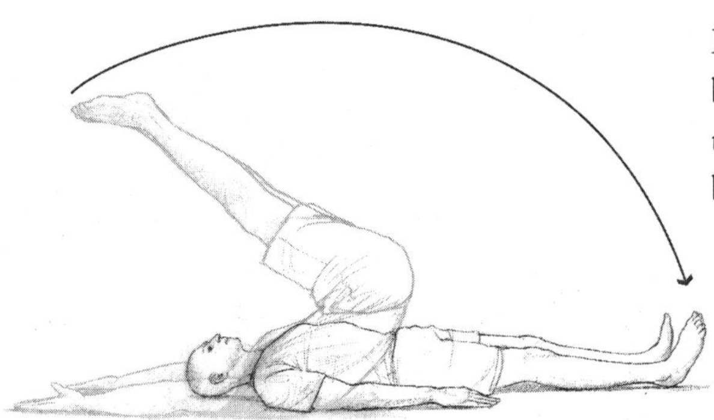

Exhale and finish lowering your body. Once you're fully lowered on the floor, bring your arms and hands back down alongside your body.

THE BEAST WITHIN

BODY POSITION Like the Crab, I rarely see this exercise taught. It is a small tragedy because it's a great exercise. You must hold your powerhouse firmly in or else your spine and hips will collapse. Keep your spine lifted. Balance your weight among your shoulders, arms, and neck—with the least amount of weight in your neck. You should feel neither pressure nor pain in your neck. You may clasp your ankle at either the same spot or with one hand higher on your leg than the other. You may also extend your ankle and point the toes of your clasped leg. Keep your knees locked and your hips square.

THE MIND IN MOTION This exercise both demands and develops flexibility, balance, coordination, and powerhouse strength. If you're lacking in any of these areas, then you probably won't be able to hold this position and your bottom will roll to the floor. Switch your legs slowly at the same time (see illustration 4). When you first try this, you may lower your top leg first and then raise your opposite leg. When you become better at this exercise, switch your legs at the same time.

CAUTIONS Leave this one out if you have neck, shoulder, hip, ankle, or back problems.

THE PUSH-UP

BENEFITS: STRENGTHENS THE ENTIRE BODY; DEVELOPS AGILITY AND FLEXIBILITY

Stand in Pilates stance. Inhale and reach your hands over your head.

Round over the front of your body to the floor as you exhale, keeping your buttocks over your heels.

Finish exhaling and reach the floor with your hands.

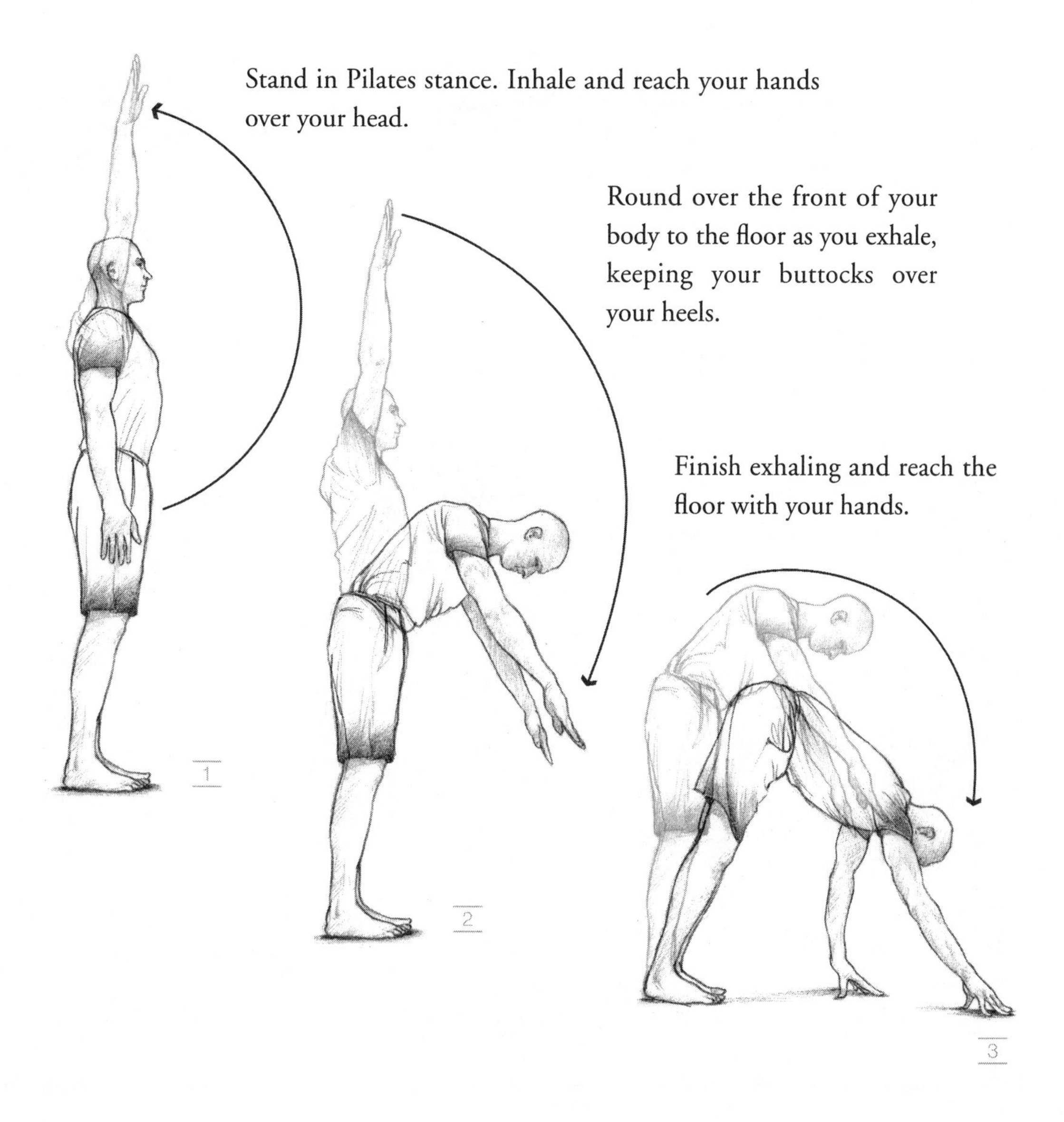

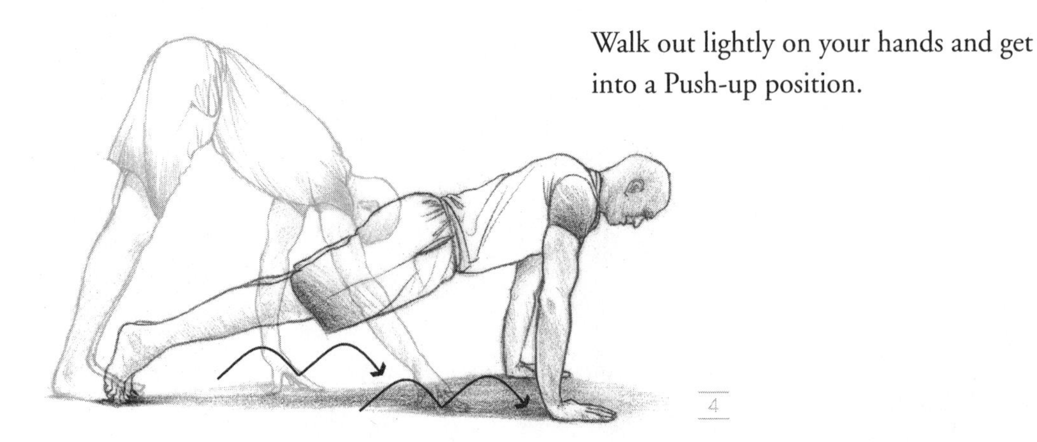

Walk out lightly on your hands and get into a Push-up position.

Inhale, look forward, and pull yourself to the floor. Exhale and lift your body up.

Perform 3 to 5 Push-ups.

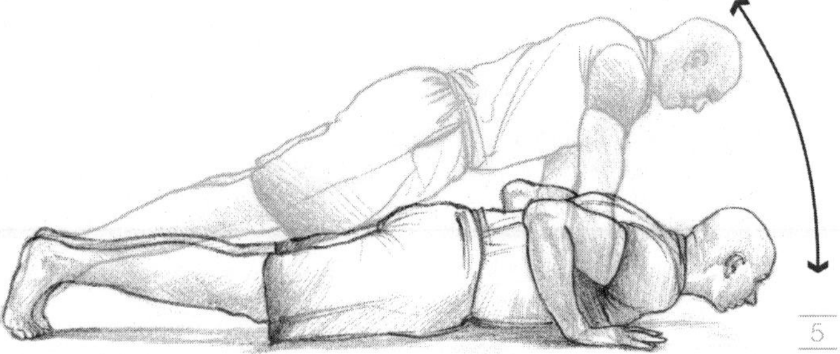

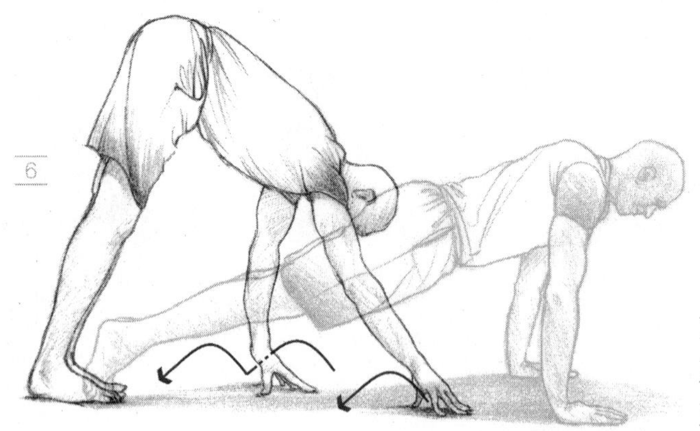

Keep your powerhouse in. Inhale and lightly walk your hands back to your feet.

Exhale and bend forward toward your legs.

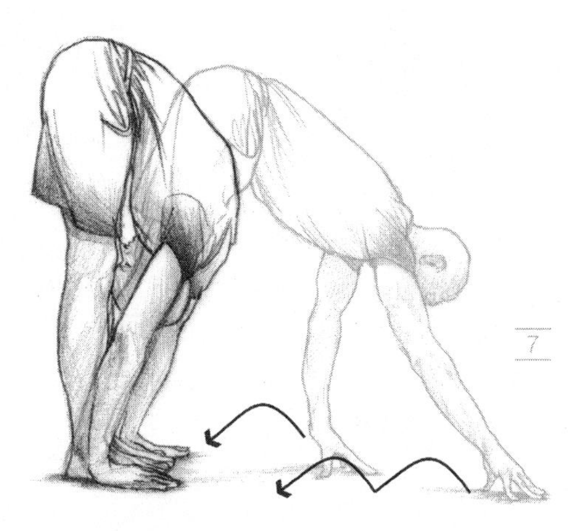

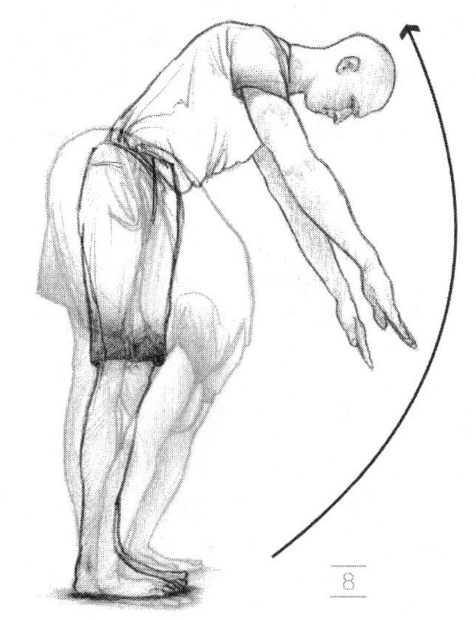

Inhale and roll your spine up one vertebra at a time. Keep your powerhouse in and your bottom over your heels.

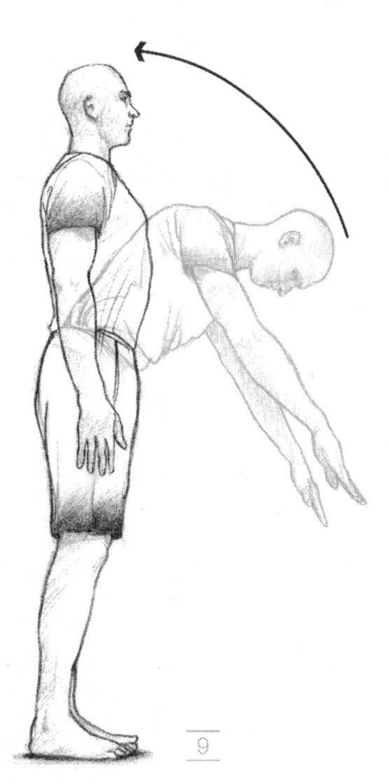

Exhale, finish rolling up, and resume Pilates stance.

THE BEAST WITHIN

BODY POSITION The Push-up is familiar to most men, but let us look at some of the finer points. When you take the Push-up position, make sure your wrists are underneath your shoulders. Lock your elbows. Screw your shoulders down into their sockets. Actively engage your back muscles in the Push-up. Keep your legs zipped together, as if you are in Pilates stance. Keep your tailbone tucked and your buttocks squeezed. Keep your powerhouse in and firm. Look slightly forward, not down. Hold your body straight and strong like a battering ram.

THE MIND IN MOTION When you round over and reach for the floor, don't jut out your bottom. Keep your bottom over your heels. If you can't reach the floor with straight legs, then bend your knees. When you walk out on your hands, move softly like a cat. When you perform the Push-ups, keep your entire body tight and engaged. Don't allow your head, hips, or lower back to sag. Don't allow your elbows to rotate out. If you follow all of these guidelines, you'll maximize the benefits of the Push-up and strengthen your entire body.

If you are recovering from an injury and have diminished strength, simply try to hold yourself in an upright position and firm up your entire body (see illustration 4). Lower your knees to the floor and take a break long before you begin to shake. Try this for 3 repetitions.

In Pilates, men often work up to performing "clapping Push-ups" and then "leaping Push-ups" (neither illustrated). Clapping Push-ups are performed by thrusting your upper body and hands off the floor, as you rise up, ya clap your hands together once. As gravity pulls you back down to the floor, you meet the floor with your hands to absorb your body weight. This helps to soften the landing, which can be hard on the wrists. In leaping Push-ups, you thrust your arms and feet off the floor and bring your entire body into the air with each repetition.

CAUTIONS If you're overweight, it's especially important to hold your powerhouse in so your weight doesn't pull on your lower back. If you have wrist problems, make fists and distribute your weight onto the first two knuckles of your fists to perform the Push-up. If it still hurts, then leave the Push-up out. Leave this exercise out if you have neck, shoulder, elbow, or back problems.

PART III

INTRODUCTION TO REFORMER ON THE MAT

The "reformer on the mat" is considered super advanced mat work. It is rarely taught, and I seldom witness Pilates practitioners or instructors performing the reformer on the mat within their own practice. There is a certain mystique to the reformer on the mat that intimidates people, but this is unwarranted.

Like the traditional mat work, the reformer on the mat are body weight-only exercises. You do not need exceptional mental faculties to conceptualize the movements. Remember, Pilates was designed to be natural for our bodies. Although the workout is difficult in its entirety, it is still based on the six principles of Pilates. It is still about contrology—control of the mind and body.

You only need to answer one question before beginning the reformer on the mat: *Are you an advanced Pilates mat practitioner?* If you can't answer yes to this question, then you're not yet ready for the reformer on the mat. First, you must master the forty exercises in the traditional Pilates mat work. My definition of "advanced" is that you can execute 99 percent of the traditional Pilates mat work with control. The 1 percent that you haven't mastered represents the small things within an exercise that are difficult for you and your body specifically. When I say "master the mat work," I am urging you to demonstrate proper control, centering, concentration, precision, flow, and breathing within your movement in all forty traditional exercises before moving on.

If you are an advanced mat practitioner, then you are ready to begin the reformer on the mat. As always, work intelligently and safely. If something hurts, then leave it out. Like the traditional Pilates mat work, these exercises are broken up into beginner, intermediate, and advanced levels, and are depicted in the complete sequential order. See the chart showing the beginner, intermediate, and advanced curriculums for the reformer on the mat available on pages 137 to 140. Use the chart as a guide for adding exercises into your practice as you did with the traditional mat work. Begin with your basic reformer on the mat exercises and add on exercises as your body absorbs the work.

I recommend that you start out by adding the beginner reformer on the mat exercises to the end of your traditional mat work. This will lengthen the time of your practice and allow your body to acclimate to more exercises. When you have incorporated the entire beginner and roughly about a third to half of the intermediate exercises into your regular practice, then you may begin to dedicate one workout a week to the reformer on the mat exclusively. When you reach this level, I recommend performing the traditional mat work one to three times a week and the reformer on the mat once a week.

The reformer on the mat exercises are named after the universal reformer, the apparatus in a Pilates studio on which they are typically performed. The apparatus is about eighty-five inches long and about fifteen inches off the ground, depending on which model a studio uses. It has a sliding carriage that rests on two tracts. The underside of the carriage, closest to the feet, is connected to four springs of equal tension. (Some companies make reformers with five springs and varying tensions.) The beginner, intermediate, and advanced levels of the reformer on the mat exercises are based on the difficulty of performing them on a universal reformer, with the help of the four springs that act as four extra muscles.

In many cases, it's more difficult to perform an exercise on the mat, because you have neither the aid of the four springs nor the structure of the reformer on which to align your body. In other cases, the instability of a moving carriage coupled with spring settings can add difficulty to an exercise, making it easier to perform on a stable floor. The Stomach Massage Round (see page 223) is a good example of the prior. On a universal reformer, your feet are resting on an elevated foot bar. In the reformer on the mat, your legs and feet extend out into space. Although the four springs of the universal reformer create resistance, it is much more difficult to perform this exercise on the mat with your feet in the air because you have to hold your legs up. The Stomach Massage Round is listed as a beginner exercise because it is considered basic when performed on the universal reformer apparatus. In other words, please note that even the basic reformer on the mat exercises are advanced and can be quite challenging.

Between the traditional mat and the reformer on the mat, there is a cornucopia of exercises for a lifetime of practice. While there are more variations of the reformer on the mat exercises than are illustrated in this book, sixty-six variations are more than enough of a challenge for most people. Don't rush through these exercises. Practice diligently and adhere to the six principles of Pilates—control, centering, concentration, precision, flow, and breathing. Over time, you will move with more assurance and strength than you ever thought possible. Enjoy the challenge!

REFORMER ON THE MAT EXERCISES

REFORMER ON THE MAT CURRICULUM

BEGINNER

1. Footwork: Toes 141
2. Footwork: Arches 143
3. Footwork: Heels 145
4. Footwork: Tendon stretch 147

1b–4b. Standing Footwork Series 149

5. The Hundred 153

20. Short Box Round 191
21. Short Box Flat 194
22. Side to Side 196

25. The Tree 203

29. The Elephant 217

32. Stomach Massage Round 223
33. Stomach Massage Hands Back 225
34. Stomach Massage Reach Up 228

56. Knee Stretches I, II and III 287
57. Running 293
58. The Pelvic Lift 295

INTERMEDIATE

ADVANCED

ADVANCED (continued)

FOOTWORK SERIES
TOES, ARCHES, HEELS, TENDON STRETCH

FOOTWORK: TOES

BENEFITS: STRENGTHENS THE LEGS AND THE POWERHOUSE

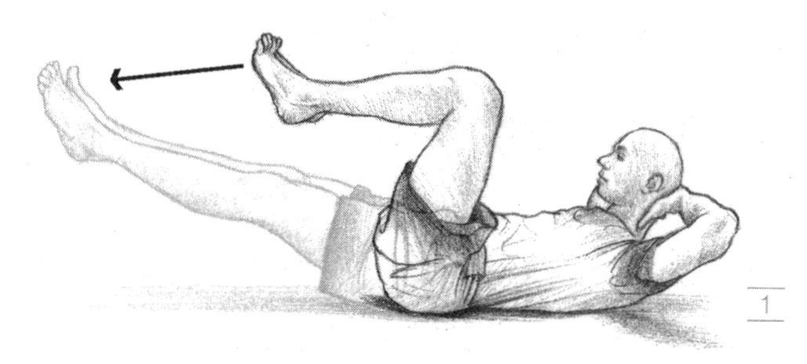

Lie on the floor with your knees bent toward your chest. Interlace your fingers behind your head and lift your shoulders off the floor using your abdominal muscles. Point your feet out in Pilates stance, with your toes pulled back. In this starting position, your knees will be apart. Keep your powerhouse in and extend your legs as you inhale.

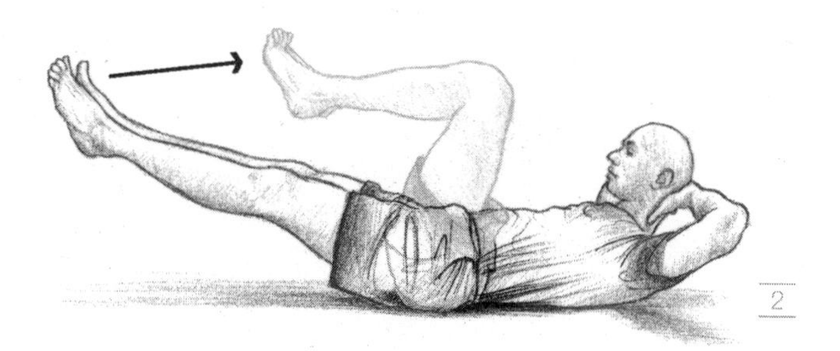

Exhale and pull your legs back in, keeping your powerhouse engaged.

Perform 10 times.

THE BEAST WITHIN

BODY POSITION From your tailbone to the tips of your shoulder blades, your spine should remain on the floor. Keep your abdominal muscles firm and in throughout the movement; don't release your powerhouse.

THE MIND IN MOTION Start out by holding your extended legs out high. As you progress, lower them to challenge the strength of your powerhouse. Do not arch your lower back. If your back hurts, try holding your legs higher or cease the exercise. Initiate the movement from your powerhouse and work both legs fully. Squeeze your buttocks firmly to assist your legs. If you have a popping hip, then either widen the turnout of your feet, or close the turnout and touch the insides of your feet together instead. If you have a knee problem, don't bring your knees in too close to your chest. You don't have to lock your knees when you extend your legs either. If you let your quads dominate the movement, your hip flexors are likely to get tight and your powerhouse won't work or benefit as much from the exercise. You also risk straining your lower back. To avoid this, it helps to focus on squeezing your inner thighs and buttocks and lengthening your hamstrings as you press your legs out.

CAUTIONS After a complete Footwork Series, your abdominal muscles will feel like they're on fire. Work up to the complete repetition count among the Footwork Series exercises to avoid fatiguing your powerhouse. Try 5 of each instead of 10. If you overwork your powerhouse, you risk hurting your back on subsequent exercises because you won't be able to control your movement. Leave this out if you have neck, shoulder, hip, knee, or back problems.

FOOTWORK SERIES
TOES, ARCHES, HEELS, TENDON STRETCH

FOOTWORK: ARCHES

BENEFITS: STRENGTHENS THE LEGS AND THE POWERHOUSE

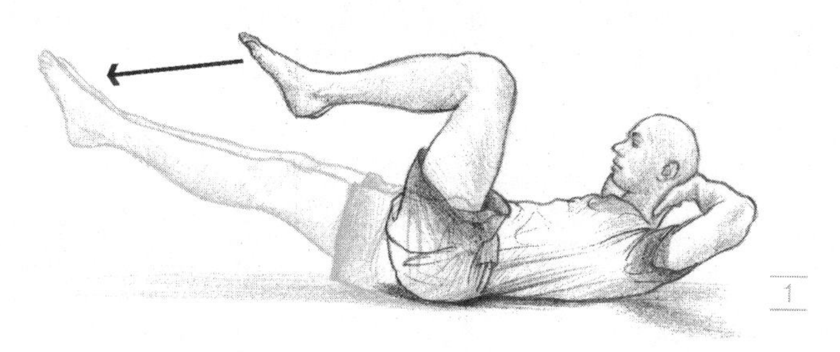

Stay in the same position that you were in for the Footwork: Toes, keep your knees, legs, and feet pressed together. Point your toes and drop your heels so that you are pushing at the arches of your feet. Engage your powerhouse. Inhale and extend your legs out.

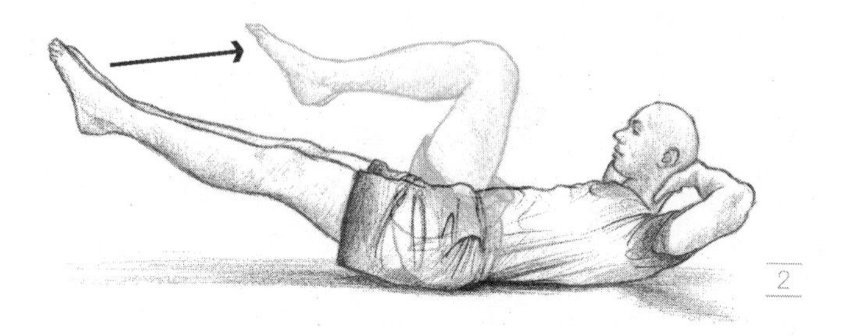

Exhale and bring your legs back to your chest.

Perform 10 times.

THE BEAST WITHIN

BODY POSITION From your tailbone to the tips of your shoulder blades, your spine should remain on the floor. Keep your abdominals firmly in throughout the movement; don't release your powerhouse. Keep your legs together.

THE MIND IN MOTION Start by holding your extended legs out high. As you progress, lower them to challenge your powerhouse strength. Do not arch your lower back. If your back hurts, try holding your legs higher or cease the exercise. Initiate the movement from your powerhouse and work both legs fully. Squeeze your buttocks firmly to assist your legs. If you have a knee problem, don't bring your knees in too close to your chest. You don't have to lock your knees when you extend your legs either. If your knees roll in as you extend your legs, try turning your feet out slightly. The turnout may open your legs a bit when you bring your knees to your chest. If you let your quads dominate the movement, your hip flexors are likely to get tired and your powerhouse won't work or benefit as much from this exercise. You also risk straining your lower back. To avoid this, it helps to focus on squeezing your inner thighs and buttocks and lengthening your hamstrings as you press your legs out.

CAUTIONS Leave this out if you have neck, shoulder, hip, knee, or back problems.

FOOTWORK SERIES
TOES, ARCHES, HEELS, TENDON STRETCH

FOOTWORK: HEELS

BENEFITS: STRENGTHENS THE LEGS AND POWERHOUSE

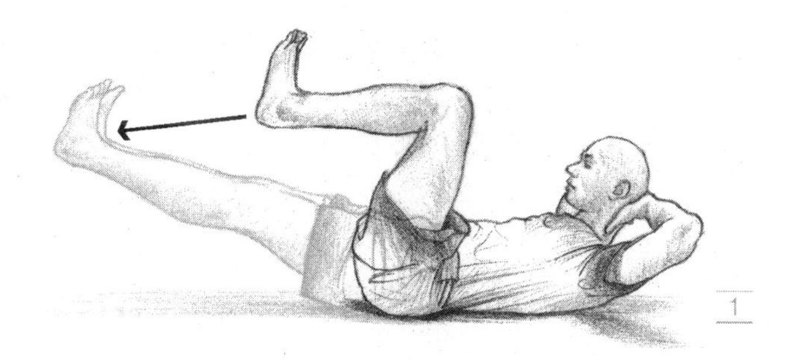

Maintain the same body position that you were in for the Footwork: Arches, keep your knees, legs, and feet pressed together. Flex your ankles and pull your toes back toward your nose. Engage your powerhouse. Inhale and extend your legs out through your heels.

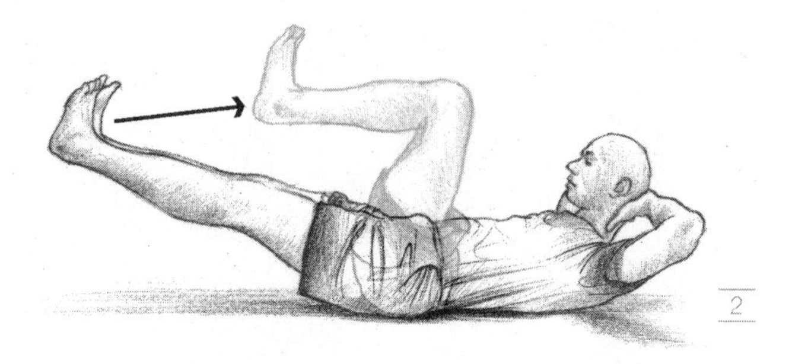

Exhale and bend your knees to your chest.

Perform 10 times.

THE BEAST WITHIN

BODY POSITION From your tailbone to the tips of your shoulder blades, your spine should remain on the floor. Keep your abdominals firmly in throughout the movement; don't release your powerhouse. Keep your ankles flexed with your toes pulled back toward your nose.

THE MIND IN MOTION Start out by holding your legs high. As you progress, lower your legs to challenge your powerhouse strength. Do not arch your lower back. If your back hurts, try lifting your legs higher or cease the exercise. Initiate the movement from your powerhouse, and work both legs fully Squeeze your buttocks firmly to assist in using your legs. If you have a knee problem, don't bring your knees too close to your chest. You don't have to lock your knees when you extend your legs either. If you let your quads dominate the movement, your hip flexors are likely to get tired and your powerhouse won't work or benefit as much from this exercise. You also risk straining your back. To avoid this, it helps to focus on squeezing your inner thighs and buttocks and lengthening your hamstrings as you press your legs out. If your knees roll in as you extend your legs, try turning your feet out slightly. The turnout may open your legs a bit when you bring your knees to your chest.

CAUTIONS Leave this exercise out if you have neck, shoulder, hip, knee, or back problems.

FOOTWORK SERIES
TOES, ARCHES, HEELS, TENDON STRETCH

FOOTWORK: TENDON STRETCH

BENEFITS: STRENGTHENS THE POWERHOUSE; LENGTHENS THE BACKS OF THE LEGS

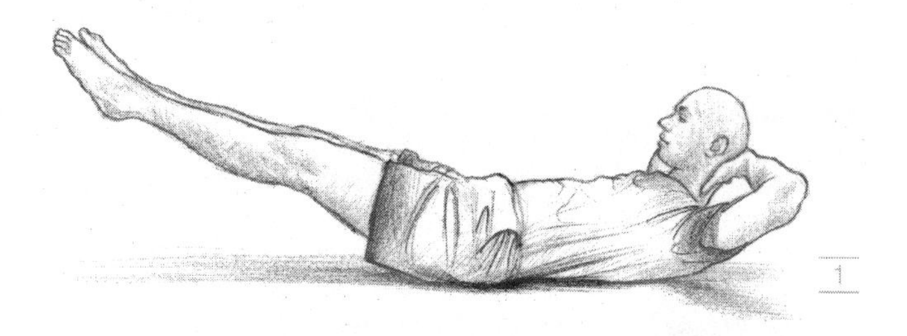

When you finish the Footwork: Heels, inhale and extend your legs out with your toes pointed and hold them there. Keep your powerhouse engaged and your legs firmly together. You may turnout your feet in Pilates stance as illustrated, or you may keep your feet together.

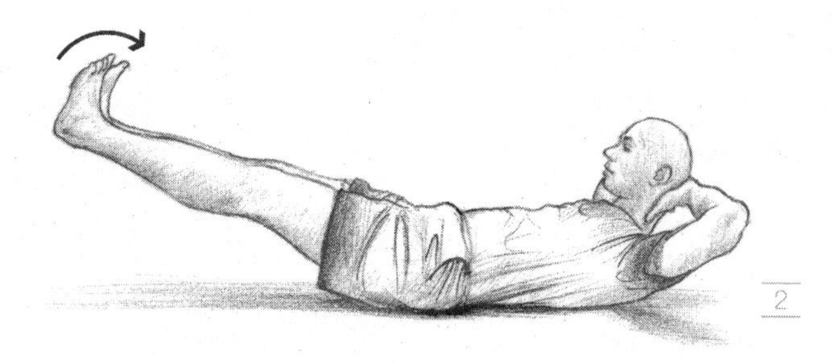

Exhale and flex your ankles, pulling your toes back toward your nose.

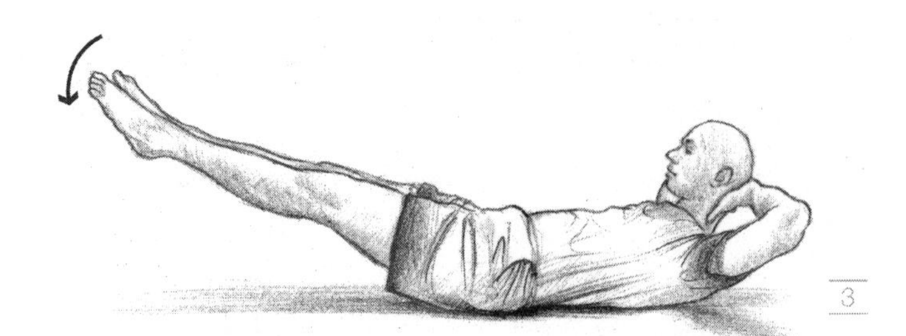

Inhale and point your toes down and away from you. Hold your powerhouse firmly in.

Perform 10 times.

THE BEAST WITHIN

BODY POSITION From the tailbone to the tips of your shoulder blades, your spine should remain on the floor. Keep your abdominals firm and down throughout the movement; don't release your powerhouse.

THE MIND IN MOTION Start out by holding your legs high. As you progress, lower them to challenge your powerhouse strength. Focus on squeezing your inner thighs and buttocks and lengthening your hamstrings as you extend and hold your legs in the air. Holding your legs out while pointing and flexing your toes can be difficult. By the end of the Footwork Series, your powerhouse may be screaming for mercy and you may find yourself anticipating the finish instead of concentrating on controlling your movement. If you release your abdominals, this can be dangerous because you risk putting strain on your lower back. Do not arch your lower back. If you begin to feel discomfort in your lower back, try the exercise with your legs higher in the air. If this doesn't alleviate your discomfort, then bend your knees and stop. Hug your shins for several seconds to release the pressure in your back.

CAUTIONS Leave this exercise out if you have neck, shoulder, hip, knee, or back problems.

STANDING FOOTWORK SERIES
TOES, ARCHES, HEELS, TENDON STRETCH

(As an alternative, all of the footwork can be performed from a standing position as well.)

STANDING FOOTWORK: TOES

BENEFITS: STRENGTHENS THE FEET, LEGS, AND POWERHOUSE; IMPROVES BALANCE

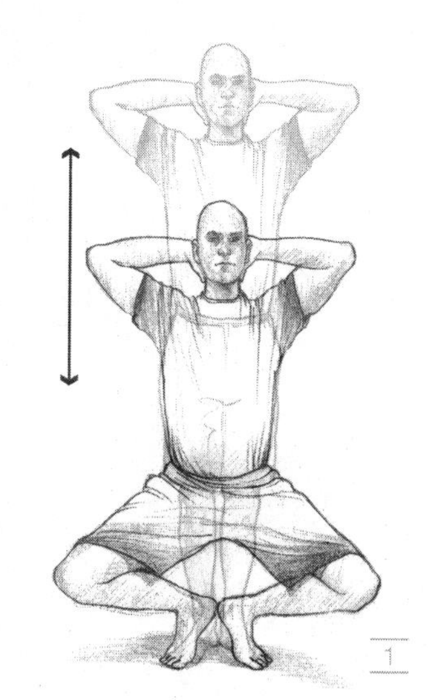

Stand in Pilates stance with your hands interlaced (or hand over hand) behind your head. Hold your elbows out to the sides and hold your neck long. Pull your powerhouse in and up. Inhale and lower yourself toward the floor. As you go down, let your heels lift and keep your knees aligned with your toes. Exhale and return to Pilates stance.

Perform 10 times.

THE BEAST WITHIN

You must hold yourself upright as you descend. Don't fall or pitch forward. As you descend, think of your thighs lengthening out of their hip sockets toward your knees. Your heels should return to the floor toward the end of your ascent to the up-right position. For an added challenge, you may keep your heels lifted for the entire ten repetitions. Your heels may come apart due to turnout, anatomical make up, or depth of descent. Lower yourself only as far as you can while maintaining control. You shouldn't feel any discomfort or pain. Leave this out if you have any hip, knee, foot, or ankle problems.

STANDING FOOTWORK SERIES
TOES, ARCHES, HEELS, TENDON STRETCH

STANDING FOOTWORK: ARCHES

BENEFITS: STRENGTHENS THE FEET, LEGS, AND POWERHOUSE; IMPROVES BALANCE

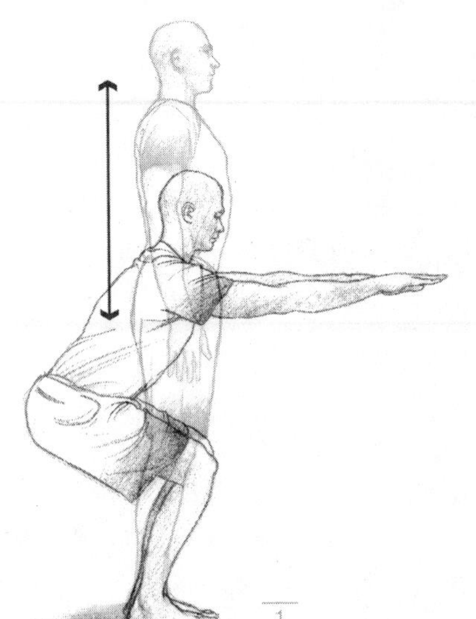

Stand up tall in Pilates stance, except bring your feet together so that they are touching and parallel to one another. Pull your powerhouse in and up. Inhale and lower yourself toward the floor, reaching forward with your arms as a counterbalance. Exhale and stand up straight.

Perform 10 times.

THE BEAST WITHIN

Imagine that you are sitting back in a chair. This image will help you keep your shins vertical as you lower your body. You want to sit more back than down. Don't round your back as you descend. At first, you may need to place your feet hip-width apart. As you become more adept at this exercise and gain better balance, bring your feet closer together. Leave this one out if you have any hip, knee, foot, or ankle problems.

STANDING FOOTWORK SERIES
TOES, ARCHES, HEELS, TENDON STRETCH

STANDING FOOTWORK: HEELS

BENEFITS: STRENGTHENS THE FEET, LEGS, AND POWERHOUSE; IMPROVES BALANCE

This is the same as the Standing Footwork for Arches, except your toes are up and you put more of your weight into your heels. Stand up tall in Pilates stance, but bring your feet parallel and together so that they are touching. Pull your powerhouse in and up. Curl your toes up and keep them up throughout the exercise. Inhale and lower your body toward the floor, reaching forward with your arms as a counterbalance. Exhale and return to an upright position.

Perform 10 times.

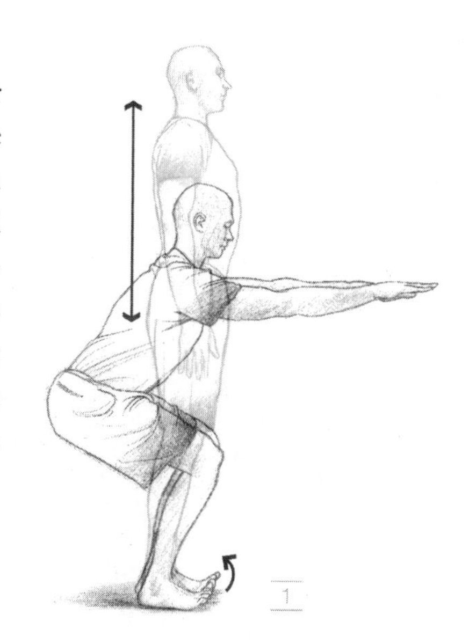

THE BEAST WITHIN

Again, imagine you're sitting in a chair. This image will help you keep your shins vertical as you lower your body. You want to sit more back than down. Don't round your back as you descend. At first, you may need to place your feet hip-width apart. As you become more adept at this exercise and gain better balance, bring your feet closer together. You may not be able to descend as low as in the Arches version because more of your weight is in your heels. Leave this out if you have any hip, knee, foot, or ankle problems.

STANDING FOOTWORK SERIES
TOES, ARCHES, HEELS, TENDON STRETCH

STANDING FOOTWORK: TENDON STRETCH

BENEFITS: STRENGTHENS THE FEET, LEGS, AND POWERHOUSE; CORRECTS POSTURE; IMPROVES BALANCE

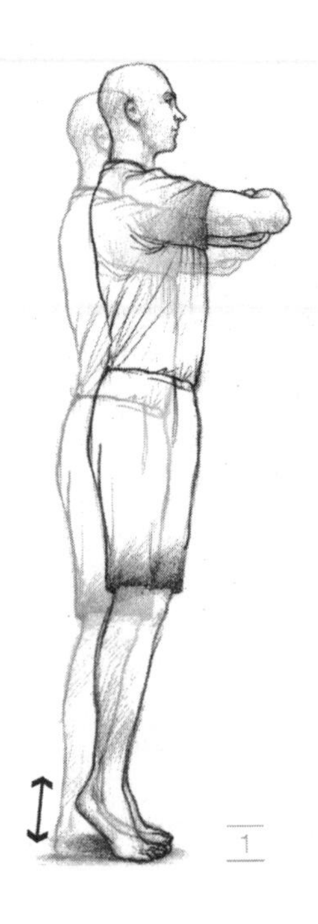

Stand in Pilates stance. Lay arm over arm and lift your arms up to shoulder height. Pull the powerhouse in and up. Inhale and lift your heels high. Exhale and lower your heels.

Perform 10 times.

THE BEAST WITHIN

Don't pitch forward. Keep your shoulders down. Maintain your balance as you lift and lower your heels. Leave this exercise out if you have any foot or ankle problems.

THE HUNDRED

BENEFITS: WORKS THE HEART, LUNGS, AND POWERHOUSE

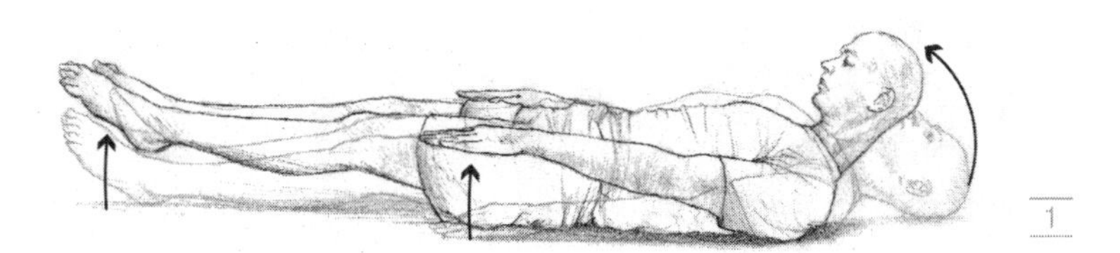

Lie on the floor with your arms alongside your body. Draw your powerhouse in. In one motion, raise your feet 2 inches off the mat, lift your hands alongside the tops of your thighs, and raise your head off the mat with your eyes focused on your toes.

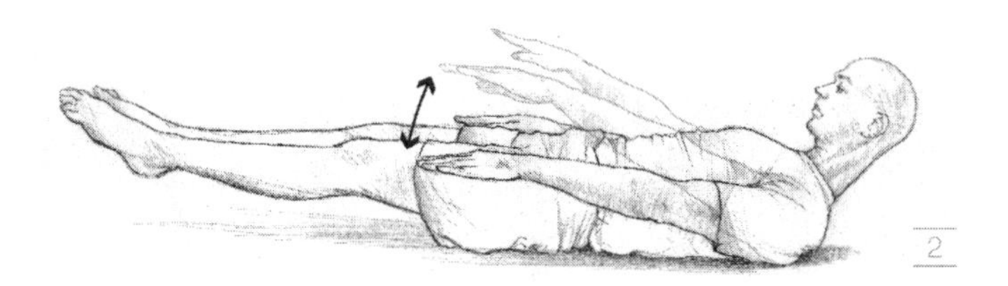

Begin pumping your arms up and down within a four-to-eight-inch range of motion. As you pump, inhale for 5 counts and exhale for 5 counts. This is 1 set. (1 set of 5 pumps inhaling and 5 pumps exhaling should take about 4 to 5 seconds.)

Perform for 10 sets.

THE BEAST WITHIN

BODY POSITION When you first begin, lift your head and your upper back up to the tips of your shoulder blades. Keep your tailbone flat on the floor. Your spine should be flat on the mat from your tailbone to the tips of your shoulder blades, but do not press down so hard that your back hurts. Keep it down with the powerhouse contraction. Imagine someone is trying to lift your feet from underneath your toes, and you are pressing down and forward through your toes to resist. This will engage your buttocks. On each exhalation, squeeze your buttocks and inner thighs and pull your stomach in. Keep your shoulders away from your ears. Keep your neck long and your feet in Pilates stance.

THE MIND IN MOTION Don't release your powerhouse as you pump. Keep it drawn in. This is the reformer on the mat version of the Hundred. If you need modifications, refer back to the Hundred in the traditional mat work. You should be capable of doing this illustrated version on page 31, if you are attempting the reformer on the mat. For an additional challenge, you may also shorten the inhalations and lengthen the exhalations (i.e., inhale for three counts and exhale for seven).

CAUTIONS The Hundred will be harder after performing the Footwork Series. Adjust your leg height to alleviate any tension in your back.

THE OVERHEAD

BENEFITS: STRENGTHENS THE POWERHOUSE, HIPS, BUTTOCKS, UPPER BODY, AND ARMS

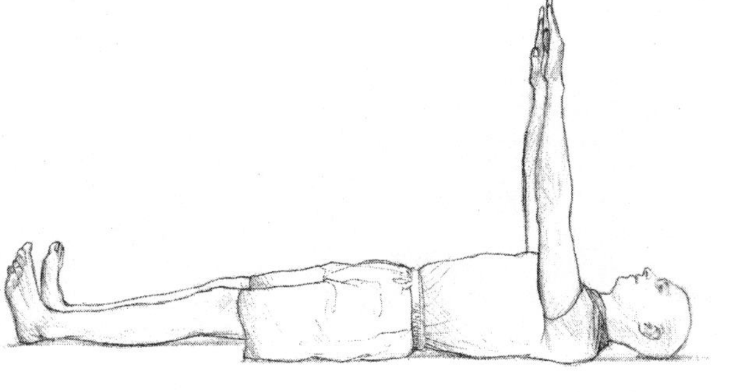

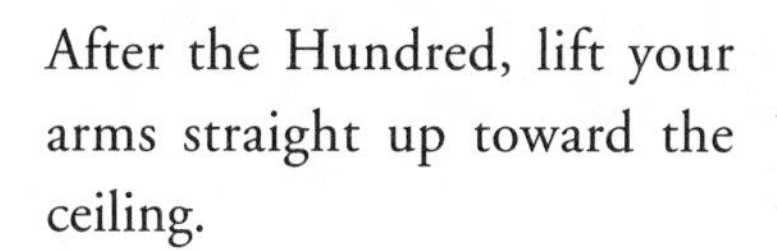

After the Hundred, lift your arms straight up toward the ceiling.

Pull your powerhouse in and inhale. Smoothly bring your arms down to the floor as you lift your legs up to a vertical position. Then press your arms down and peel your spine up off the floor one vertebra at a time.

Keep your spine and hips lifted and bring your legs just a hair above parallel to the floor.

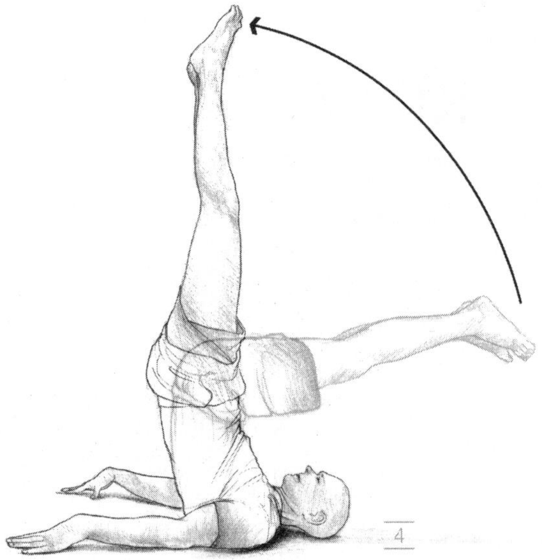

Exhale, squeeze your buttocks, and bring your legs back up toward the ceiling. Keep your toes above the area between your sternum and eye line when your feet are in the air.

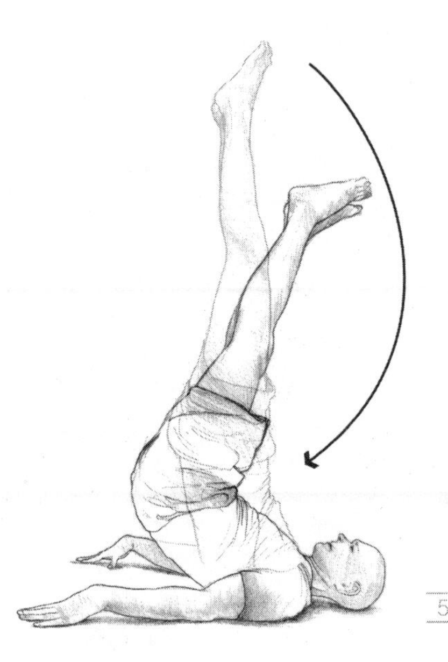

Inhale and roll your spine down to the floor. Again, keep your toes above the area between your sternum and eye line as you roll yourself down.

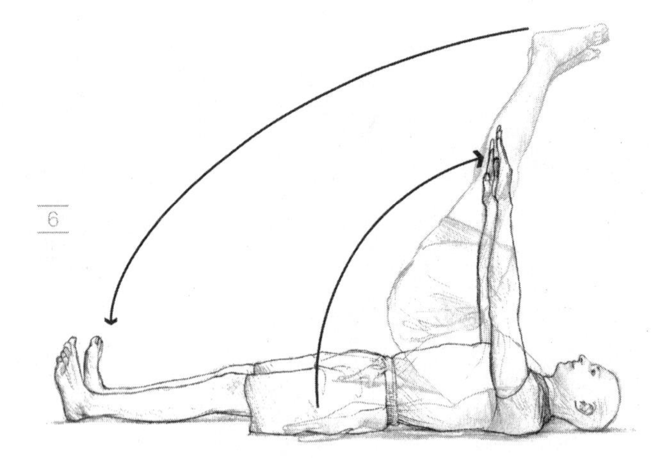

Begin exhaling when your hips and tailbone touch the floor. When your hips touch the floor, lower your legs and lift your arms simultaneously.

Perform 4 times.

THE BEAST WITHIN

BODY POSITION Keep your shoulders pulled down and away from your ears throughout the exercise. Keep your legs together and your neck long.

THE MIND IN MOTION The universal reformer archival photos of Joseph Pilates show this exercise to be the Roll Over (from the traditional mat work) as done on the reformer. Today, as in Joseph Pilates's day, the body is lifted into the air similarly to the traditional mat exercise called the Jackknife. If you find it easier to control, bring your body up (as in illustration 3), and then roll your spine down. If you'd like the challenge, then jackknife your legs into the air as depicted on the previous page. In either case, remember that you must still control the movement. To avoid relying on momentum in step 2, make sure your arms are pressed down on the mat before peeling your hips off the floor.

CAUTIONS Men tend to forget about their powerhouses and throw their body over and up with momentum and upper body strength. If you are overweight, you may find it difficult to lift your hips up with control. Skip this exercise if this is a problem for you. Leave this out if you have neck, shoulder, elbow, back, or hip problems.

COORDINATION

BENEFITS: IMPROVES COORDINATION OF BREATH AND MOVEMENT; STRENGTHENS THE POWERHOUSE, LEGS, AND ARMS

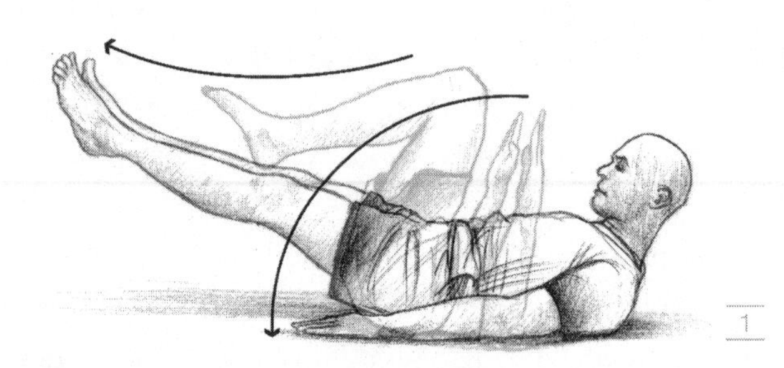

After the Overhead, keep your elbows down and bring your forearms vertical to the floor. Bring your knees inward to your chest. Lift your head in the chin-to-chest position. Pull your powerhouse in. Keep your shoulders down and away from your ears. Inhale and straighten your arms and legs, keeping your legs in the air.

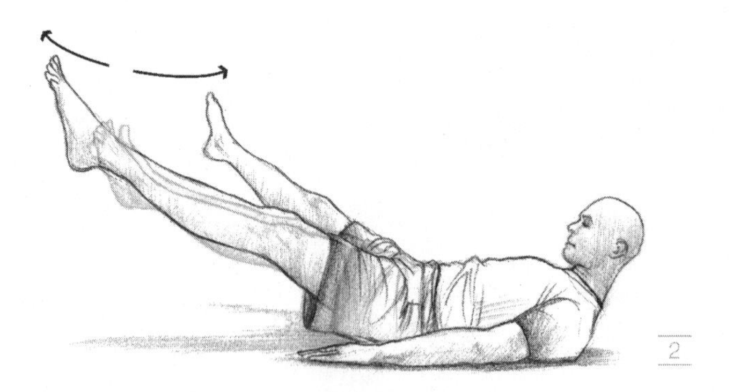

Open your legs. Keep your abdominals firm and hold your breath.

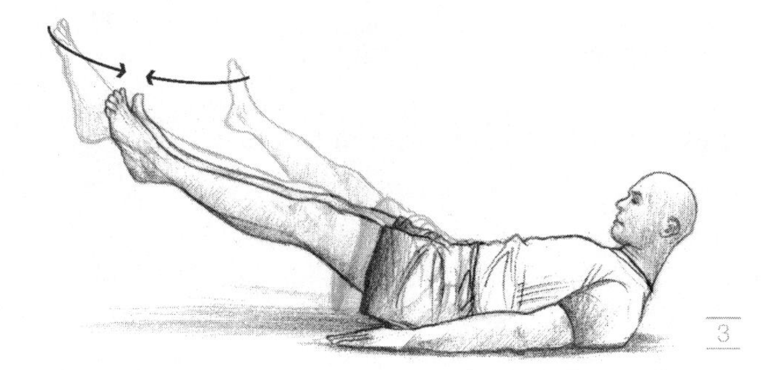

Close your legs and continue to hold your breath.

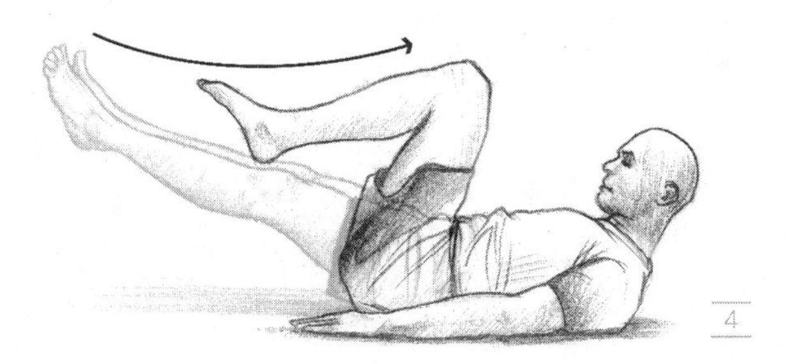

Begin exhaling and bring your knees back to your chest. Keep your tailbone down.

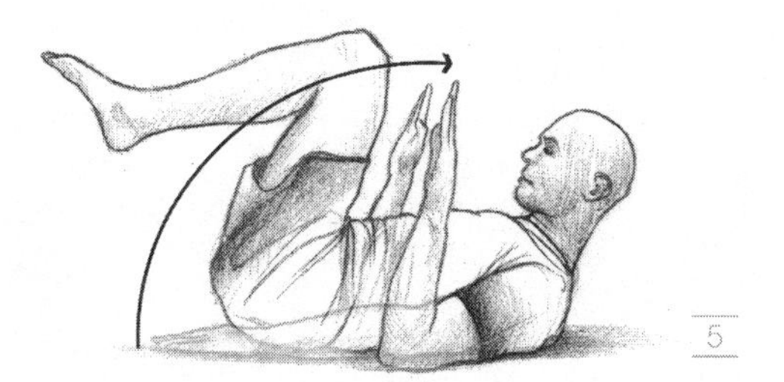

Finish exhaling and bend your arms, bringing your forearms back to the vertical position.

Perform 5 times. Only add the "changement" flutter kicks (described in the following section) in the last 2 repetitions, if you decide to perform them.

THE BEAST WITHIN

BODY POSITION Keep your spine anchored on the floor, from your tailbone to the tips of your shoulder blades. Keep your powerhouse firm throughout the exercise.

THE MIND IN MOTION Don't release your powerhouse when you extend your legs. Do not let your lower back arch. To maintain control and avoid back pain, you may extend and hold your legs higher off the floor.

For a bigger challenge, you may add eight changement repetitions when your legs are straight. A changement is simply a tight flutter kick of the feet over and under each other. The archival reformer photos show Joseph Pilates executing this exercise with fists and his head down throughout the exercise. Keeping your head down will make this exercise more difficult; your upper body will want to come up or your lower back will want to arch. But if you do it correctly, keeping your head down will deepen the work into your lower powerhouse. Making fists will yield a feeling of strength throughout your body.

CAUTIONS If this aggravates your neck and/or shoulders, lower them to the floor. Leave this exercise out if you have neck, shoulder, elbow, or back problems.

ROWING INTO THE STERNUM

BENEFITS: STRENGTHENS THE POWERHOUSE; LENGTHENS THE LEGS AND BACK; OPENS THE CHEST AND SHOULDERS

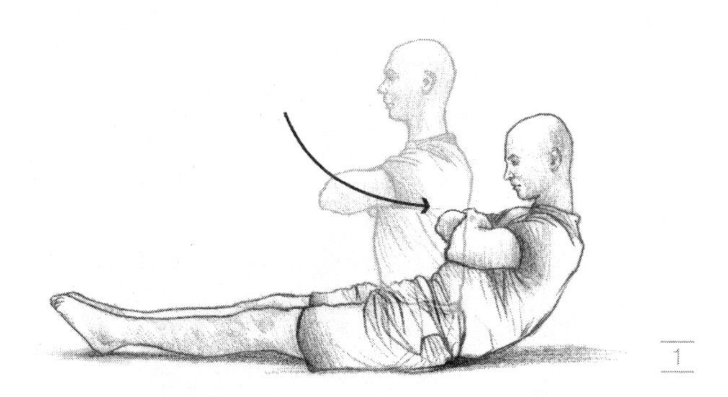

After the Coordination, sit up tall with your legs straight in front of you. Point your toes forward and down. Make fists and push the knuckles of your two fists together. Touch the knuckles of your pointer and middle fingers to your sternum, with your thumbs facing down. Pull your powerhouse in. Inhale and begin rolling your spine one vertebra at a time down to floor. Stop at about your mid-back or slightly before.

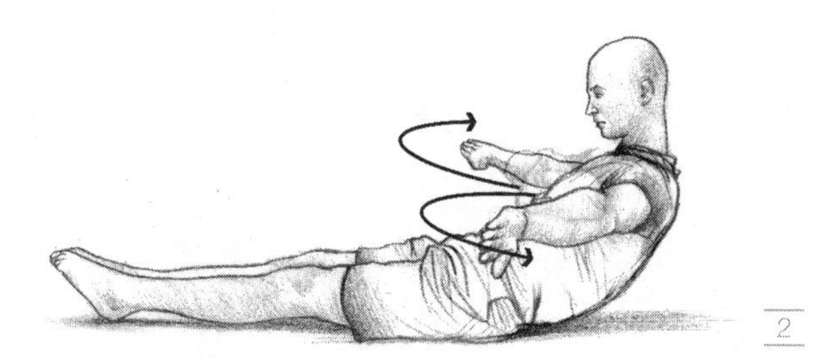

Exhale as you open your hands, with your thumbs still down, and straighten your arms out to the sides.

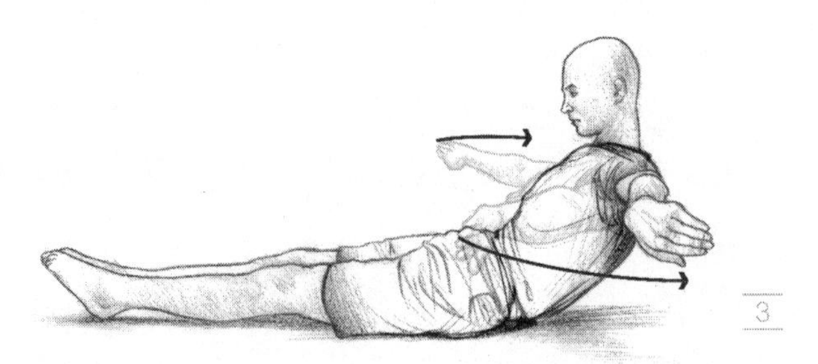

Inhale and push your straight arms back behind you, keeping them parallel to the floor, while holding the rest of your body in the same position. Keep your shoulders down and your powerhouse in.

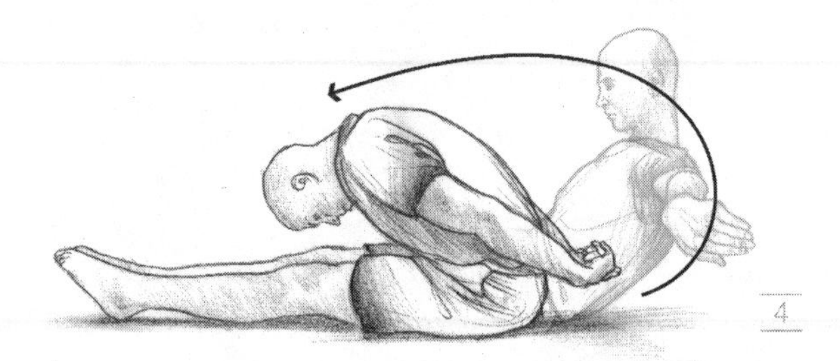

Bring your forehead to your knees and clasp your hands behind your back as you exhale. Lift your powerhouse in and up.

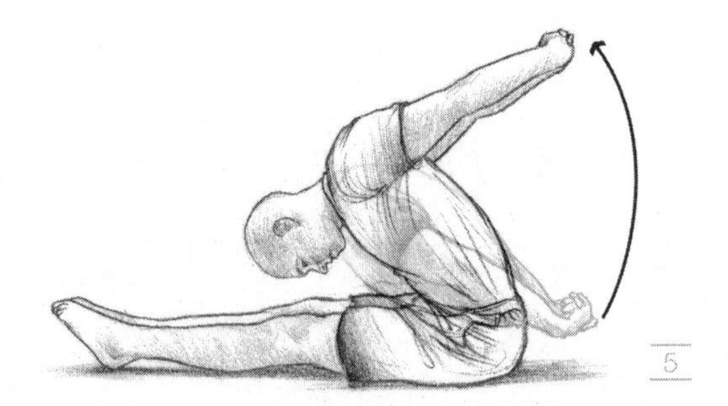

Inhale and lift your straight arms and clasped hands as high as you can. Keep your powerhouse lifted in and up.

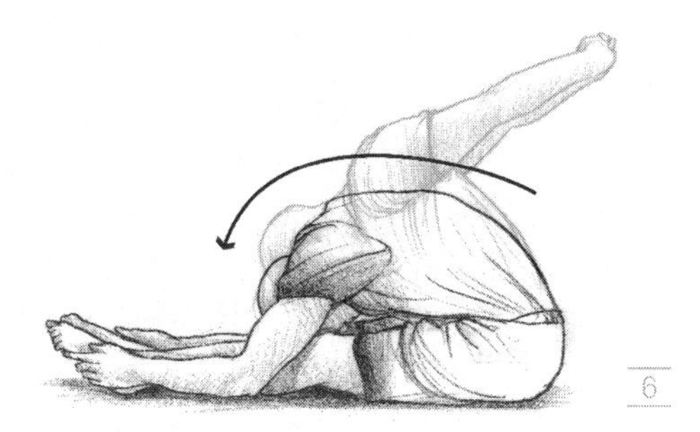

Release your hands out to the sides and fold them into a forward bend as you exhale.

Perform 3 times.

THE BEAST WITHIN

BODY POSITION Keep your powerhouse tightly in, your spine long, and your legs anchored to the floor throughout the exercise.

THE MIND IN MOTION The first repetition will teach you how far you can roll down while still maintaining control of your body throughout the exercise. If you roll back too far, you will find it difficult to bring your forehead to your knees, and your feet will rise off the floor. When you reach your hands behind you (see illustration 3), keep your shoulders down and your toes pointed forward to help anchor your body. Keep your arms either parallel to the floor or higher as you push them behind you; don't drop them down. It is not necessary to clasp your hands when they are behind you. If tightness prevents you from clasping your hands behind your back, then reach your straight arms with open palms up as high as you can behind you and alongside your body as you bring your forehead to your knees (see illustration 5). Hold your powerhouse in throughout the movement, and keep it lifted in and up off your legs in the final step (see illustration 6).

CAUTIONS Men frequently have tight backs and shoulders. Limit the range of motion of your arms or leave this exercise out if you have shoulder problems. Leave it out if you have back problems.

ROWING 90 DEGREES

BENEFITS: STRENGTHENS THE POWERHOUSE; LENGTHENS THE SPINE AND LEGS; OPENS THE CHEST AND SHOULDERS

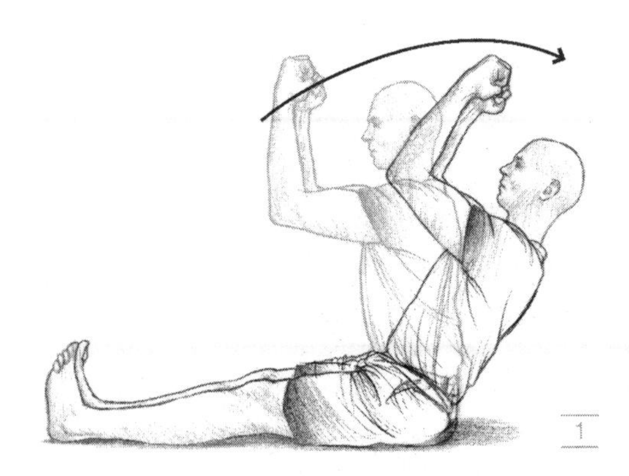

1

After Rowing into the Sternum, sit up tall with your legs straight and your ankles flexed. Bend your arms so that your upper arm is parallel to the floor and your elbow forms a right angle. Squeeze your buttocks and pull your powerhouse in. Inhale as you pivot backward from your buttocks, while maintaining a straight spine.

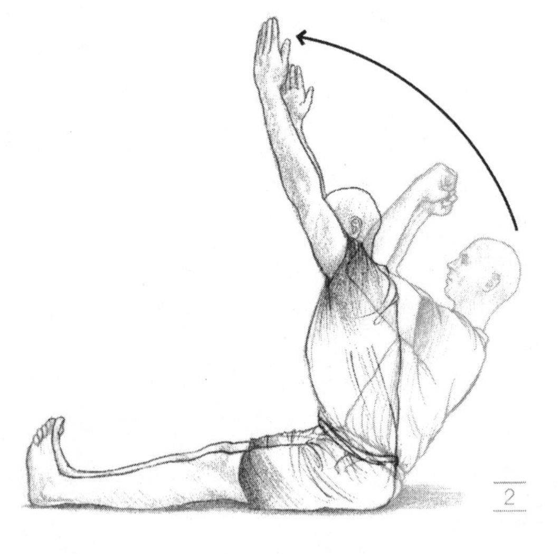

2

Begin exhaling and pivot back to a sitting up tall position, reaching your arms high toward the ceiling. Keep your spine long.

Continue exhaling as you lengthen upward and fold your body forward as far as possible. Keep your powerhouse lifted.

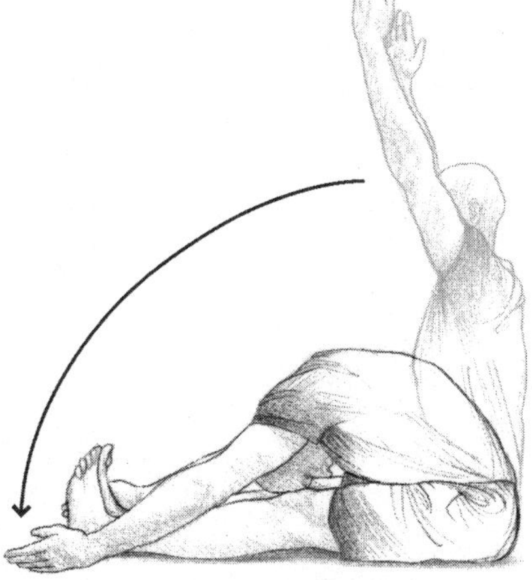

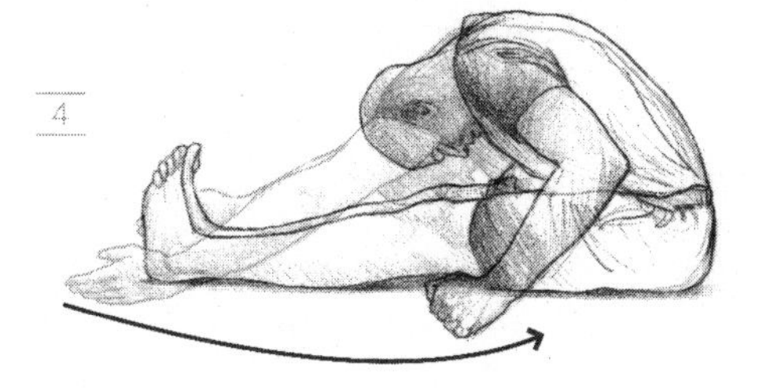

Inhale and run your arms alongside your body toward your rear.

Clasp your hands behind you. Keep your powerhouse pulled in and up.

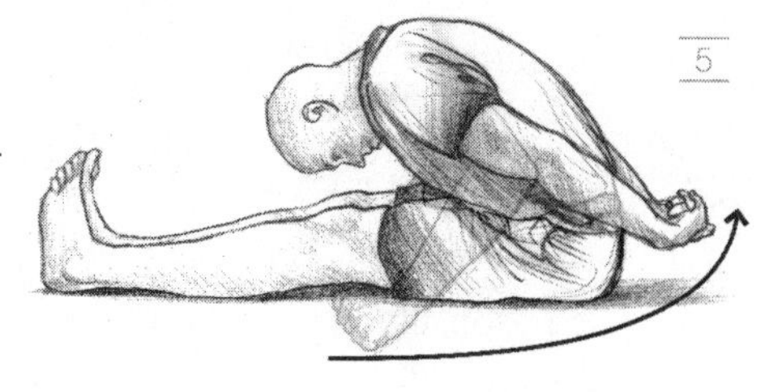

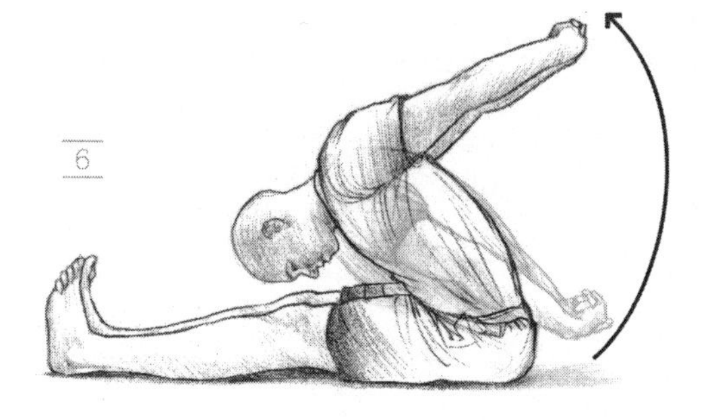

Reach straight arms high into the air behind you.

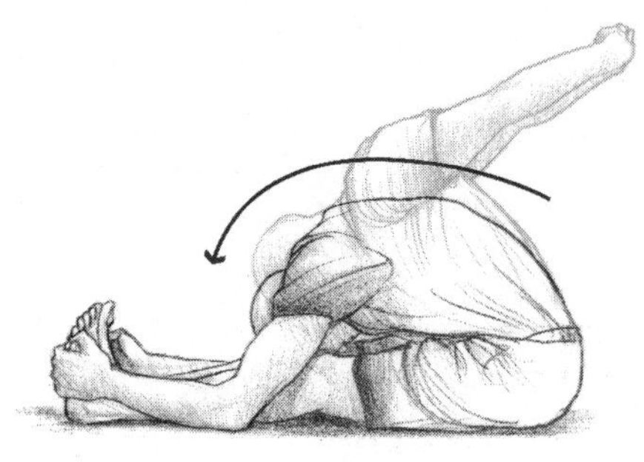

Exhale and reach your arms around as you fold into a forward bend. Keep your powerhouse lifted into your spine.

Perform 3 times.

THE BEAST WITHIN

BODY POSITION Sit up as tall as possible. Squeeze your buttocks. You may keep your hands in fists or flat with open palms during this exercise. Anchor your legs to the floor.

THE MIND IN MOTION Your range of motion backward will be small. Neither arch your spine nor hinge on any one spot in your spine when you pivot backward on your sit bones; maintain an upright posture throughout the exercise. When you straighten your arms to come back up and forward, lift out your hips and stay as tall as possible. Don't release the powerhouse; keep it in the entire time. As in Rowing into the Sternum, you don't have to clasp your hands when they are behind you.

Old photos of Joseph Pilates show that when he performed this exercise on a reformer, he rolled backward as well, which looks like the spinal movement in Rowing into the Sternum. It is easier and feels great, so feel free to try this variation.

Men typically have a limited range of motion due to stiff backs and legs. This is a fantastic exercise for helping men lengthen their bodies.

CAUTIONS Proceed slowly if you have neck, shoulder, or back problems. Leave this exercise out if these problems are severe. It's important that you to listen to your body and act accordingly.

ROWING FROM THE CHEST

BENEFITS: STRENGTHENS THE POWERHOUSE; LENGTHENS THE SPINE

Sit up tall after Rowing 90 Degrees. Bend your elbows and align your hands by your chest as in the Push-up position. Pull your powerhouse in and squeeze your buttocks. Inhale and straighten your arms out so that your hands are roughly at eye level.

1

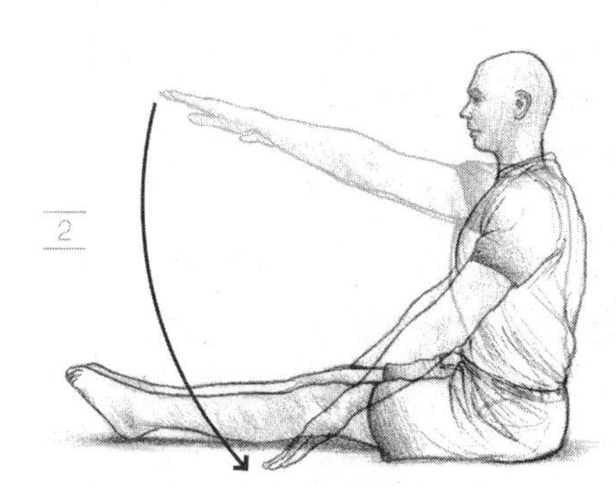

2

Exhale and lower your straight arms to the floor. Lift yourself up slightly by flexing your buttocks as your fingertips lightly touch the floor.

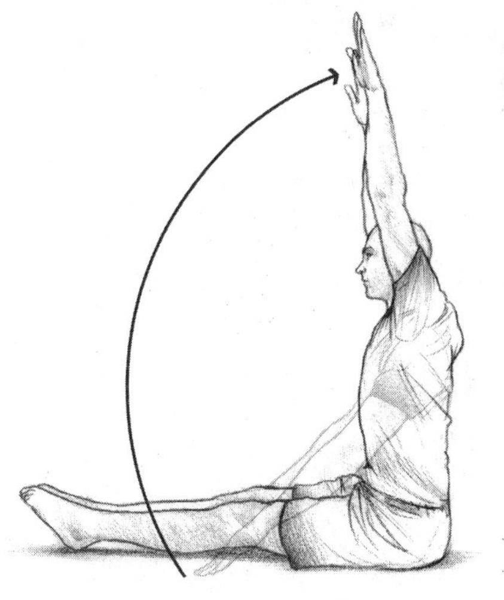

Inhale and lift your arms toward the ceiling.

3

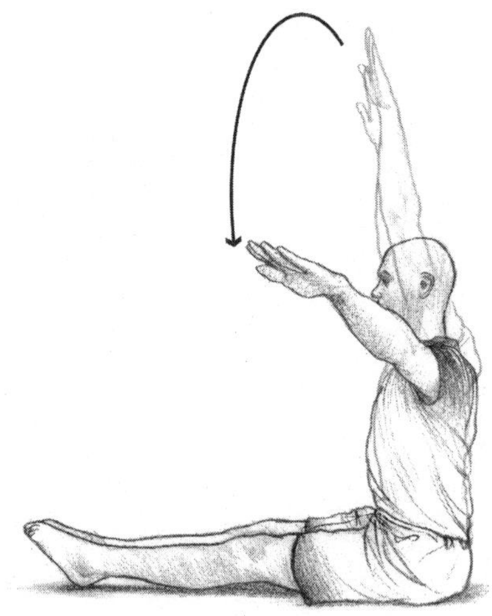

Exhale and press your arms down to your sides.

Perform 3 times.

THE BEAST WITHIN

BODY POSITION Keep your powerhouse in firmly. Keep your spine lifted throughout the movement. The Rowing Series is about developing and maintaining a long spine and a strong powerhouse. This exercise demonstrates this well. Keep your eyes focused in front of you with the crown of your head reaching for the ceiling.

THE MIND IN MOTION For an extra lift in your spine, press your fingertips into the mat when your hands are down (see illustration 2), and flex your buttocks. Do not let the movement of your arms change your seated position. If your lower back is rounded, you may bend your knees to sit up tall. You may extend your arms higher in the first movement so your biceps are at eye level (see illustration 1). Just remember not to shrug your shoulders up when you extend your arms out in step 1. If you can't keep your shoulders down in step 3, bend your elbows slightly to help pull them down.

CAUTIONS Leave this exercise out if you have shoulder problems.

ROWING FROM THE HIPS

BENEFITS: LENGTHENS THE SPINE AND LEGS; STRENGTHENS THE POWERHOUSE

Sit up tall and then bring your chin to your chest. Place your hands on the floor. Lengthen your spine and pull your powerhouse in and up. Keep your ankles flexed.

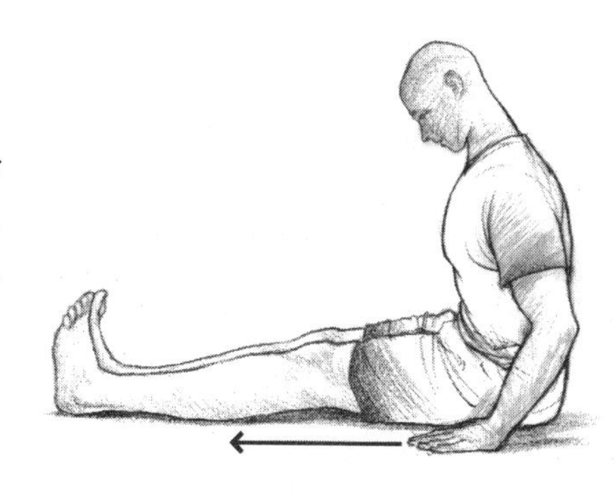

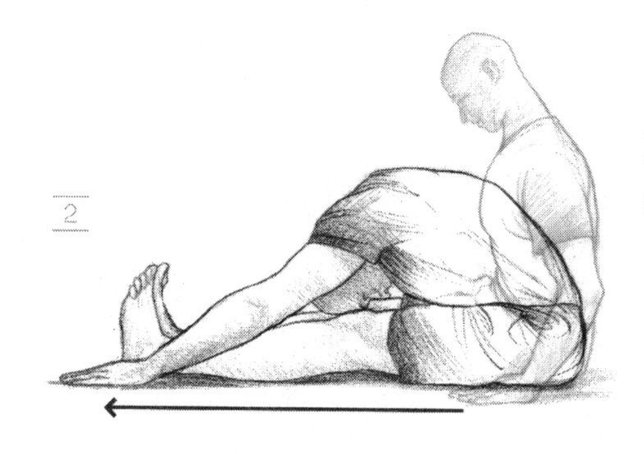

Inhale as you slide your hands forward on the floor. Keep your powerhouse lifted in and up.

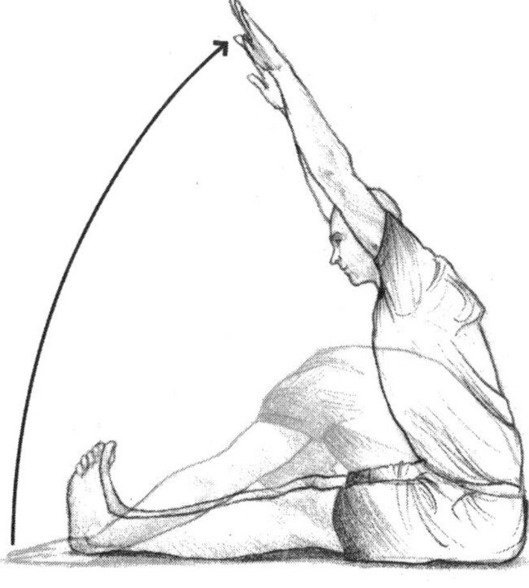

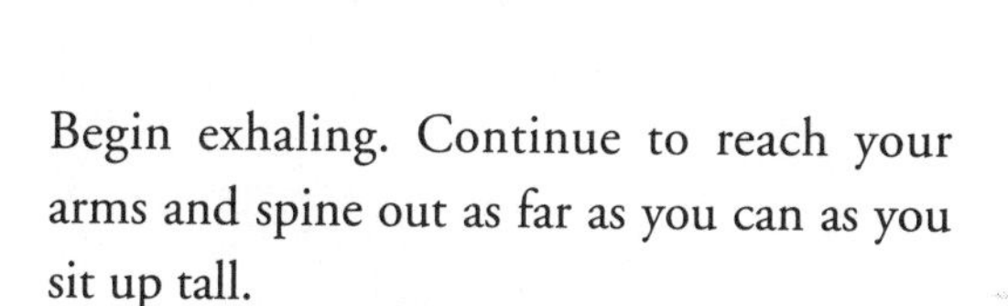

Begin exhaling. Continue to reach your arms and spine out as far as you can as you sit up tall.

Finish exhaling and sit up as tall as possible with your arms reaching up toward the ceiling.

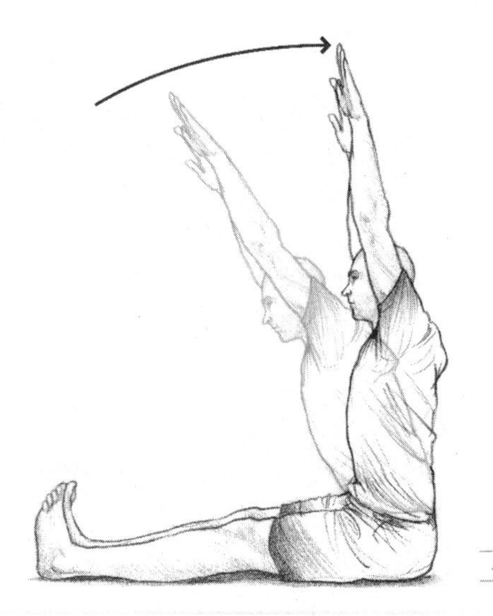

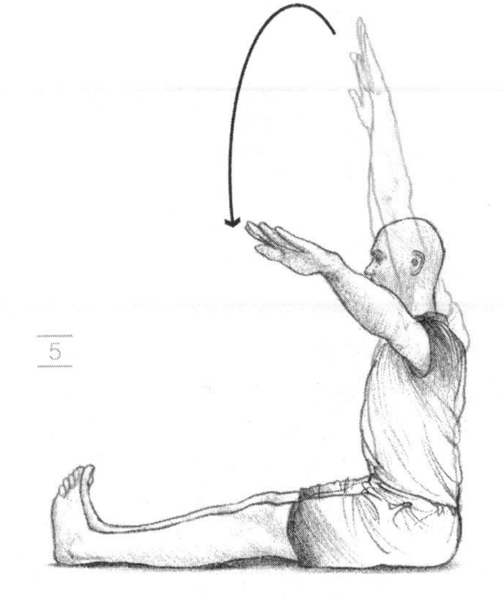

Maintain a firm powerhouse as you inhale and press your arms down to your sides; place your hands back on the floor.

Perform 3 times.

THE BEAST WITHIN

BODY POSITION This is a great exercise for men with tight backs and legs. Sit up tall with your chin to your chest. Keep your feet flexed, your legs straight, and your spine long throughout.

THE MIND IN MOTION Reach as far forward as you can from your lower abdominals when your hands slide forward on the floor. Continue to reach as far as possible as you sit up tall. Lift your spine up from your sit bones as you press your hands down in step 5. Keep your powerhouse firmly in throughout the movement.

To try an older version of this exercise, you may keep your hands on the floor as you sit up tall in step 3. Your shoulders will automatically settle into place. Once you are sitting upright, then you may raise your arms toward the ceiling (see illustration 4). You may also execute your breathing differently. Try exhaling when you first slide out, inhaling as you sit up and exhaling as you press your hands down to the sides.

CAUTIONS Proceed slowly or leave this exercise out if you have neck, shoulder, back, or hamstring muscle problems.

THE SHAVE

BENEFITS: LENGTHENS YOUR SPINE, LEGS, AND ARMS; WORKS YOUR UPPER BACK AND POWERHOUSE

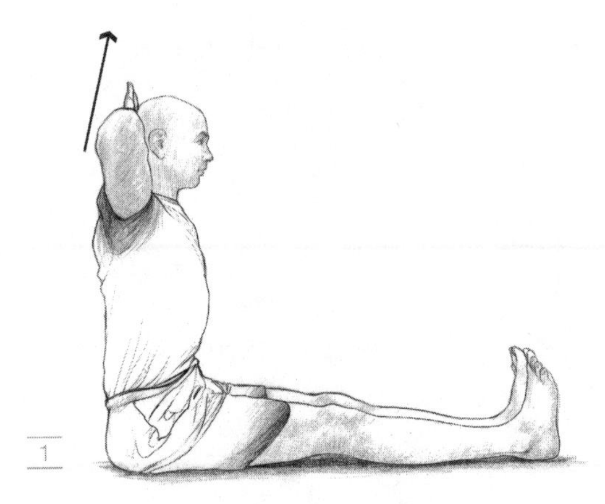

Remain sitting up tall after Rowing from the Hips, keep your legs together. Form the shape of a diamond with your two thumbs and index fingers of each hand; place this "diamond" on the back of your head or neck. Pull your powerhouse in and up.

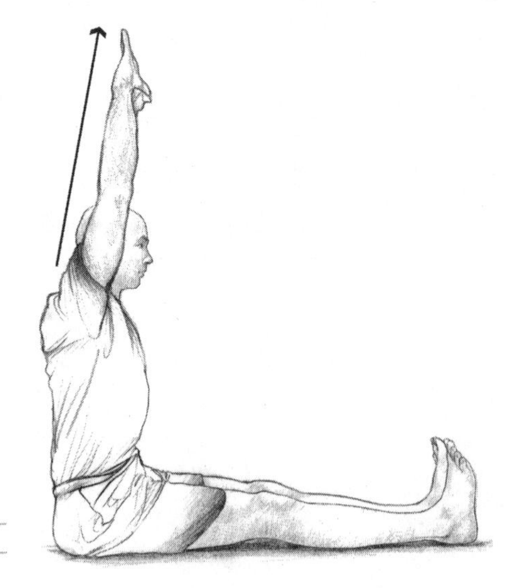

Inhale and straighten your arms toward the ceiling, while maintaining the diamond shape between your hands. Exhale and return to the starting position.

Perform 5 times.

THE BEAST WITHIN

BODY POSITION Today, this exercise is commonly performed in the cross-legged position on the reformer. I've illustrated Joseph Pilates's straight legs variation because it helps to feel lifted in the spine and stronger in the powerhouse. Also, men often have difficulty sitting cross-legged due to tight hips and knees. You may sit either way. If you sit with straight legs, keep both legs active by squeezing your buttocks and lifting up your kneecaps by flexing your quadriceps (the muscles on the tops of your thighs).

THE MIND IN MOTION As your hands "shave" upward, keep your shoulders down and away from your ears. This is difficult for men with tight upper backs and shoulders. Leaning slightly forward may make it easier. Tightness in your hamstrings and lower back might cause you to bend your knees slightly when you pitch forward. This is fine. If your lower back rounds in this position, you may bend your knees to help you sit up tall. Without the benefit of the universal reformer's spring resistance, you must create muscular tension from your powerhouse through your shoulders and arms up to your fingertips as you raise them up. When your hands return to the back of your head, pull your shoulder blades together and down. This may cause just your thumbs to separate, which is okay.

CAUTIONS Leave this exercise out if you have neck or shoulder problems.

THE HUG

BENEFITS: STRENGTHENS THE BACK, SHOULDERS, AND CHEST; WORKS THE POWERHOUSE AND ARMS

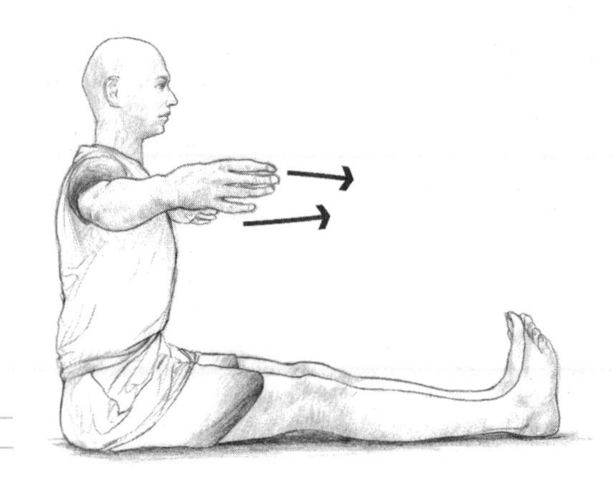

Remain sitting upright after the Shave and hold your arms out to the sides. Bend your elbows slightly with your palms facing each other. Pull your powerhouse in and up.

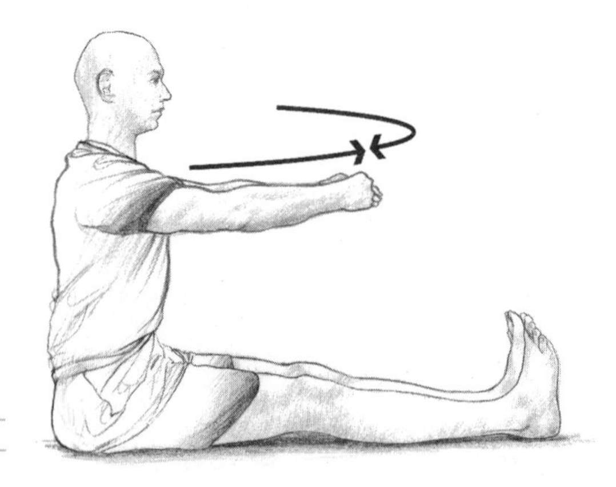

Inhale and bring your hands together as if you are hugging a barrel, while creating tension in your arms, chest, and back. Exhale and return to the starting position.

Perform 3 times, then perform 3 more times with a reversed breathing pattern (exhale then inhale).

THE BEAST WITHIN

BODY POSITION Keep your shoulders down and away from your ears. Don't arch your spine. You may perform this exercise with open hands (as illustrated on page 174) or with closed fists. Maintain the same slight bend in your elbows throughout the exercise. You must engage your powerhouse and squeeze your buttocks to effectively lift up your torso from the base of your spine.

THE MIND IN MOTION Concentrate on actively working your back, arms, shoulders, and chest muscles with a firm powerhouse throughout the exercise. If tightness in your lower back keeps it rounded, then bend your knees slightly to help you sit up tall. As in the Shave, you can perform this exercise in the cross-legged position.

CAUTIONS Leave this exercise out if you have neck or shoulder problems.

THE SWAN

BENEFITS: LENGTHENS THE SPINE; STRENGTHENS THE ENTIRE BACK, ARMS, AND BUTTOCKS

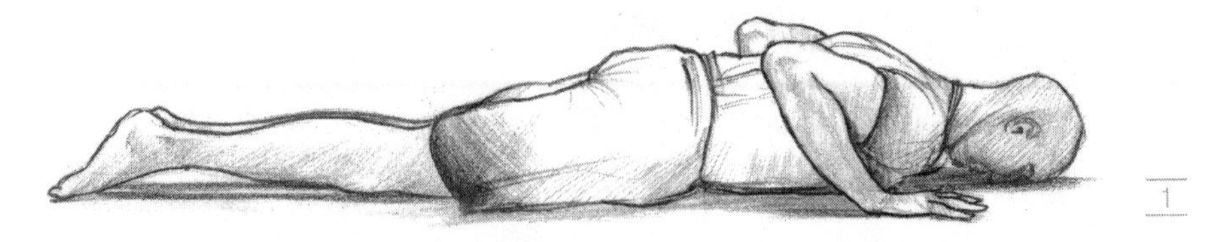

After the Hug, turn over onto your stomach. Place your forehead on the mat and your hands under your shoulders.

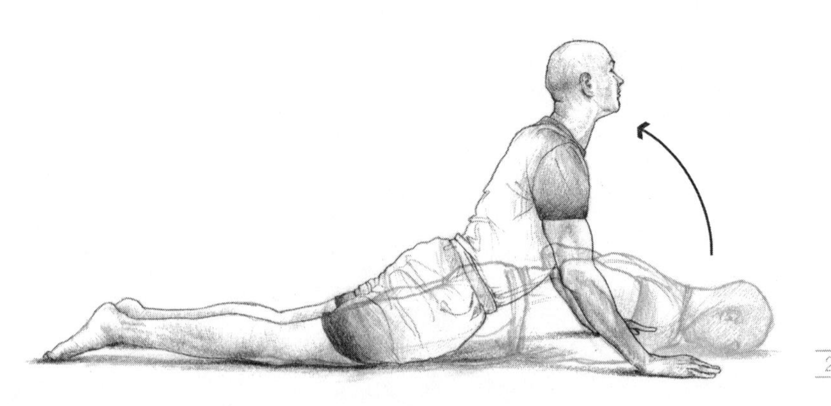

Inhale as you draw your powerhouse in, while squeezing your buttocks and lifting your chest high into the air. Keep your shoulders down and back.

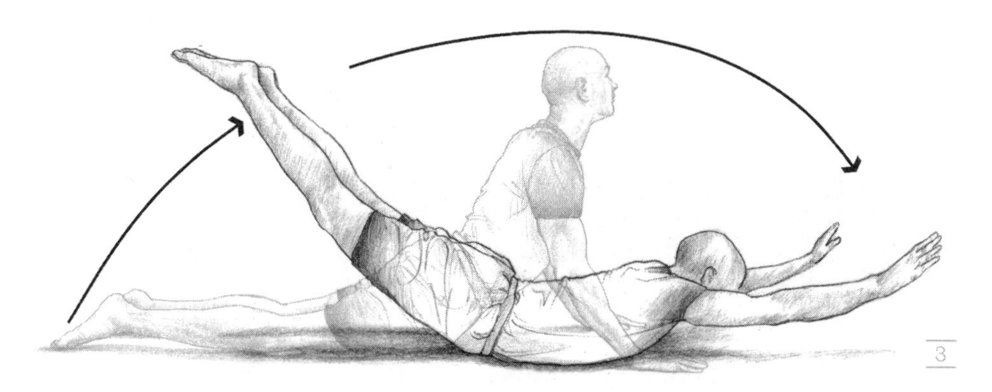

Shoot your hands forward and up as you rock forward and exhale.

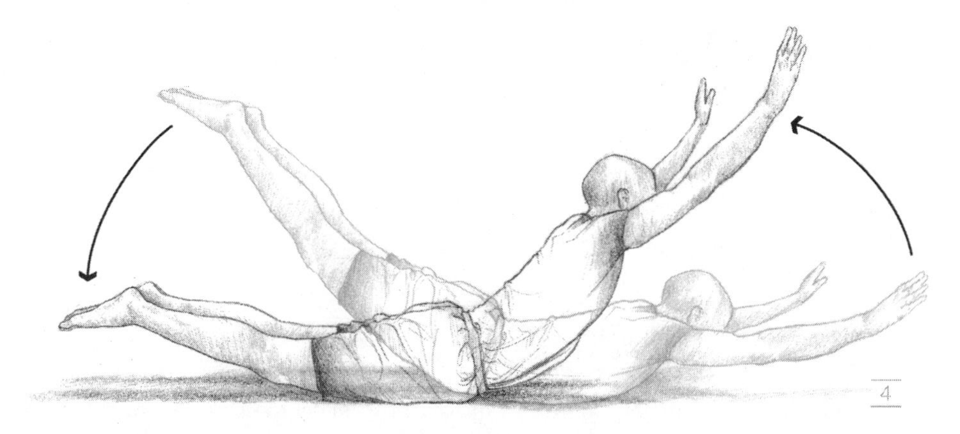

Inhale as you lift your chest and rock backward.

Perform 6 times.

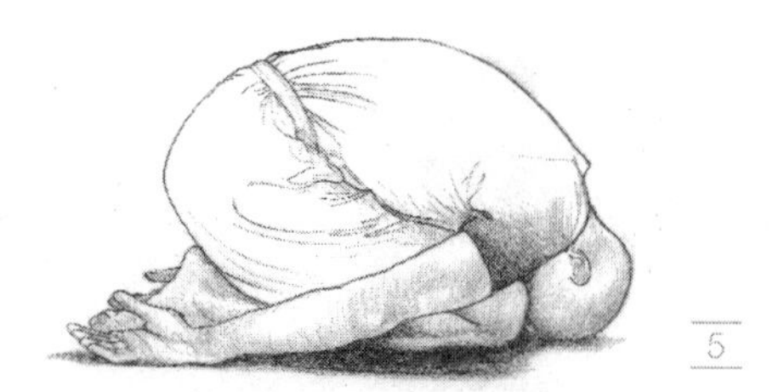

Sit back on you heels with your forehead touching your knees. Breathe while you are in this position to release your back muscles.

THE BEAST WITHIN

BODY POSITION This is the exact same exercise as the Swan Dive from the traditional mat work (see page 63); it appears here because it's also performed on the reformer. To begin, lift your upper body as high off of the mat as you can. Think of your entire spine and body lengthening into a back bend as you lift your breastbone upward. It helps if you squeeze your buttocks firmly and imagine someone pulling your feet out from your hips.

THE MIND IN MOTION If necessary, you may practice holding the up right position in step 2 for several workouts. This will let your body open up and get stronger before you attempt the rocking. If the straight arm variation is too difficult, then come up onto your forearms—instead of your hands—for a reduced back bend.

During the movement, you may also keep your hands palm up—as if you just dunked a basketball and are hanging backward from the rim. You may also rock with your arms out to the sides instead of forward. If your arms are out to the sides, try rotating your palms up when your chest is lifted and palms down when your legs are lifted. Don't hinge or sink into any single spot in your back. At the end, if sitting back on your heels hurts your knees (see illustration 5), turn onto your back and hug your legs into your chest by holding the backs of your thighs.

CAUTIONS The Swan is not particularly friendly to the male anatomy, so adjust accordingly before rocking. If you have tightness in your back, hip flexors, and shoulders (as men typically demonstrate), you'll find the initial lift up difficult. Leave this exercise out if you have neck, shoulder, rib, back, hip, or knee problems.

PULLING STRAPS

BENEFITS: STRENGTHENS THE ARMS, LEGS, BACK, BUTTOCKS, AND POWERHOUSE; DEVELOPS FLEXIBILITY OF THE SPINE

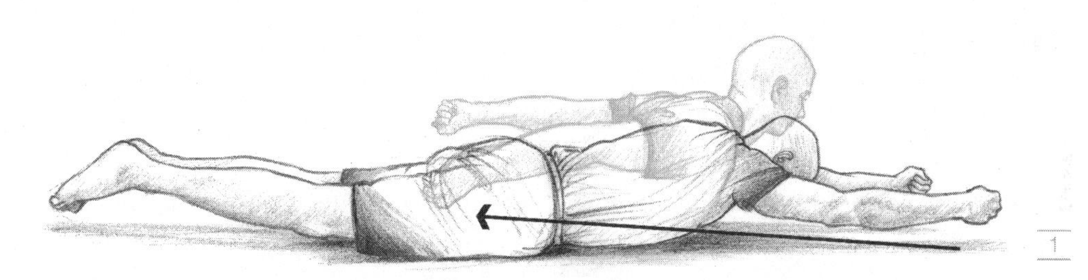

After the Swan, lie facedown on the floor with your neck long and your head slightly lifted. Reach out in front of you with loosely clenched fists, with the palm side of each fist facing each other. Look at the floor. Keep your feet on the floor or elevated slightly. Pull your powerhouse in and engage your buttocks. Simultaneously inhale and pull your fists alongside your body until they are behind you. As you pull your arms behind you, lift your chest up off the floor.

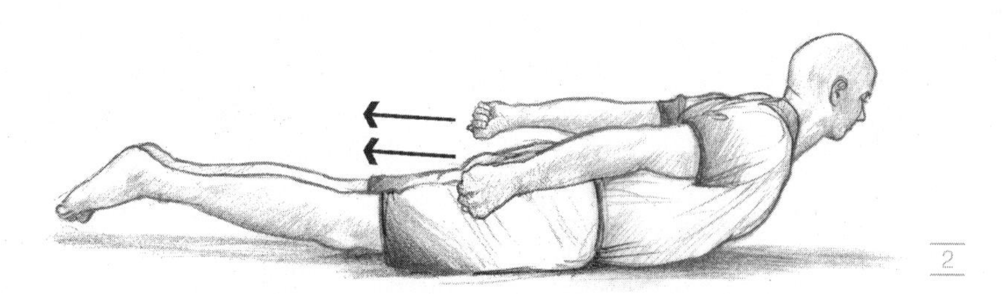

Hold your breath in this position for a second or two. Contract your fists, arms, back, buttocks, and powerhouse, squeeze your legs together.

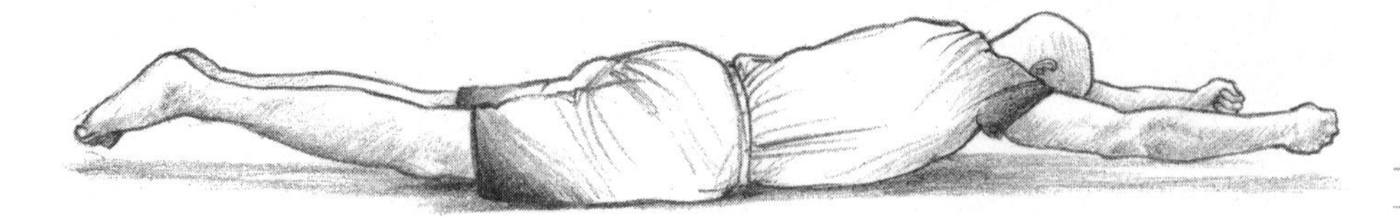

Exhale and return to the starting position.

Perform 3 times.

THE BEAST WITHIN

BODY POSITION Lengthen your body and reach out.

THE MIND IN MOTION Pull your powerhouse in firmly, squeeze your buttocks tightly, and keep your fists tight as you lift up your sternum/diaphragm region off the floor. Thrust your chest out. Your feet may be down or slightly lifted off the floor. Concentrate on actively working your arms and legs. Keep your powerhouse and buttocks engaged until you arrive back in the starting position.

CAUTIONS Leave this exercise out if you have neck, shoulder, elbow, rib, back, or knee problems.

PULLING "T" STRAPS

BENEFITS: STRENGTHENS THE LEGS, BUTTOCKS, BACK, ARMS, AND POWERHOUSE; OPENS THE CHEST; STRETCHES THE SHOULDERS

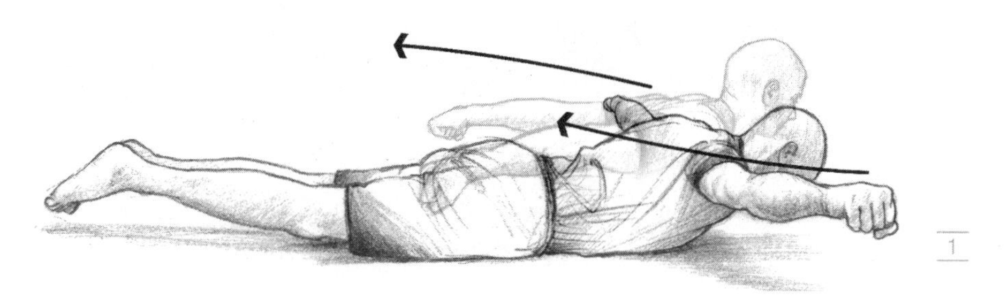

1

After the Pulling Straps exercise, remain in the same facedown position. Bring your arms out to the sides and keep your neck long. Your body should resemble the letter "T." Inhale and pull your powerhouse in and squeeze your buttocks. Pull your arms back and together, keeping them parallel to the floor as you lift your chest into the air.

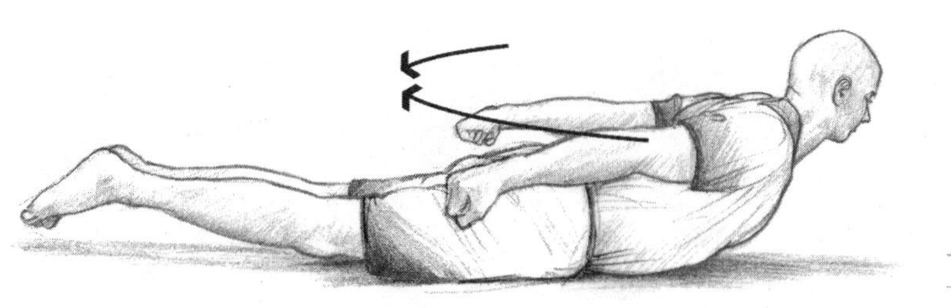

2

Hold this position for a second or two.

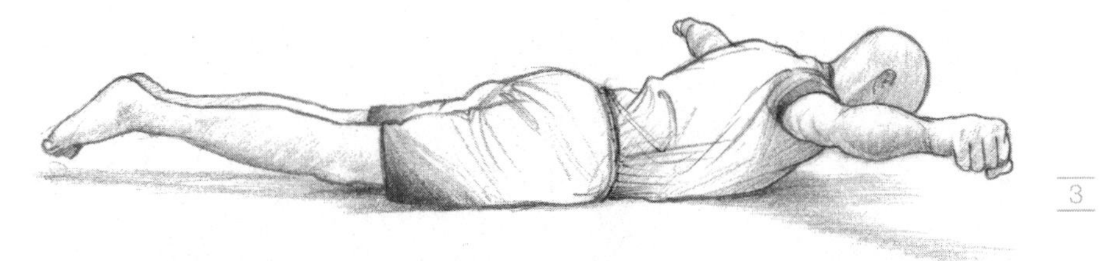

Exhale and return to the starting position.

Perform 3 times.

THE BEAST WITHIN

BODY POSITION As in Pulling Straps, you must lengthen your entire spine. Don't hinge on any one spot in your back.

THE MIND IN MOTION Pull your powerhouse in firmly, squeeze your buttocks strongly, and keep your fists tight as you lift up the sternum/diaphragm region off the floor. Engage your back and thrust your chest out. Your feet may be down or slightly lifted off the floor.

CAUTIONS Leave this out if you have neck, shoulder, rib, back, or knee problems.

THE BACKSTROKE

BENEFITS: STRENGTHENS THE POWERHOUSE, LEGS, BUTTOCKS, UPPER TORSO, AND ARMS

I love this exercise. It reminds me of the long forgotten elementary Backstroke that I learned as a boy scout.

After Pulling "T" Straps, turn over onto your back. Pull your powerhouse in and bend your knees to your chest. Bend your elbows out at the sides and bring the knuckles of your two fists together. Your thumbs should be facing your chest and the backs of your fists lightly resting on your forehead. Using your powerhouse, lift your shoulders off the floor until your upper body is resting on the tips of your shoulder blades. Inhale and straighten your arms and legs up toward the ceiling. Keep your fists together and your legs together.

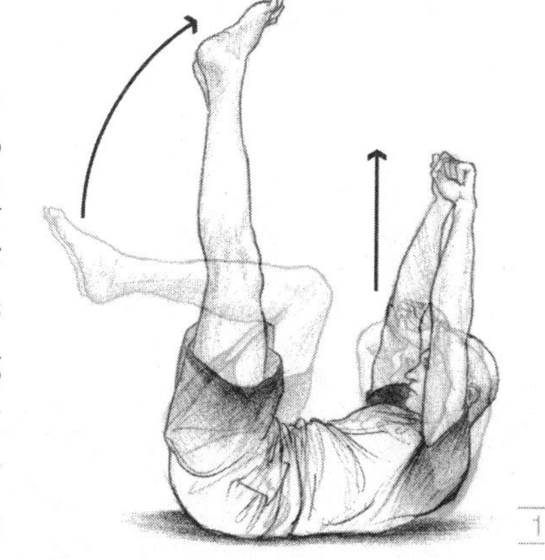

Exhale as you open your arms about 6 to 12 inches outside of shoulder-width and your legs about 6 to 12 inches outside of hip-width.

2

Inhale and sweep your arms and legs down and away from your upper body (as if you were propelling yourself backward in water). Keep your powerhouse in and your body tight. Hold this position for 3 counts.

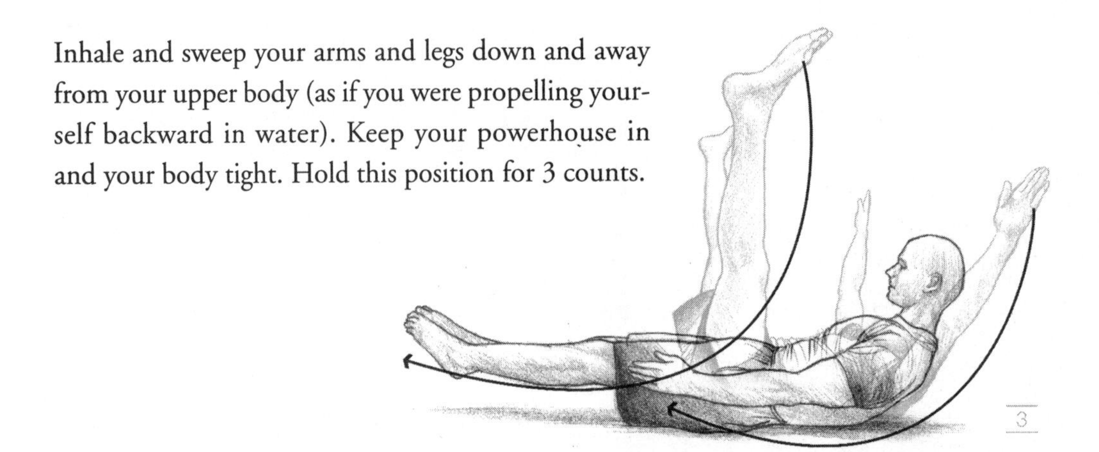

Exhale and bend your knees to your chest as you bring your fists back to your forehead.

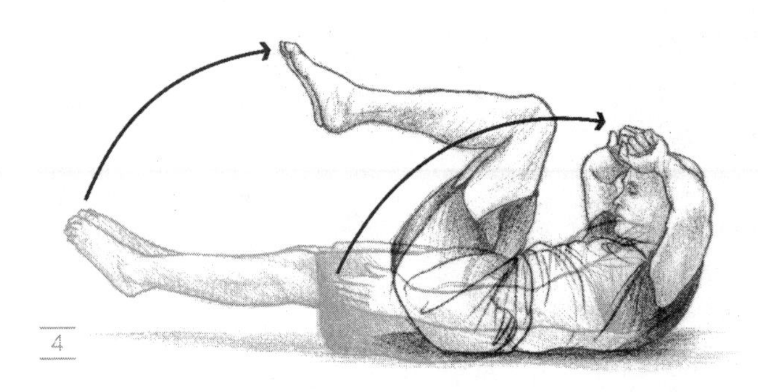

Perform 3 times. Reverse the exercise sequence for 3 repetitions. When performing this exercise in reverse, extend your arms and legs as per illustration 4—inhale and hold your breath and body firmly for 3 counts. After 3 counts, exhale and open your arms and legs, bring them up toward the ceiling, close your arms and legs, and then bend your knees and elbows to return to the starting position.

THE BEAST WITHIN

BODY POSITION To begin, keep your spine on the floor from your tailbone to the tips of your shoulder blades. Keep your neck long.

THE MIND IN MOTION If your neck fatigues, lower it to the floor. If your back begins to ache, hold your legs at a higher angle off the floor or stop the exercise. Don't let your stomach release as you circle your legs around; keep your powerhouse firm and tight. You may keep your hands open or in fists. On a universal reformer, your hands would be above your thighs when your legs are together in step 3. In this variation, with my hands pressing firmly against the sides of my legs (as illustrated), I am stimulating the strength benefits of the original version of the Double Leg Stretch. If you ever get the opportunity to try this exercise on a reformer in a studio, you'll find that placing your hands along the sides of your legs will allow the reformer's straps, which are behind your shoulders, to clear your shoulders without hindering your upper body movement.

CAUTIONS Men tend to throw their arms and legs around too quickly, losing their connection to the powerhouse. Simply keep the movement smooth and steady. You should feel your whole body moving in unison, as if you were propelling yourself in water. Leave the Backstroke out if you have neck, shoulder, or back problems.

THE TEASER

BENEFITS: STRENGTHENS THE POWERHOUSE; DEVELOPS BALANCE AND COORDINATION

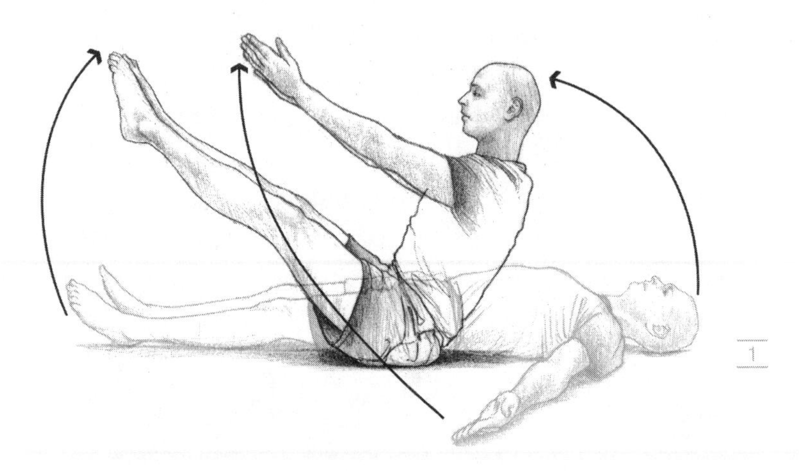

As in Teaser III from the traditional mat work (see page 95), pull your powerhouse in as you inhale and fold your body up, creating the letter "V" with your legs and torso. Ideally, your arms should be parallel to your legs.

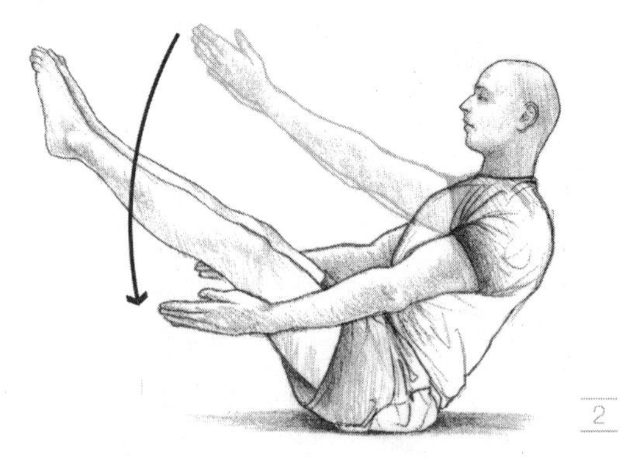

Exhale and lower your arms.

Inhale and lift your arms in a slow, controlled fashion.

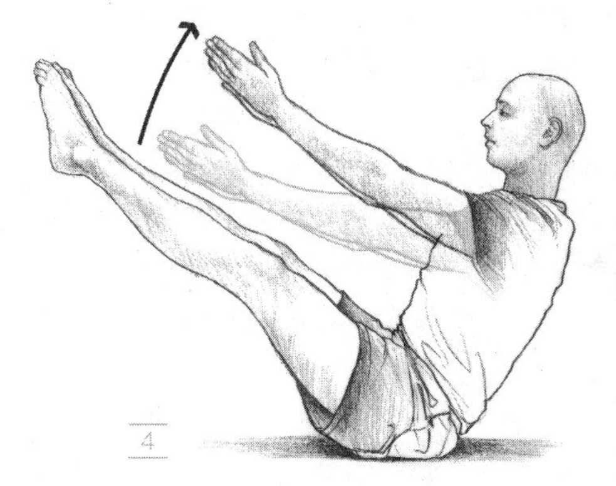

Finish inhaling while lifting your arms back to their starting position.

Lower and lift your arms three times (as illustrated).

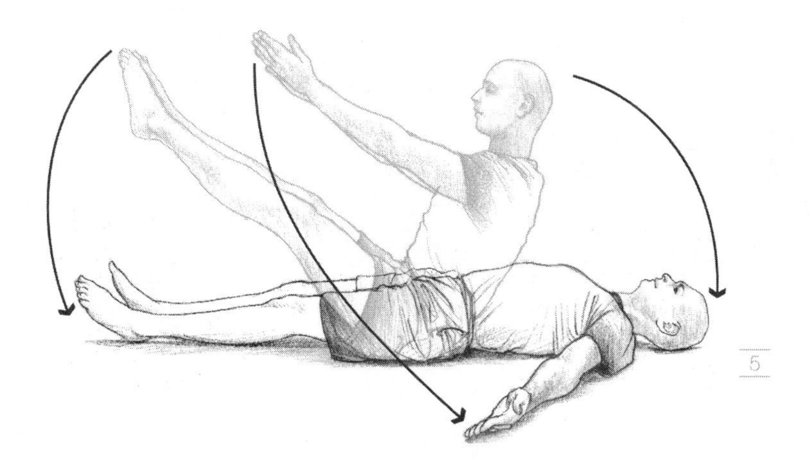

Exhale and roll your body down to the floor with control.

Perform the entire sequence 3 times.

After lowering and lifting your arms, you may perform arm circles on the second repetition. Simply reach your fingers forward with your palms up and circle your arms from your shoulders. On the third repetition reverse the arm circles.

THE BEAST WITHIN

BODY POSITION Focus on keeping your long spine and your powerhouse strong as you control the movement.

THE MIND IN MOTION Do not throw yourself up into the Teaser position. Roll up with control. You may need to bend your knees to your chest and then straighten them out when you first lift your legs in the air. If your lower back sags while holding your legs straight, you may perform this exercise with bent knees throughout. It is more important to keep your lower back lifted than to have straight legs. With practice, you'll eventually be able to straighten your legs as well. Don't arch your back. Your arms and thighs should be parallel before you lift your arms toward the ceiling. Keep your abdominals in. If you have straight legs, you may turn your feet out so your hip flexors stay relaxed. If your lower back hurts, lower yourself to the mat and hug your shins to relieve the pressure. When lifting or circling your arms, don't lower your elbows behind your hips. After the final circling, you may "shave" the back of your head (see the Shave exercise on page 172).

CAUTIONS Leave the Teaser out if you have neck, shoulder, hip, or back problems. If you experience discomfort in your tailbone during this exercise, place a thin rubber pad underneath your tailbone or leave the exercise out entirely.

HORSEBACK

BENEFITS: STRENGTHENS THE ARMS, UPPER BODY, POWERHOUSE, AND LEGS

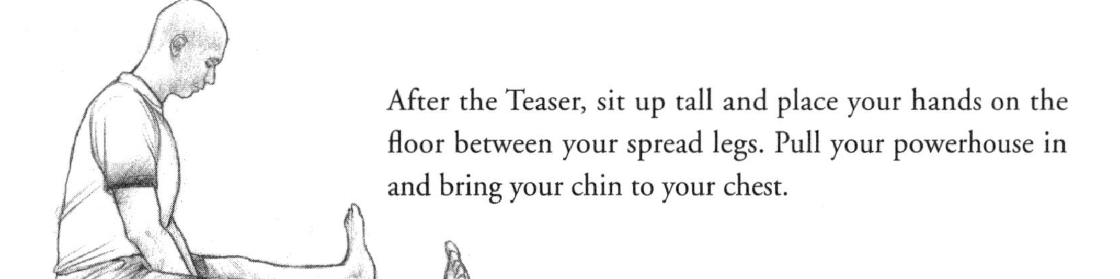

After the Teaser, sit up tall and place your hands on the floor between your spread legs. Pull your powerhouse in and bring your chin to your chest.

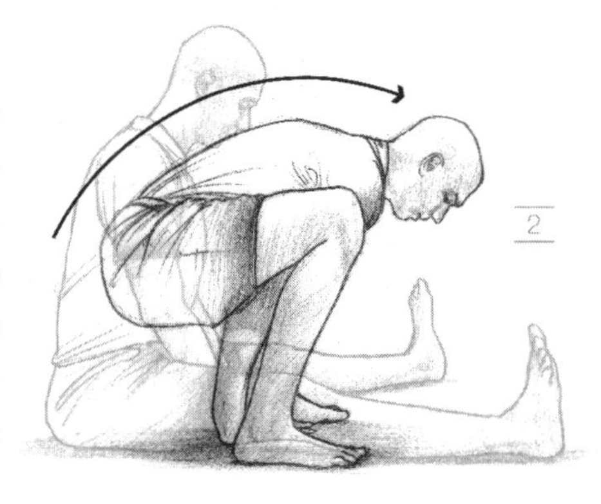

This step is optional. If you have enough upper body strength and control, you may proceed directly to the next step (see illustration 3). Come up into a squatting position with your feet alongside your hands and your bottom in the air. (You may need to place your hands outside of your legs to come up into a squat and then place them back in between your legs.)

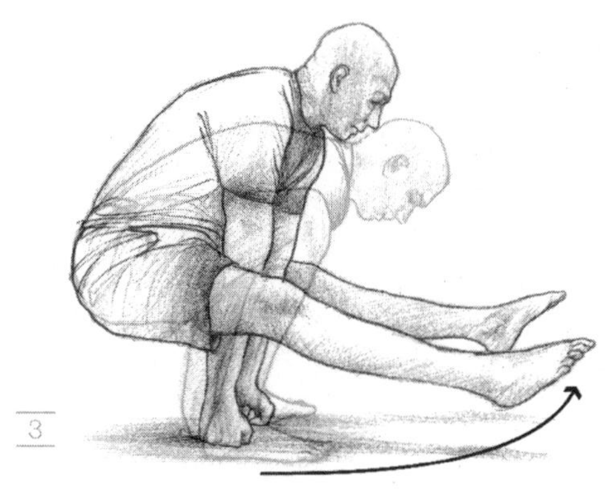

Lean your body weight onto your hands. Inhale and straighten your arms as you lift your straight legs off the floor. Keep your powerhouse in and up as you hold this position for two full breaths. Finish by lowering yourself down to the starting position.

Perform 1 to 3 times.

THE BEAST WITHIN

BODY POSITION Sit up tall with your legs straight.

THE MIND IN MOTION The Horseback is a challenging exercise. When you are able to perform the Horseback with ease, you'll know that you have made some serious strength gains in your body. I've demonstrated this exercise in three steps to make it easier. If you are strong enough, you may skip the bent knee step (illustration 2) and lift your straight legs and body directly off the floor. I've also demonstrated this exercise with fists because it is easier on my wrists. Lock your elbows when you straighten your arms. Try to straighten your legs completely and point your toes. If you find it too difficult to straighten your arms, you may try using bent arms from the optional step 2. With your elbows bent, position your legs until your hamstrings and inner thighs rest lightly on the backs of your arms. Engage your powerhouse and quadriceps to straighten your legs off the mat. You may not be able to straighten your legs, but try to get your feet in the air. This bent arm variation will still challenge your strength.

Instead of holding the position for two breaths, you may simply lift and lower yourself in one motion. If your wrists hurt when you lean your body weight forward into your hands, try lifting up on fists or use the optional second step. Men typically have the strength to lift their bodies up but lack the combination of powerhouse, quadriceps strength, and balance necessary to properly perform this exercise.

CAUTIONS Leave the Horseback out if you have neck, shoulder, wrist, elbow, back, or hip problems. You will find this exercise difficult to impossible if you are overweight.

SHORT BOX ROUND

BENEFITS: STRENGTHENS THE POWERHOUSE; LENGTHENS THE SPINE

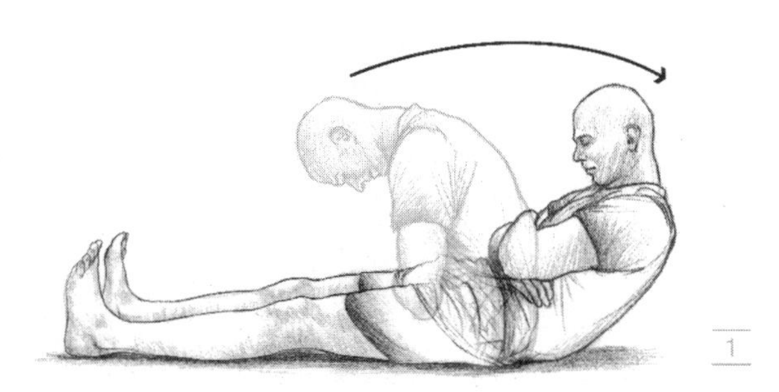

After the Horseback, sit up tall with your ankles flexed and hip-width apart. Bring your chin to your chest. Pull your powerhouse in and round your upper body slightly forward. Fold your forearms on top of each other against your stomach, with your hands on your lower waist. Keep your shoulders down. Inhale as you begin to roll down to the floor—one vertebra at a time.

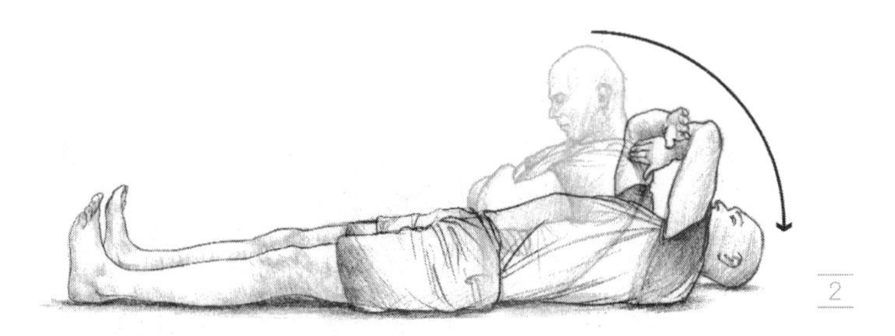

Begin exhaling about halfway down. When your spine is all the way down, reach your bent arms over your head.

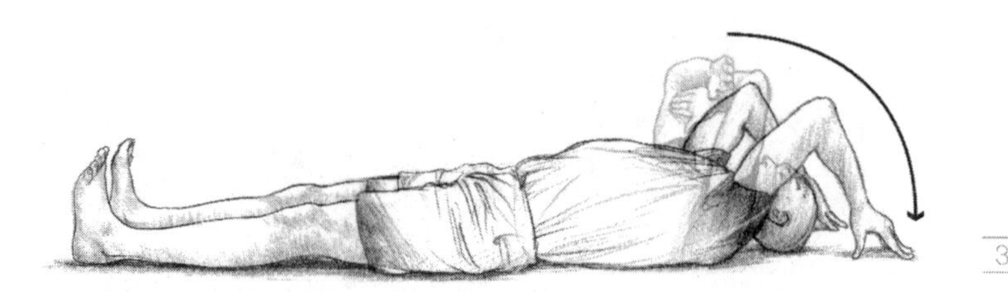

Touch your fingertips on the floor behind your head.

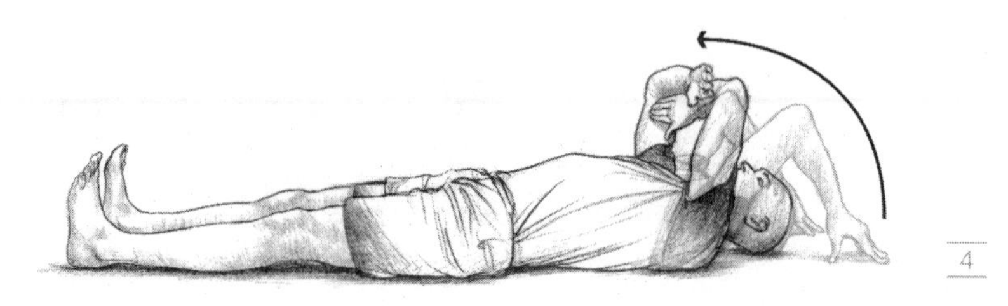

Refold your arms and bring them back to your stomach.

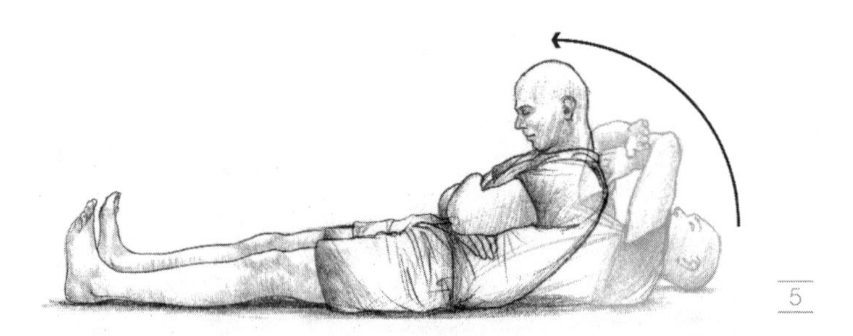

With your arms folded on your stomach and your chin to your chest, inhale as you begin to roll your vertebra up one at a time. Keep your powerhouse pulled in.

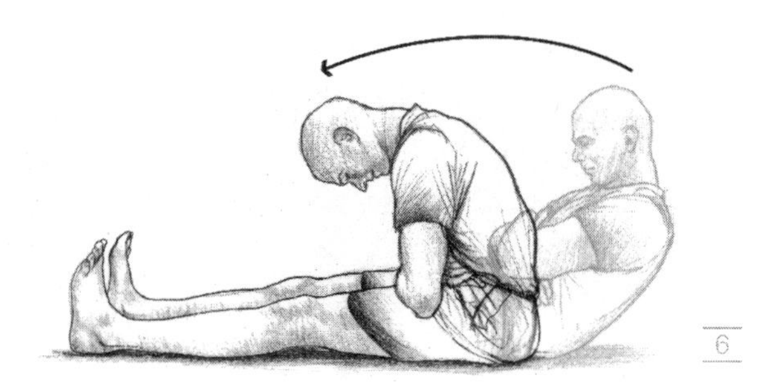

Begin to exhale as you round up and over into the starting position.

Perform 5 times.

THE BEAST WITHIN

THE MIND IN MOTION This exercise is quite similar to the Roll Up in the regular mat work. Articulate your vertebra down to the floor one at a time. Keep your powerhouse drawn firmly in. When you bring yourself upright and over, keep your spine long and your powerhouse active—don't left it release—to ensure that your spine doesn't collapse under the weight of your upper body. You may perform this exercise with your hands, instead of your forearms, on your stomach. The function of the hands or forearms is to alert you, should you either push your abdominals out or release them as you move. When you're on your back with your fingertips on the floor behind your head in step 3, you may arch your back slightly and place the crown of your head on the floor.

CAUTIONS Leave this exercise out if you have neck, shoulder, or back problems.

SHORT BOX FLAT

BENEFITS: STRENGTHENS THE POWERHOUSE, LEGS, AND BUTTOCKS; LENGTHENS THE SPINE

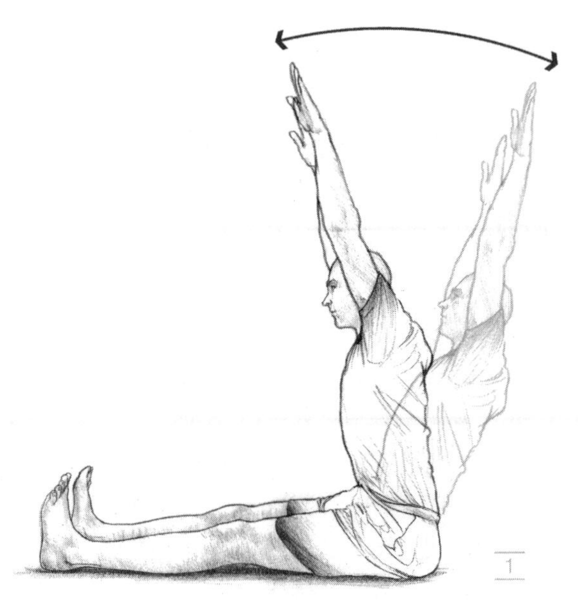

After the Short Box Round, sit up tall with your arms straight up in the air, and your legs straight and hip width apart. Pull your powerhouse in and up. Squeeze your buttocks. Inhale and lean back from your sit bones in one straight line. Exhale and return to the starting position.

Perform 5 times.

THE BEAST WITHIN

BODY POSITION Keep your spine tall; don't arch it. Don't allow the lift of your arms to change the position of your spine. Sit up tall on your sit bones. Hold your stomach firmly in.

THE MIND IN MOTION Pivot backward from where your sit bones meet the floor. If you only have a small range of motion, honor it by demonstrating fantastic control. If you can't sit up tall and your lower back is rounded, bend your knees slightly to help straighten it. With bent knees, you will have an even smaller range of motion. (Posture is becoming a common problem for men, who often lean against stationary objects when they stand or slouch when they sit.) For an easier variation, try placing your hands with interlaced fingers behind your head, instead of holding your arms straight out in the air. If you have shoulder problems, you may cross your arms in front of your chest with your hands resting lightly on the opposite shoulders.

CAUTIONS Leave this exercise out if you have neck, shoulder, hip, or back problems.

SIDE TO SIDE

BENEFITS: STRENGTHENS THE POWERHOUSE, LEGS, AND BUTTOCKS; LENGTHENS THE SIDES, LEGS, AND SPINE

After the Short Box Flat, remain in the same starting position and pitch forward until your shoulders are just in front of the area where your thighs meet your hips. Pull your powerhouse in and squeeze your buttocks. Inhale and reach over to your right as far as you can, while keeping the opposite hip down. Squeeze your buttocks again and return to the starting position as you exhale.

Repeat on the left side. Perform for a total of 3 times on each side.

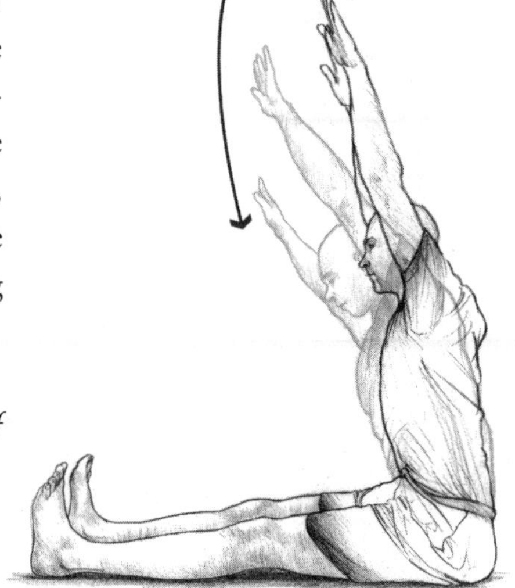

THE BEAST WITHIN

BODY POSITION It is most important to sit up tall. Keep your spine long. Keep your arms equidistant from your head throughout the exercise. Don't let your shoulders move or your arms meander toward your ears. Lock your elbows and knees. You may bend your knees, if it helps you sit up taller. Keep your shoulders down. You may bend your elbows, if it helps to keep your shoulders down.

THE MIND IN MOTION Reach tall from the base of your spine up through the crown of your head. Keep your hips down and maintain the slight forward pitch. Keep your powerhouse drawn tightly in. As in the Short Box Flat, you may place your hands with your fingers interlaced behind your head and your elbows out to the sides, instead of extending your arms straight out overhead. With your hands behind your head, you may also try another variation. Try to touch your right knee with your right elbow and your left knee with your left elbow as you reach over to either side; don't let your chest collapse forward as you do this. Due to tightness or weakness, men tend to bend their knees, lift their arms minimally, bend their elbows, or collapse in the lower backs. If you focus on anchoring your body down as you stay lifted while moving with control, you should be able to perform this exercise well.

CAUTIONS Leave this exercise out if you have neck, shoulder, or back problems.

TWIST AND REACH

BENEFITS: STRENGTHENS THE WAIST AND POWER-HOUSE; LENGTHENS THE SPINE AND LEGS

After the Side to Side, sit up tall again with your arms straight up toward the ceiling. Squeeze your buttocks and pull your powerhouse in and up. Inhale. (Move slowly through this exercise to correlate your breathing and movement as instructed.)

1

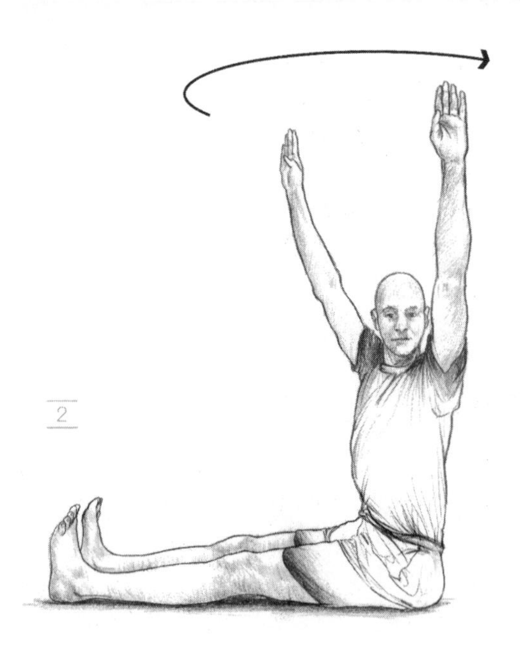

Exhale and twist your torso at the waist to your left.

Inhale, pivot back on your squeezed bottom while still facing left, and stretch your body out long.

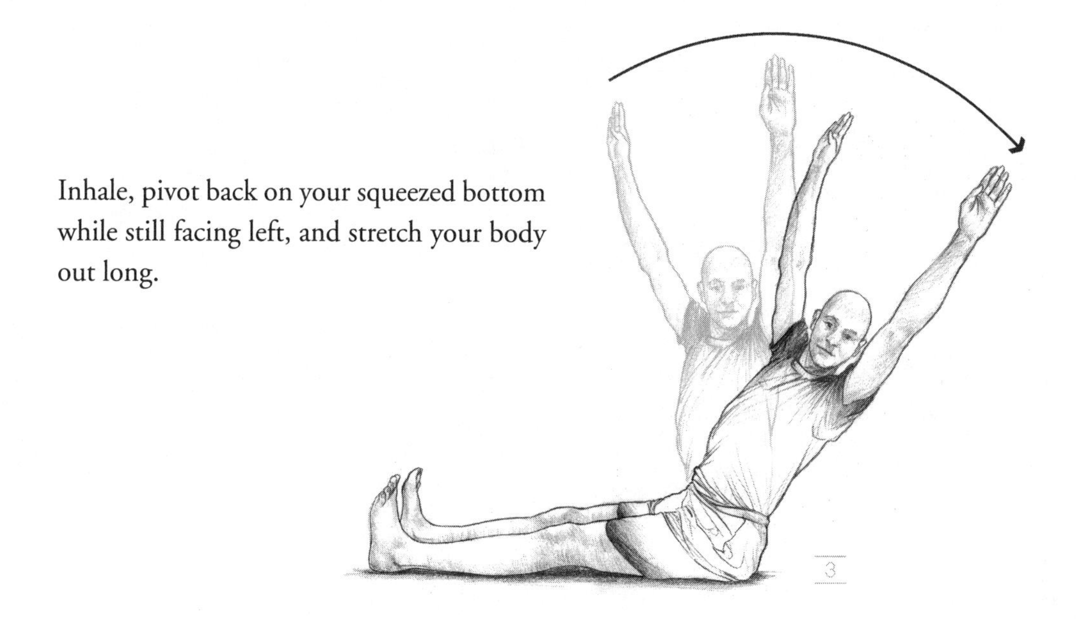

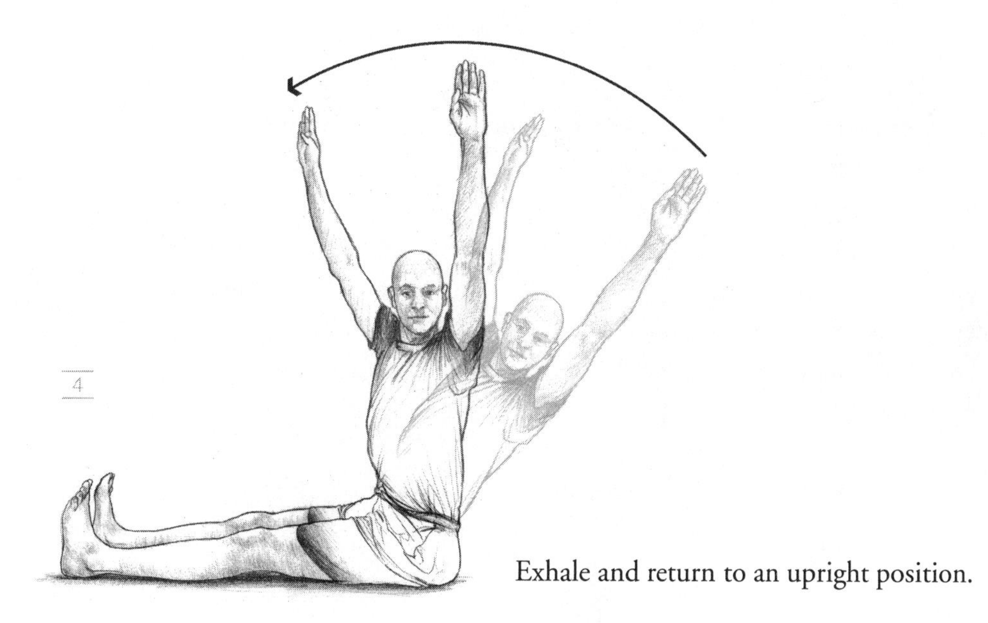

Exhale and return to an upright position.

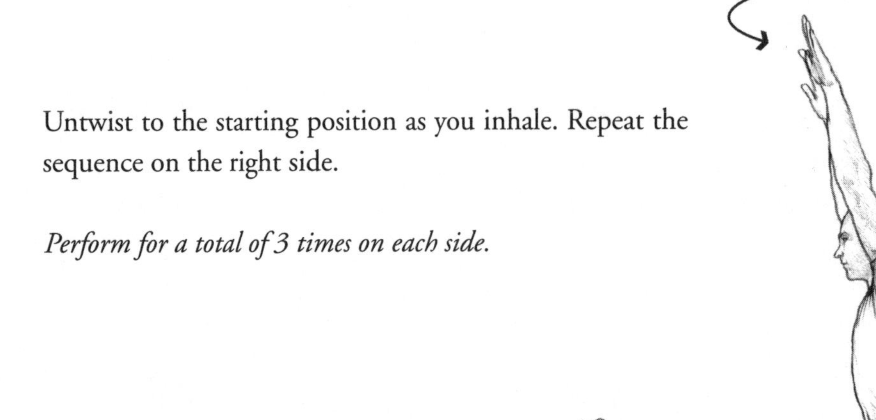

Untwist to the starting position as you inhale. Repeat the sequence on the right side.

Perform for a total of 3 times on each side.

THE BEAST WITHIN

BODY POSITION Keep your spine tall, but don't arch it. Don't let the arm lift change the shape of your spine.

THE MIND IN MOTION When you twist your torso, keep your stomach in and let nothing below your waist move. This is a *spinal* rotation, so don't let your hips shift. Keep your arms equidistant from your head as you reach back. Keep your elbows and knees locked, although you may bend your elbows slightly to help pull your shoulders down. Don't release your stomach. You will probably have a small range of motion, which is fine. You may also perform this exercise with your fingers interlaced behind your head. Do not rush through this exercise. The inhalations and exhalations will probably take longer than the actual physical movement, so proceed slowly in order to match your breathing with your movement.

CAUTIONS Leave this out if you have neck, shoulder, hip, or back problems.

AROUND THE WORLD

BENEFITS: STRENGTHENS THE POWERHOUSE AND WAIST; LENGTHENS THE SPINE AND LEGS

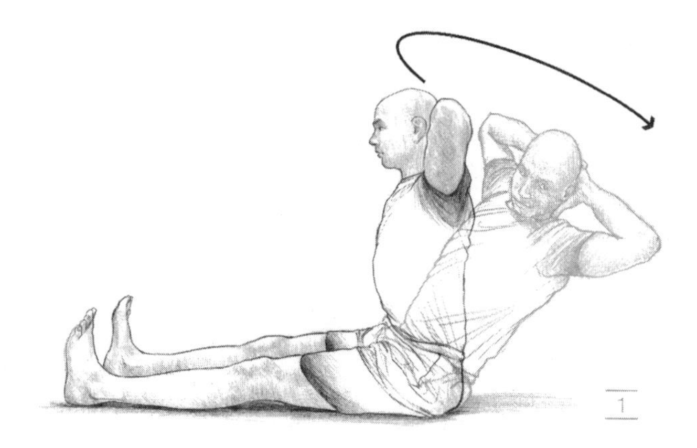

The Around the World is just a step more advanced than the Twist and Reach. Sit up tall and pull your stomach in. Squeeze your buttocks. Exhale as you twist from the waist to your left. Inhale and hinge out from your buttocks as you did in the Twist and Reach.

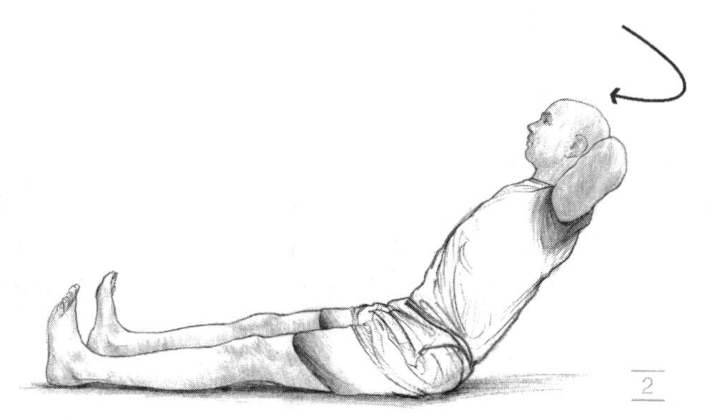

Untwist your body toward your right side. Keep your powerhouse in.

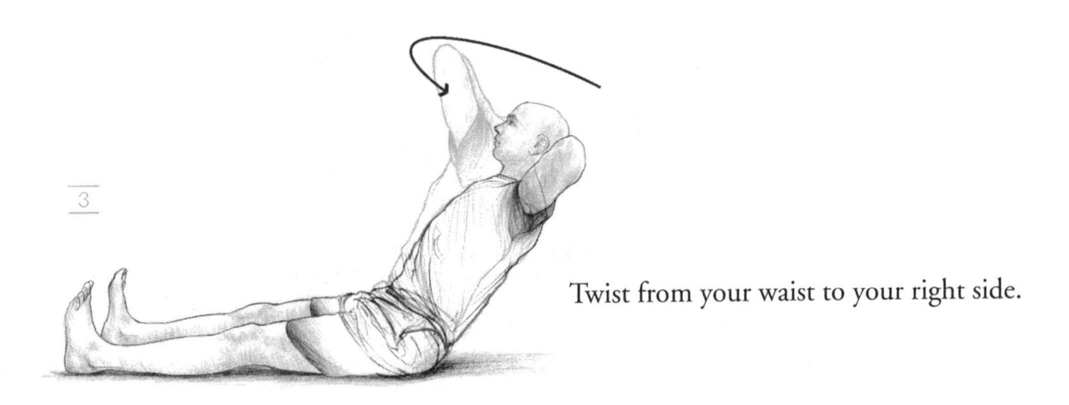

Twist from your waist to your right side.

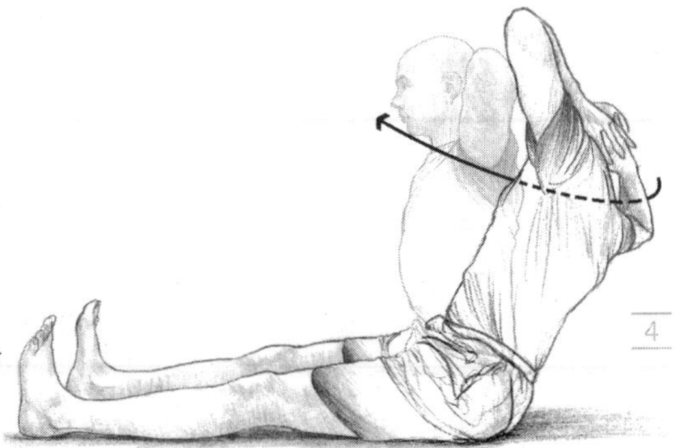

Exhale as you return to an upright position. Inhale as you untwist to face forward.

Repeat the sequence starting with a right twist.

THE BEAST WITHIN

BODY POSITION Keep your spine tall and strong; don't arch it.

THE MIND IN MOTION When you twist your torso, keep your stomach in and let nothing below the waist move. This is a spinal rotation, so don't let your hips shift. Hold your neck tall throughout the movement. If you need to bend your knees slightly to sit up tall, then do so. Your back should not hurt. Don't release your stomach. Your range of motion will probably be small.

CAUTIONS Leave this exercise out if you have neck, shoulder, or back problems.

THE TREE

BENEFITS: LENGTHENS THE SPINE AND LEGS; STRENGTHENS THE POWERHOUSE; OPENS THE HIPS

Sit up tall and extend your left leg out on the floor in front of you. Hold your hands under your right leg on the lower portion of the back of your thigh. Keep your elbows out and your shoulders down. Pull your powerhouse firmly in and up. Extend (or kick) your right leg up 3 times, and hold it up there on the third extension.

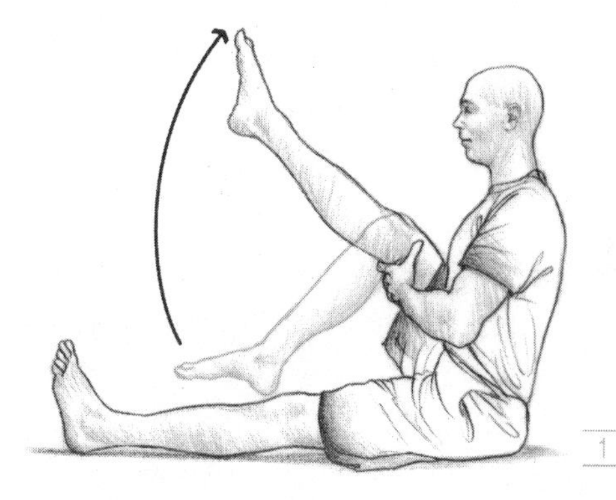

1

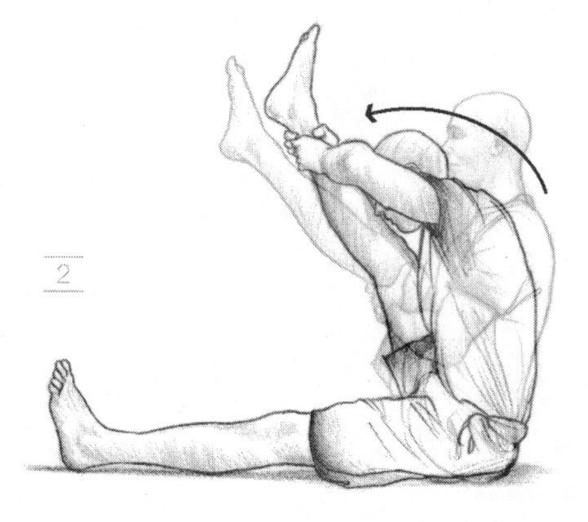

2

Walk your hands up your straight leg and grasp as high up as possible. Ideally you want to grasp your ankle—or, for a greater stretch—your toes with a flexed ankle. Without pulling your right leg, lengthen your spine and place your stomach onto your thigh, your chest onto your knee, and your forehead onto your shin.

Inhale as you pivot on your buttocks and bring your leg to a vertical 90-degree position.

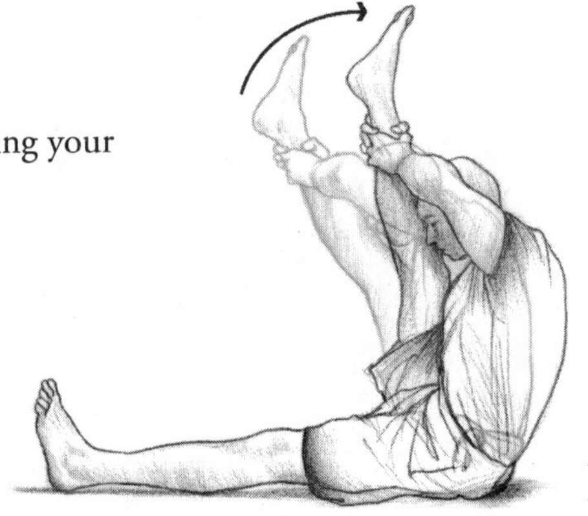

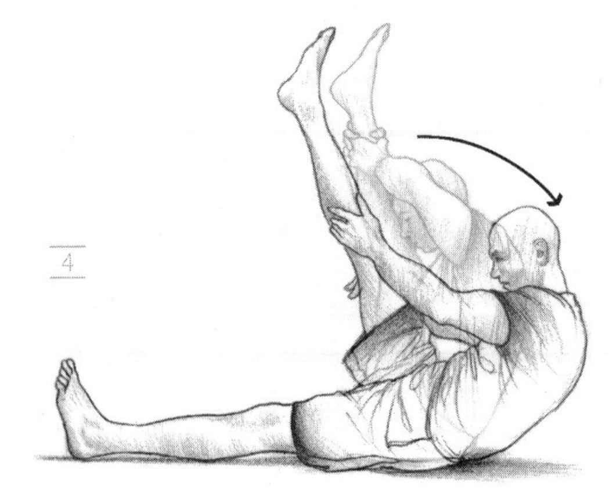

Roll your vertebrae down onto the floor as you walk your hands down the back of your leg. Begin exhaling when your spine is about halfway down.

Finish exhaling as you lay your spine down on the floor with your right leg still raised at 90 degrees.

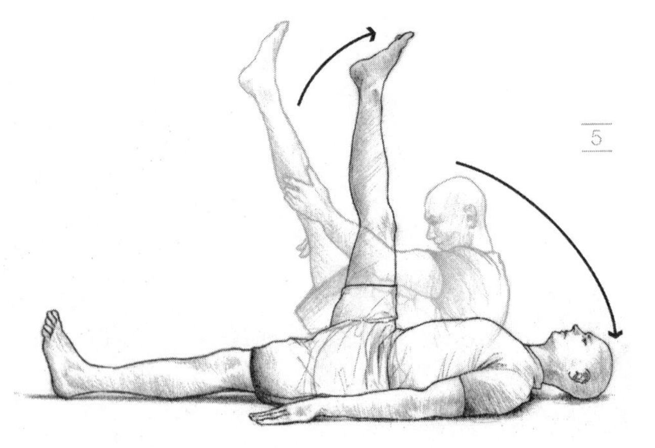

Inhale, pull your powerhouse in, and begin to roll your spine off the floor. Reach your hands past your lifted leg, and then walk them up the back of your leg (not illustrated).

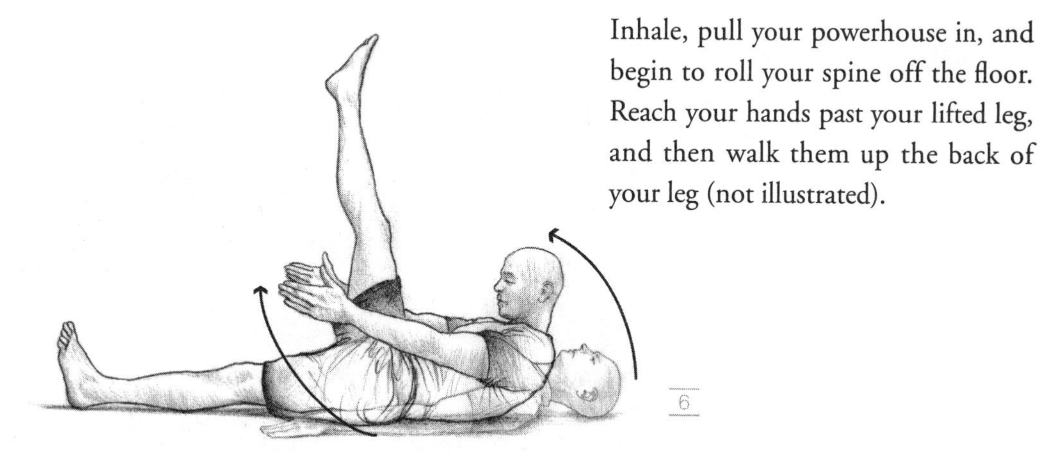

Begin exhaling before you're halfway up. Lift your spine up as tall as you can and finish your exhalation.

Perform twice or perform only once and proceed to the Leg to the Side version (see The Tree: Leg to the Side) with the same leg. Repeat the entire sequence with the opposite leg.

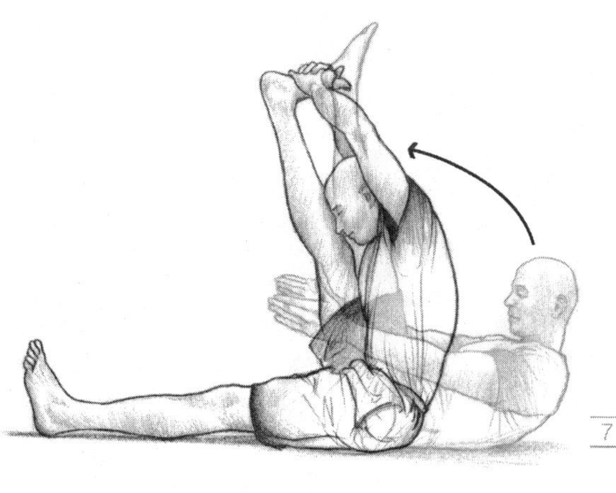

THE TREE: LEG TO THE SIDE

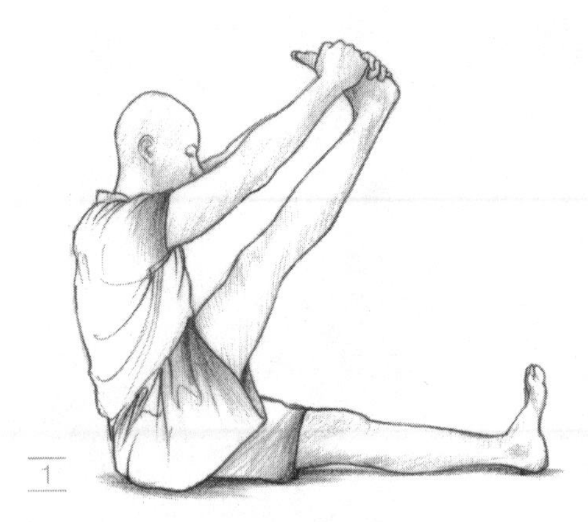

Consider this Leg to the Side variation a continuation from the first Tree exercise. Lift your spine tall. Take hold of your right foot, ankle, or leg—depending on your flexibility. Inhale and hold your powerhouse in.

Exhale. Release your left hand to your left side and adjust your right hand to grasp the inside of your foot or leg. Holding the inside of your foot or leg, lift your leg up and begin to bring it out to the side.

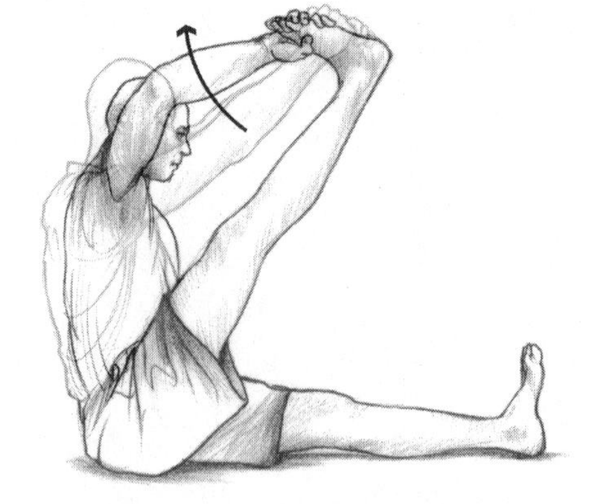

Inhale and continue to bring your right leg out to the side. Exhale and roll your spine down to the floor, while maintaining your right leg out to the side.

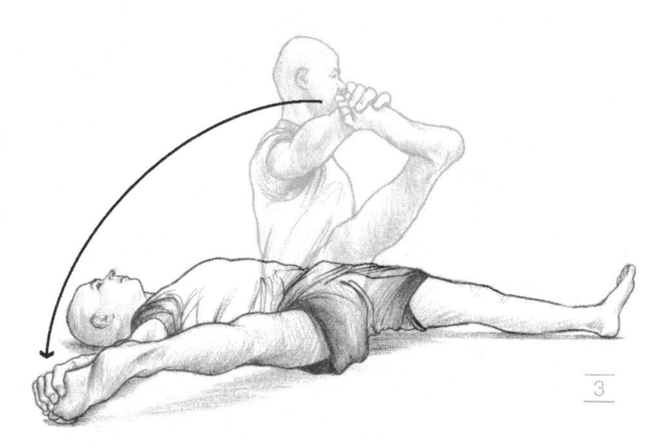

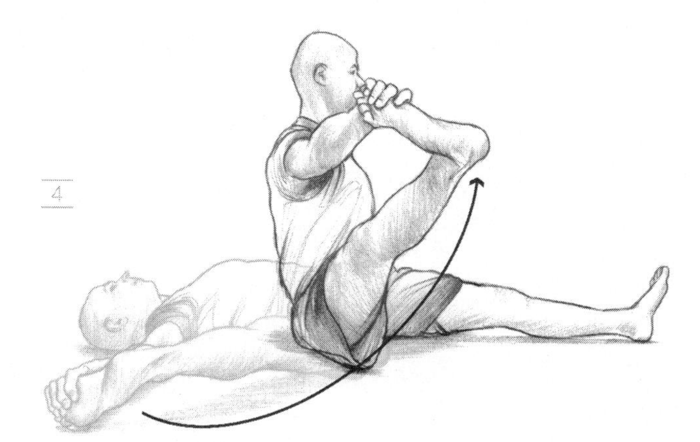

Inhale. Roll your spine up until you are again sitting up tall. Begin exhaling as you begin to peel off the floor.

Finish exhaling, bring your leg in front of you, and lift your spine against your raised leg.

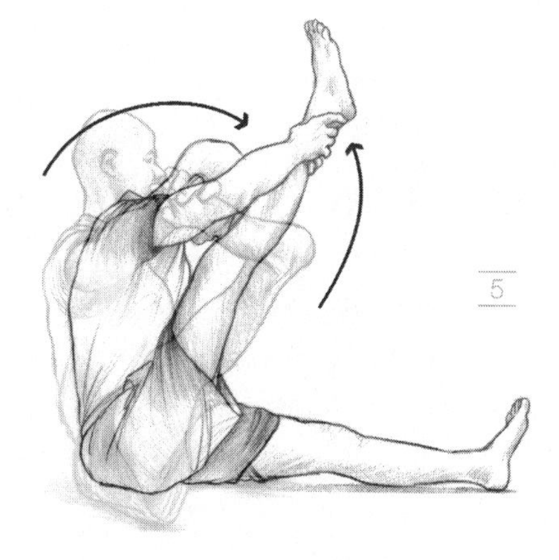

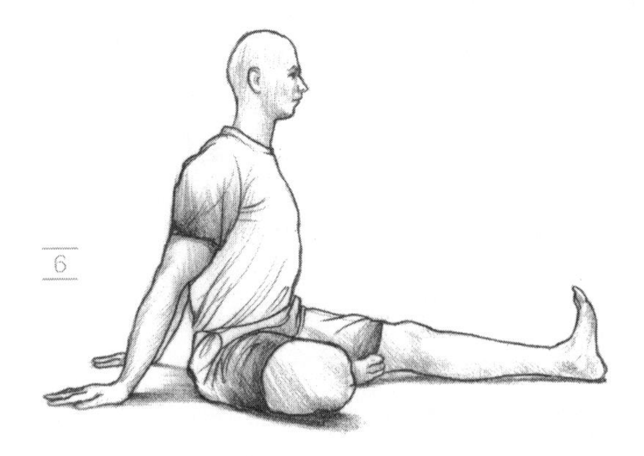
6

Lower your right leg and bend your right knee so that your right foot rests against the inside of your left leg. Place your hands on the floor behind you and inhale as you lift your spine up. Pull your powerhouse in.

Exhale and lengthen your body over your straight left leg. Keep your powerhouse lifted.

Repeat the entire sequence with your left leg.

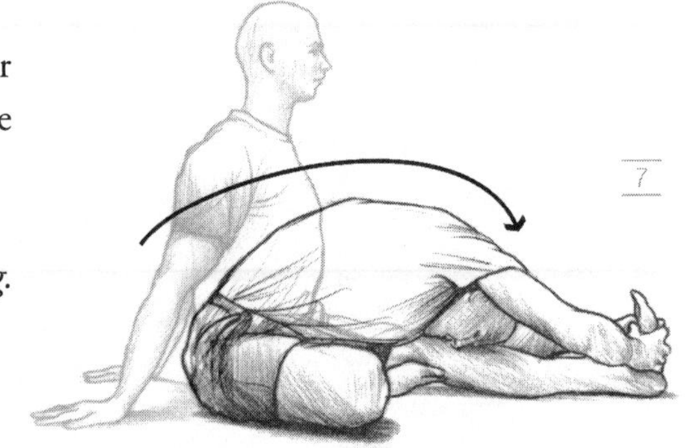
7

THE BEAST WITHIN

BODY POSITION The Tree is designed to lengthen the spine. It is not a hamstring stretch. If your hamstrings are tight, you'll find it difficult to lengthen your spine. It is important that you sit up tall, even if that means elevating your leg only a little off the floor; do not force your leg any higher if doing so hinders you from sitting up tall. If your lower back sags, it is usually because of a tight hamstring, tight lower back, and/or disengaged powerhouse. To sit up taller, lower the elevated leg and pull your powerhouse firmly in. Keep your hips square.

THE MIND IN MOTION FOR THE TREE Do not hold your raised foot/leg with your hand as you lower your spine to the floor. Walk your hands down. It is generally a good idea to walk only two fingers of each hand down and up your leg as you descend and ascend from the floor. This makes you use your powerhouse to control your movement, instead of relying on the strong upper body muscles that men typically have.

If you can sit up tall with your straight leg against your forehead, then try sliding your forehead up your shin toward your foot while keeping your chin in. Focus on lengthening your spine out from your hips as you reach the crown of your head toward the ceiling. Try this with a flexed ankle to make it even harder. Keep your powerhouse firm throughout the movement.

MIND IN MOTION FOR THE LEG TO THE SIDE VARIATION Hold your leg or foot, depending on your level of flexibility. Your hips should remain square throughout the exercise. When your leg is out to the side and your back is on the floor (step 3), keep your opposite hip down. If you find it difficult to roll up with your leg out to the side, bring your leg in front of you as in the standard Tree (see page 203). Lengthen from the base of your spine when you stretch forward in step 7.

CAUTIONS If you have tightness in your back and hamstrings, you won't be able to lift your leg very high or easily lengthen your spine at first. Focus on sitting up tall instead. Proceed slowly or leave this exercise out it you have neck, knee, or back problems.

THE LONG STRETCH

BENEFITS: STRENGTHENS THE ENTIRE BODY

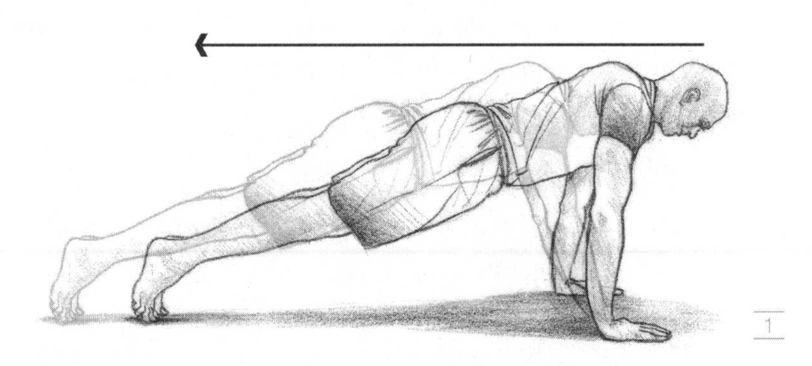

Assume a Push-up position. Pull your stomach to your spine. Tuck your tailbone and squeeze your buttocks. Inhale and push your body backward by sliding on your feet.

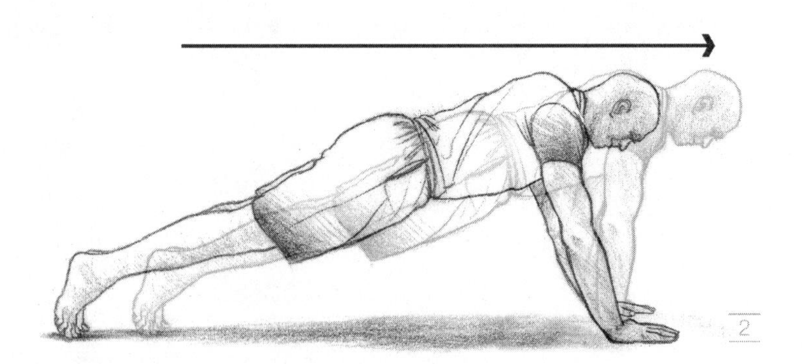

Keep your entire body rigid and exhale as you pull your body forward, sliding forward on your feet.

Perform 5 times.

THE BEAST WITHIN

BODY POSITION When you take the Push-up position, tuck your tailbone under, squeeze your bottom, and firmly hold your navel to your spine. Keep your spine long. Lock your elbows and knees. Keep your shoulders down and away from your ears.

THE MIND IN MOTION You may slide both backward and forward on the balls of your feet, or slide backward on the Balls and then slide forward on your toes. With practice, you will discover the best method of sliding for you. An easier way to slide forward is to flip onto the tops of your toes, but there is a tendency to sink into the lower back. If you choose this option, be certain to maintain your rigid body position. Don't let your lower back sink. Don't release your stomach. You may want to wear socks to facilitate sliding. Men tend to do well with exercises that use the Push-up position. Think of your body as a battering ram and take out the castle gate!

CAUTIONS Leave this exercise out if you have neck, shoulder, wrist, elbow, back, knee, foot, or ankle problems. If you are overweight, you have a higher risk of injuring your lower back; be extra careful not to release your powerhouse.

THE DOWN STRETCH

BENEFITS: STRENGTHENS THE ARMS, LEGS, SHOULDERS, BACK, BUTTOCKS, AND POWERHOUSE; DEVELOPS FLEXIBILITY IN THE SPINE; OPENS THE CHEST

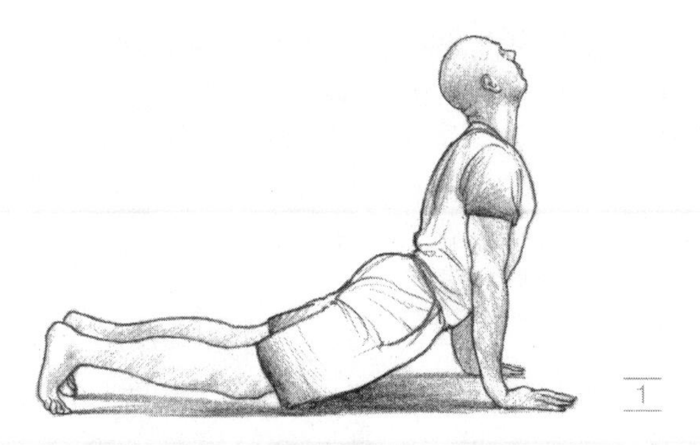

1

After the Long Stretch from the Push-up position, look up at a spot on the ceiling and lift your sternum toward that spot. Your hips will automatically lower when you look up. Squeeze your buttocks. Keep your arms and legs as straight as possible. Keep your shoulders down and back.

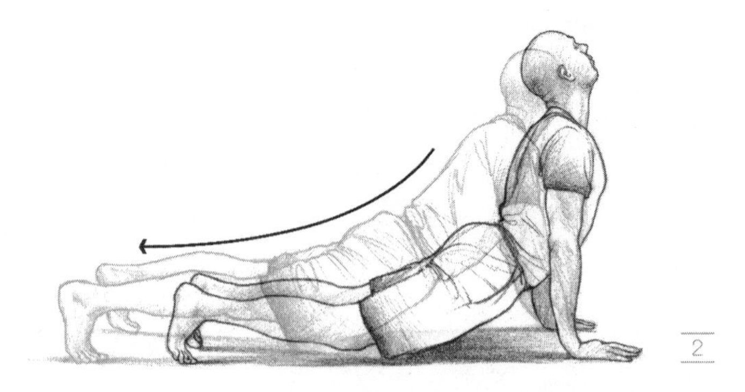

2

Hold your powerhouse in as you inhale and slide your feet backward along the floor.

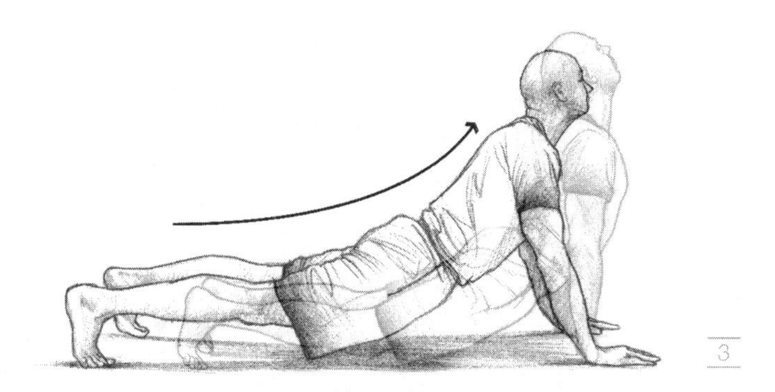

Exhale as you slide forward to the starting position. Pull your powerhouse in and up. Keep your chest lifted.

Perform 3 times.

THE BEAST WITHIN

BODY POSITION Wear socks to help you slide back and forth along the floor. Squeeze your buttocks hard, and focus on reaching your sternum toward the ceiling throughout the exercise to prevent your lower back from sinking. Squeezing your bottom will also help you stretch and open your hip flexors. Keep your arms locked and legs straight.

THE MIND IN MOTION You may slide both backward and forward on the balls of your feet, or slide backward on the balls and then slide forward on your toes. With practice, you will discover the best method of sliding for you. An easier way to slide forward is to flip onto the tops of your toes. You may make this exercise easier by simply holding the starting position for a few breaths. If you choose to slide, start with a small range of back and forth motion. If your back tightens up when you squeeze your buttocks, sit back on your heels with your forehead on your knees as you would at the end of the Swan (see page 176). Men tend to have a small range of motion in their backbends; do not force the movement. You may also do this exercise with your knees down on the mat. It is gentler on the lower back.

CAUTIONS Leave this out if you have neck, shoulder, wrist, back, knee, ankle, or weight problems.

THE UP STRETCH

BENEFITS: STRENGTHENS THE ARMS, UPPER BODY, POWERHOUSE, LEGS, AND BUTTOCKS

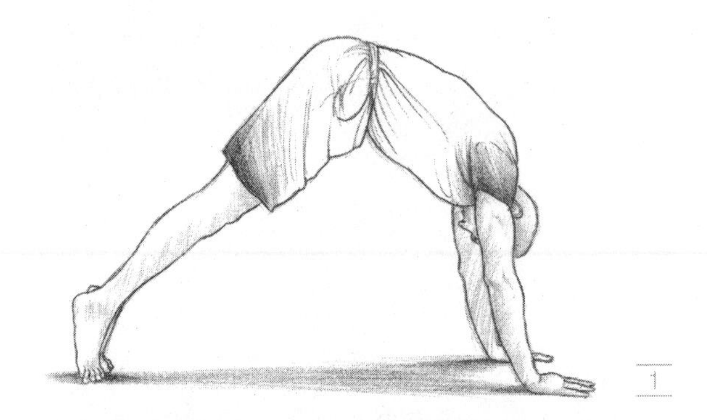

After the Down Stretch, exhale and lift your buttocks high into the air with your back rounded. Distribute more weight in your hands than in your feet. Pull your powerhouse in and up.

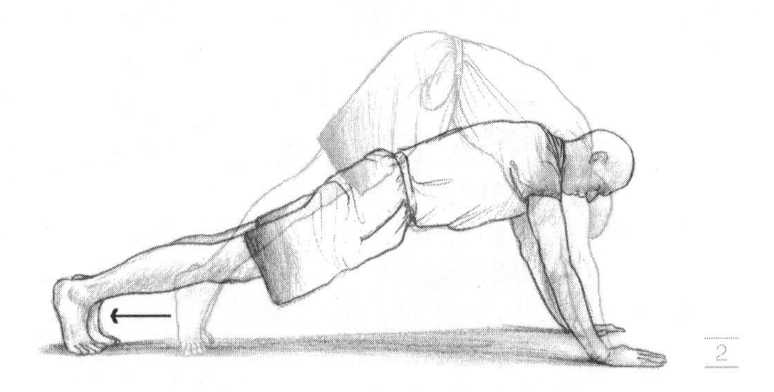

Inhale and slide your feet out until your body is in a Push-up position, but keep your shoulders behind your hands instead of over them. Your tailbone should be tucked, and your buttocks should be engaged.

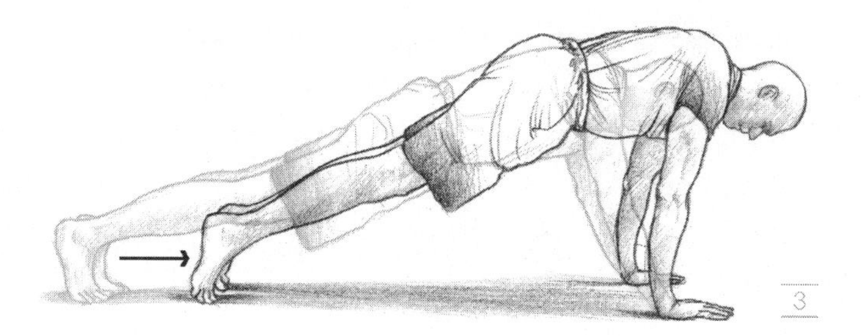

Slide forward on your feet until your shoulders are above your hands. Begin to exhale as you round your back up.

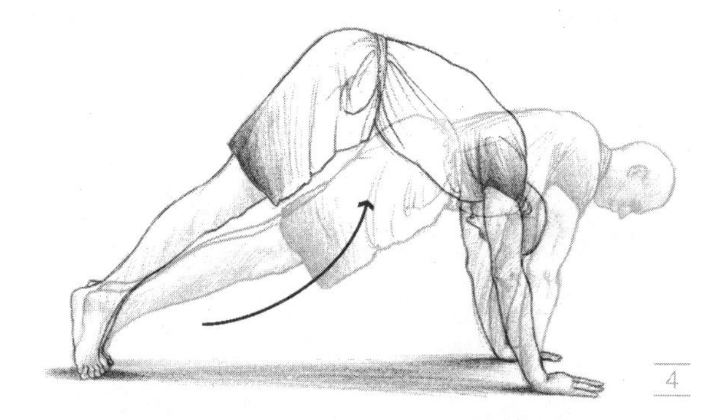

Finish exhaling as you pull your powerhouse in, round your back high into the air, and look to your navel—until you're in the starting position again.

Perform 4 times.

THE BEAST WITHIN

BODY POSITION Follow instructions in illustration 1.

THE MIND IN MOTION Wear socks to help you slide. You may slide both backward and forward on the balls of your feet, or slide backward on the ball, and then slide forward on your toes. With practice, you will discover the best method of sliding for you. An easier way to slide forward is to flip onto the tops of your toes, but there is a tendency to sink the lower back. If you choose this option, be certain to maintain your rigid body position. Throughout the Push-up portion of this exercise (see illustrations 2 and 3), keep your tailbone tucked under, squeeze your buttocks hard, and keep your powerhouse drawn in. Your body should form one rigid line during this Push-up phase; don't arch your lower back. Don't slide backward too far or you risk sinking into your lower back. Keep your arms and legs straight throughout the exercise.

CAUTIONS Leave this out if you have neck, shoulder, wrist, elbow, back, hip, knee, foot, or ankle problems.

THE ELEPHANT

BENEFITS: STRENGTHENS THE POWERHOUSE; LENGTHENS THE SPINE AND LEGS

Stand on your heels with your hands shoulder-width apart on the floor. Pull your powerhouse in and up as you round your back. Look at your navel. Push through your heels and keep your toes lifted.

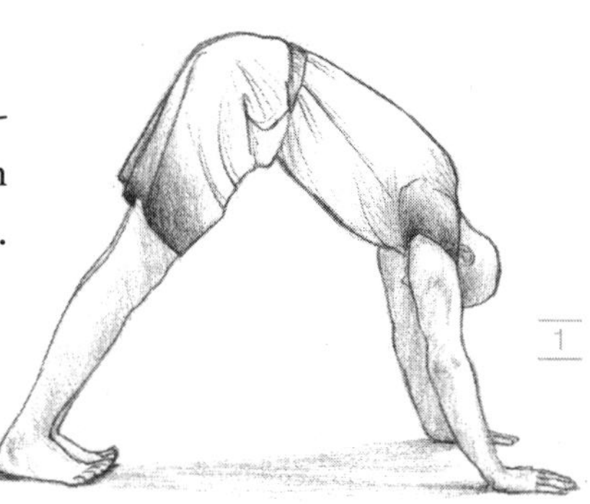

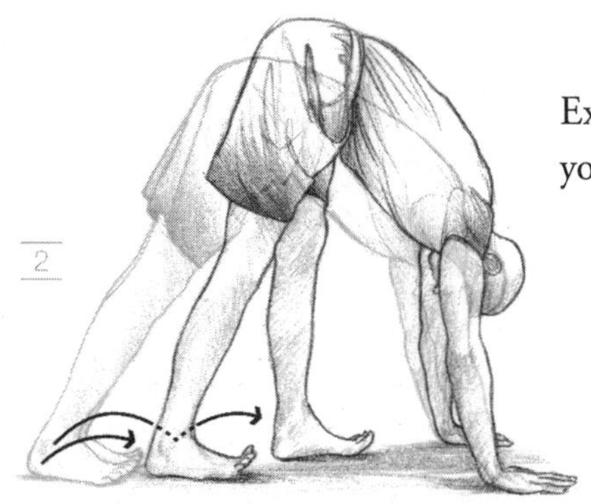

Exhale and walk your feet forward while keeping your toes lifted. Keep your legs and arms straight.

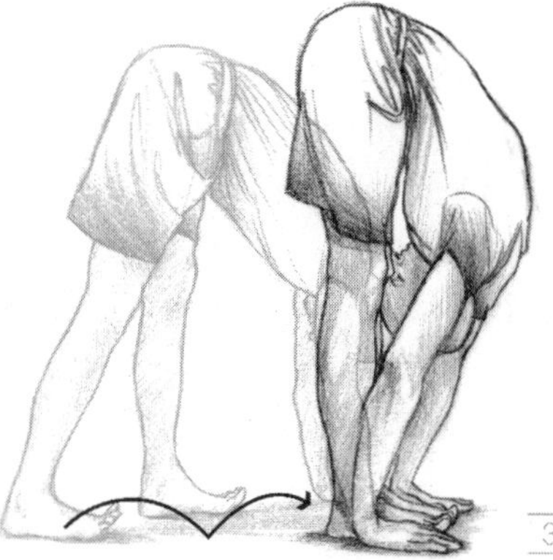

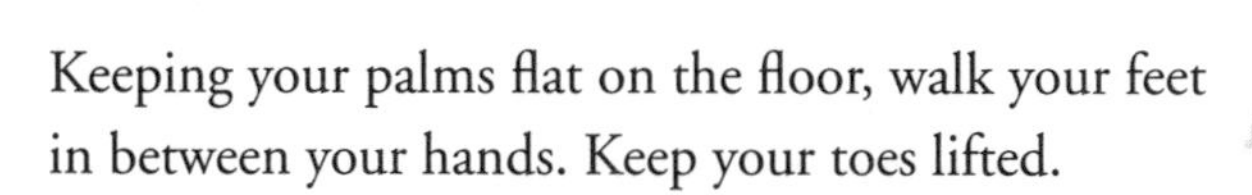

Keeping your palms flat on the floor, walk your feet in between your hands. Keep your toes lifted.

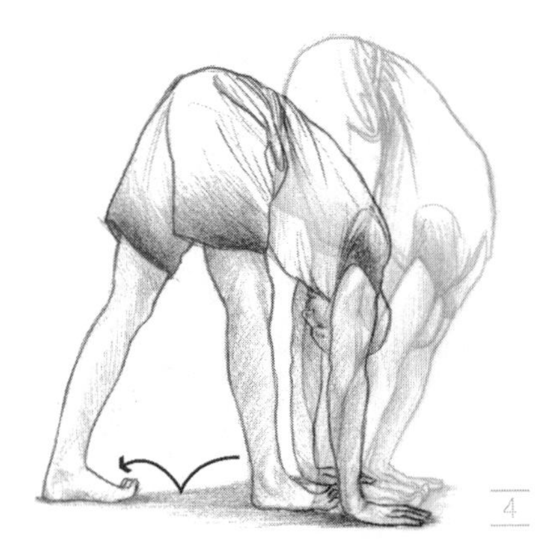

Inhale and keep your powerhouse in as you walk your feet back away from your hands. Keep your toes up.

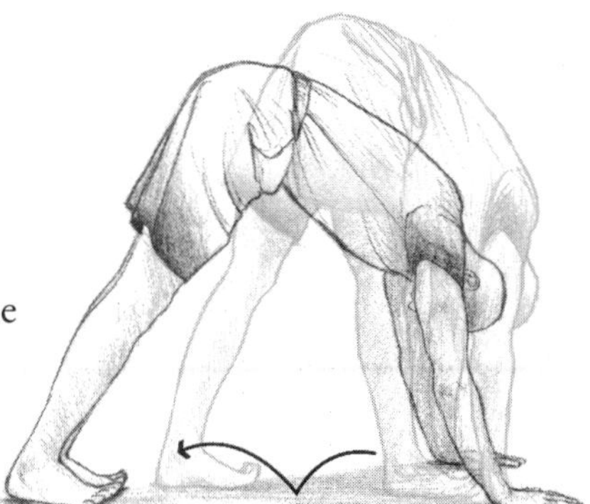

Continue walking your feet back until you are in the starting position.

Perform 5 times.

THE BEAST WITHIN

BODY POSITION Do not release your stomach during this exercise; keep your powerhouse engaged. Keep your palms flat on the floor and your legs straight. Don't bend your knees. Keep your toes lifted.

THE MIND IN MOTION Look at your navel as you walk. Men tend to be stiff in their legs and backs, so walk only as far forward as you can, while maintaining straight arms and legs. Illustrated here is the more commonly used and modern-day version of the Elephant, which begins with a rounded back. Another version is performed with a flat back, which you can try by pushing your hips back and up. Your back will appear flatter. (If you're familiar with yoga, this variation resembles the yoga posture called Downward Dog.)

Your breathing may not be as smooth as the illustrations depict. If you need to take more breaths than instructed, then do so, but be aware of keeping your powerhouse in and up.

CAUTIONS Leave this out if you have neck, shoulder, wrist, or back problems.

ARABESQUE

BENEFITS: STRENGTHENS THE ARMS, SHOULDERS, POWERHOUSE, LEGS, AND BUTTOCKS; OPENS THE HIP; LENGTHENS THE LEGS

Begin the Arabesque in the Elephant position. Round your back and pull your powerhouse in and up. Place your hands shoulder-width apart. You may place your feet together or shoulder-width apart.

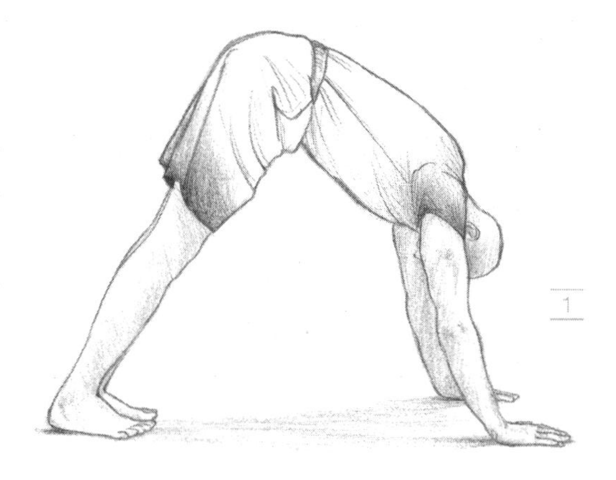

1

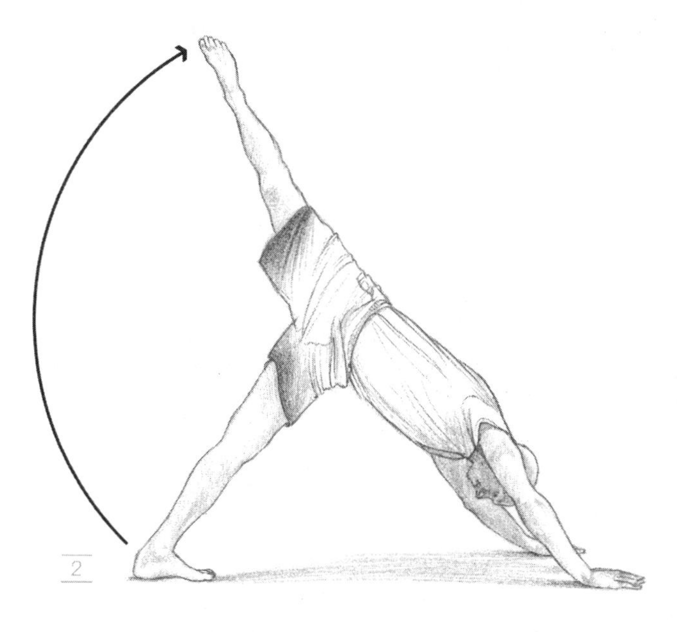

2

Inhale and bring a straight right leg with pointed toes to the ceiling. Simultaneously open your right hip as you push your hips back and up. Your back will naturally straighten. Hold this Arabesque position for a breath or two. Exhale and lower your leg to the starting position. Repeat with your left leg.

Perform the whole sequence 2 times—twice for each leg.

THE BEAST WITHIN

BODY POSITION You may keep your hips square while reaching your leg behind you (not illustrated), or you may open your hip and try reaching for the ceiling with your toes (see illustration 2). Keep your shoulders square throughout the movement.

THE MIND IN MOTION You may simply hold the Arabesque position with the heel of your supporting leg pressed into the floor, or you may lift and lower your supporting heel—inhaling as your heel rises and exhaling as you press it into the mat. All variations of this exercise are effective and challenging. Try to maintain a straight line from your hands through your shoulders to your hips. As in the Elephant, you may also start with your back straight (instead of rounded); achieve this position by lifting your hips back and up while both legs are on the floor. Your back will flatten. Don't bend your elbows or knees. Keep your powerhouse lifted into your spine and don't drop your ribs. Your hands should make full contact with the floor. Men tend to have tight, weak hips. The illustrated version will help you regain mobility and strength in your hips. It may take you some time to strengthen your hips enough to hold your leg up for the suggested duration in step 2.

CAUTIONS Leave this exercise out if you have neck, shoulder, wrist, back, knee, hip, or ankle problems.

THE LONG BACK STRETCH

BENEFITS: LENGTHENS THE SPINE; STRENGTHEN THE ARMS, SHOULDERS, LEGS, HIPS, BUTTOCKS, AND POWERHOUSE

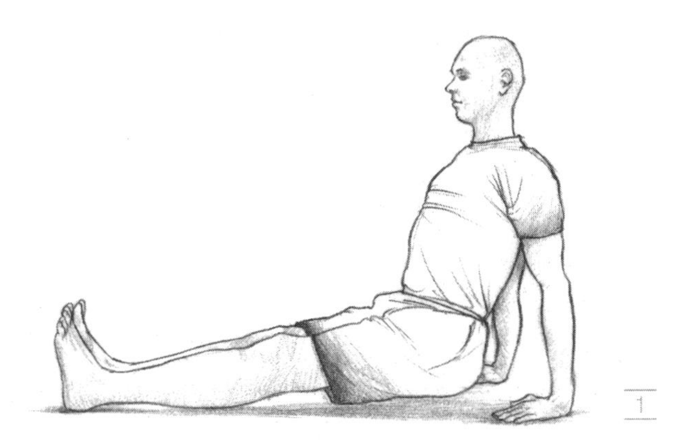

After the Arabesque, turn over and sit up tall on your bottom. Keep your legs straight and the palms of your hands flat on the floor slightly behind your hips. Keep your spine long. Pull your powerhouse in and up. Straighten your arms and lift your bottom off the floor as you exhale.

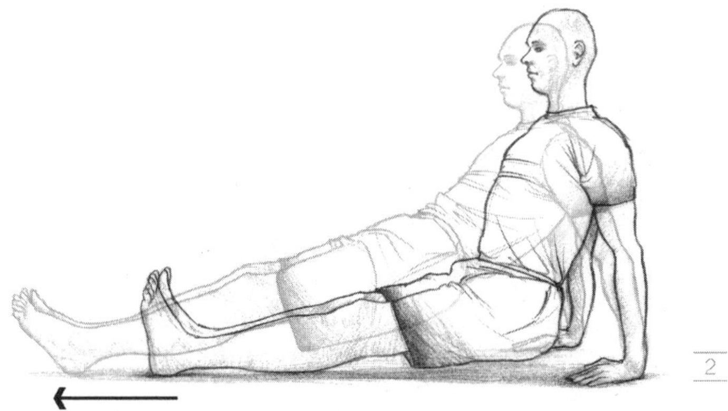

Inhale and slide your feet away from your hands as you lift your bottom higher into the air.

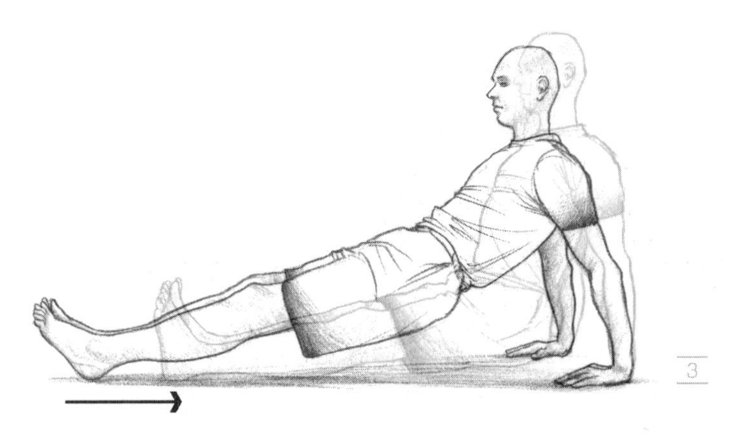

Keep your bottom lifted as you exhale and slide your body back into the starting position.

Perform 3 repetitions.

THE BEAST WITHIN

BODY POSITION You may also perform this exercise on your knuckles with clenched fists. Wear socks to help you slide. Keep your arms and legs straight. Don't allow your head to "turtle" down into your shoulders. Keep the crown of your head reaching for the ceiling and your eyes looking forward throughout the exercise.

THE MIND IN MOTION Keep your powerhouse engaged throughout the movement. Don't let your chest cave inward. Men typically have the requisite upper body strength for this exercise but lack the mobility and powerhouse strength to lift their hips very high.

CAUTIONS Leave this exercise out if you have neck, shoulder, wrist, elbow, back, hip, knee, ankle, or foot problems. This long list of body parts is a testimony to how fully you work your body during the Long Back Stretch and—for that matter—the entire reformer on the mat.

STOMACH MASSAGE ROUND

BENEFITS: STRENGTHENS THE POWERHOUSE AND LEGS; LENGTHENS THE SPINE; DEVELOPS BALANCE

After the Long Back Stretch, bend your knees to your chest with your feet lifted off the floor. Keep your heels together and your toes apart. Line your knees up with your toes. Touch the floor lightly with your fingertips and bring your chin to your chest. Round your back and keep your spine long.

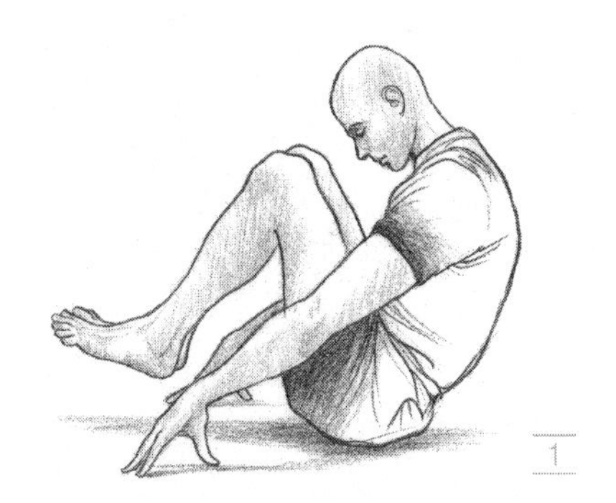
1

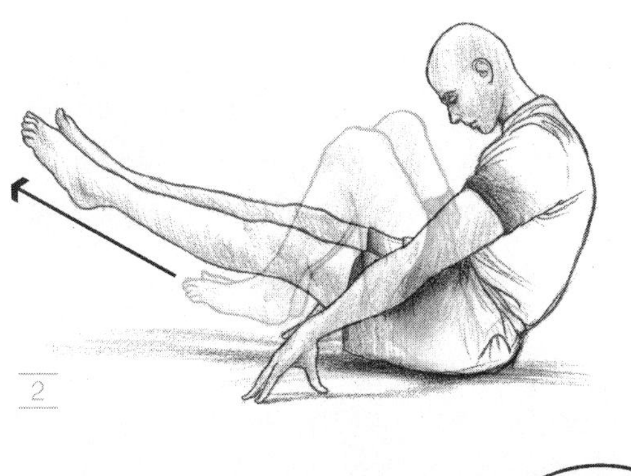
2

Inhale and extend your legs out while holding your powerhouse in.

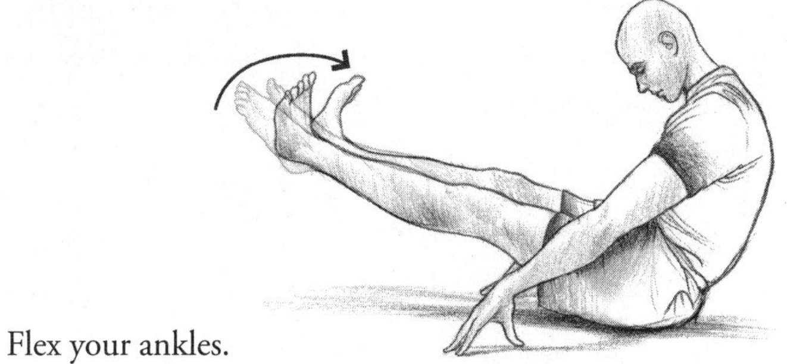
3

Flex your ankles.

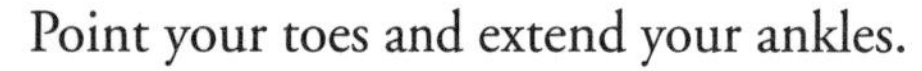

Point your toes and extend your ankles.

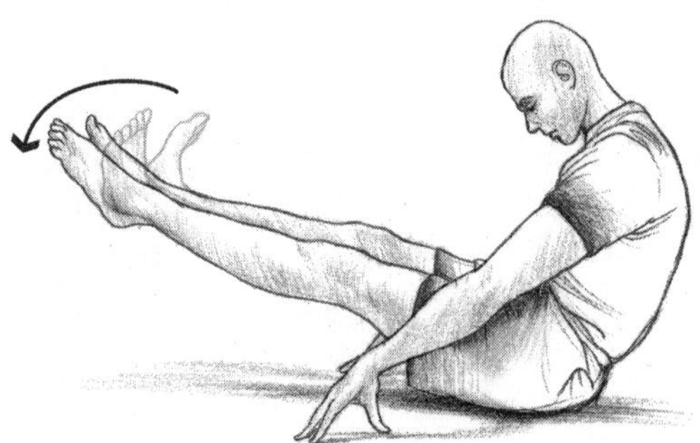

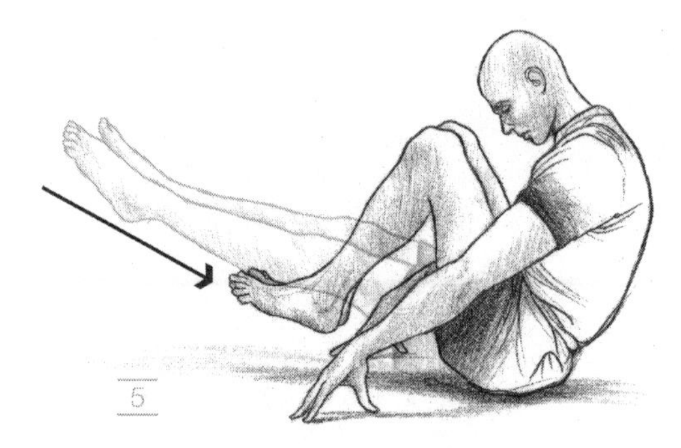

Pull your legs back to your chest as you exhale.

Perform 10 times.

THE BEAST WITHIN

BODY POSITION Hold a strong powerhouse. Keep your neck long. When you pull your legs in steps 1 and 5, bring your thighs in as close to your chest as possible. The starting position is quite similar to Rolling Like a Ball from the traditional mat work (see page 41).

THE MIND IN MOTION Don't lean back when you extend your legs. Don't sink into your lower back. Instead, picture the top of your head continuing the "C" shape of your spine, pointed in the same direction as your feet. You may extend your legs at a higher angle to make it easier on your back. When you extend your legs, squeeze your inner thighs and lengthen your hamstring muscles.

CAUTIONS This exercise can easily strain your hip flexors. If your hip flexors cramp, lie down and massage the area with your thumbs. If you begin to feel discomfort in your back, then lie down and hug your shins with your knees to your chest. Proceed slowly or exclude this exercise if you have back, knee, or hip problems.

STOMACH MASSAGE HANDS BACK

BENEFITS: OPENS THE CHEST; STRENGTHENS THE UPPER BACK, POWERHOUSE, AND LEGS; IMPROVES YOUR BALANCE

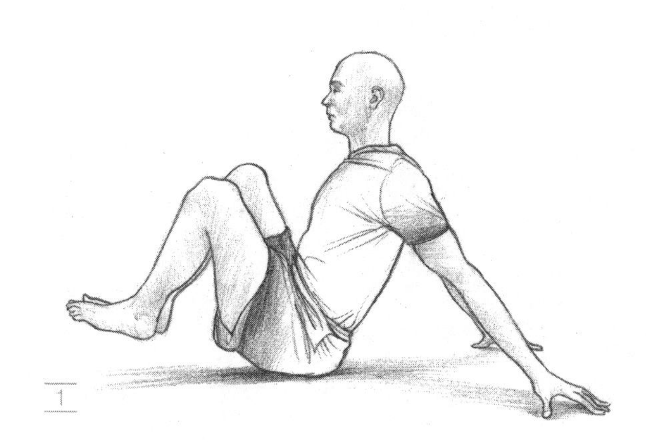

After the Stomach Massage Round, reach your arms behind you with your fingertips on the floor. Squeeze your shoulder blades together. Keep your neck long and your shoulders pulled down and back. Bring your thighs to your chest. Hold your heels together and your toes apart with your feet off the floor. Align your knees with your toes. Pull your powerhouse in and up.

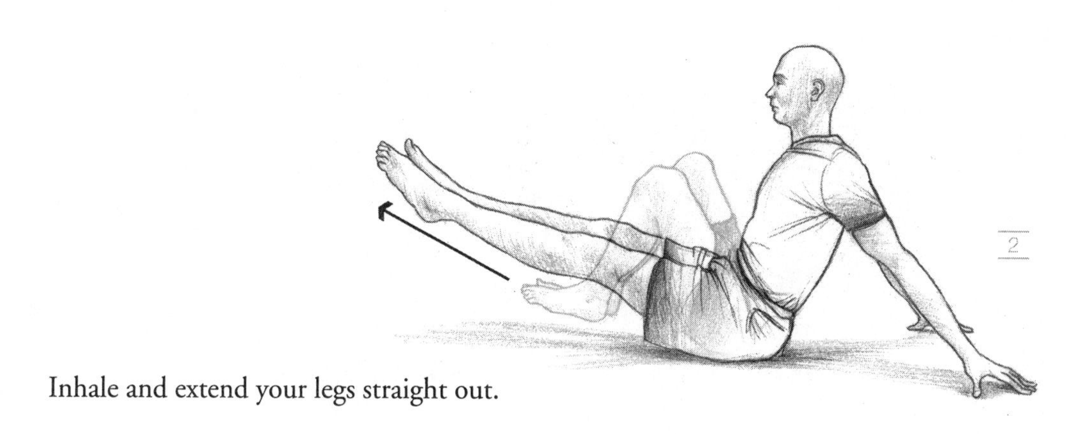

Inhale and extend your legs straight out.

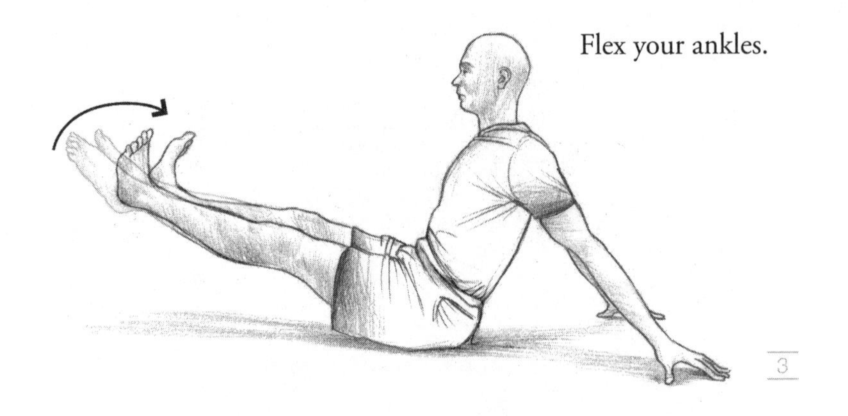

Flex your ankles.

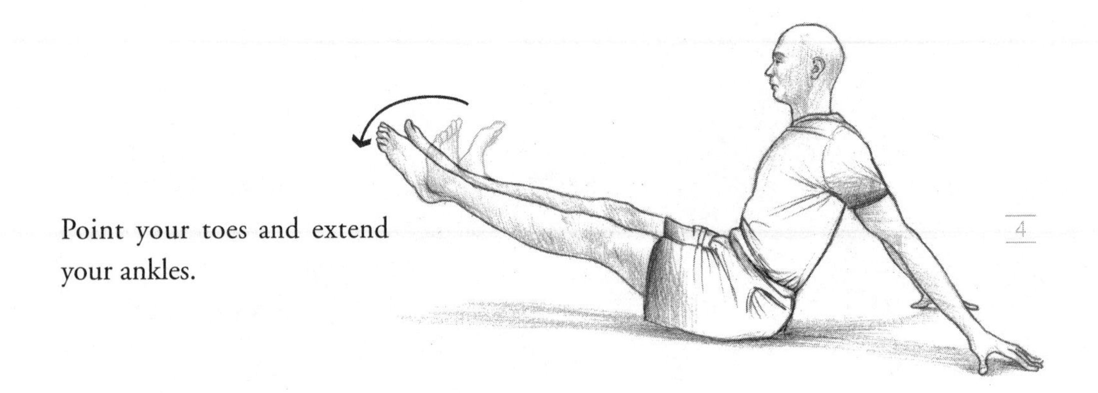

Point your toes and extend your ankles.

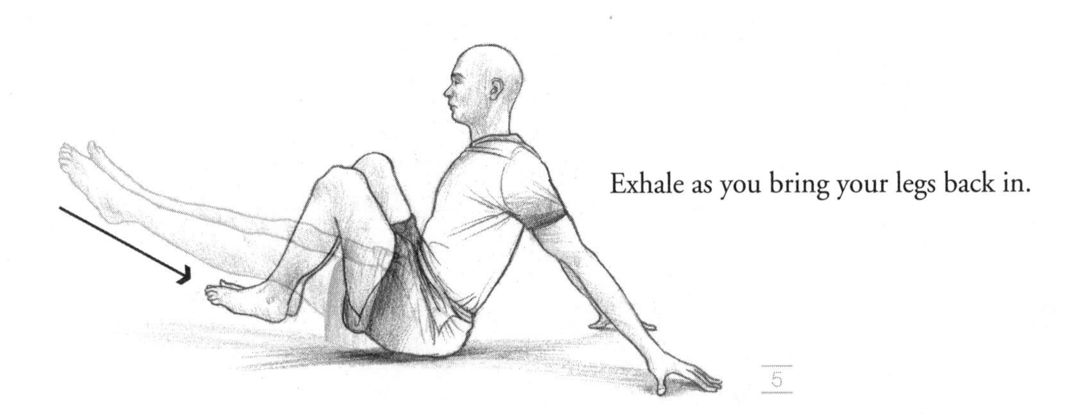

Exhale as you bring your legs back in.

THE BEAST WITHIN

BODY POSITION Sit up with a tall spine. Keep your upper body lifted and your neck long; don't collapse in your chest. You may start out by performing this exercise with your hands flat on the floor; as you become stronger, progress to placing just your fingertips on the floor.

THE MIND IN MOTION Don't let your upper body wobble, shift, lean, or move at all when you extend your legs. Extend your legs at an angle that you can control without any discomfort in your back. When you extend your legs, squeeze your inner thighs. Don't release your powerhouse during the exercise. Don't sink your neck and head into your shoulders. Bring your thighs as close to your chest as possible at the beginning and end of each repetition.

CAUTIONS If you have stiffness in your legs and back (a common problem for men), you will have difficulty keeping the integrity of the upper body position. This exercise can easily strain your hip flexors; be sure to stop if they begin to cramp. If you begin to feel discomfort in your back, then lie down and hug your shins with your knees to your chest. Proceed slowly or leave this exercise out if you have shoulder, wrist, back, knee, or hip problems.

STOMACH MASSAGE REACH UP

BENEFITS: DEVELOPS BALANCE; STRENGTHENS THE POWERHOUSE AND LEGS

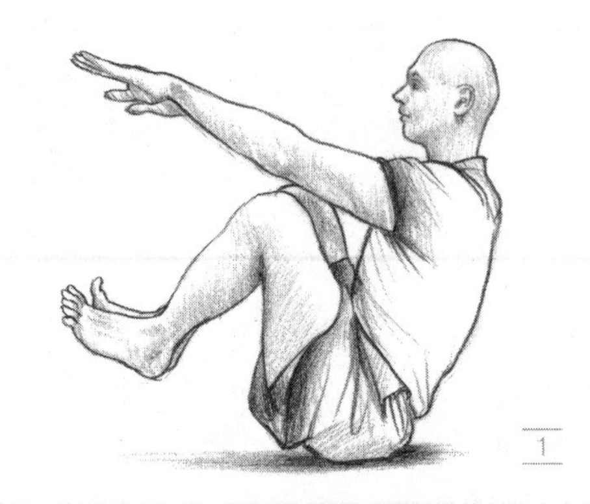

1

Following the Stomach Massage Hands Back, reach your arms forward and take the position of a bent leg Teaser.

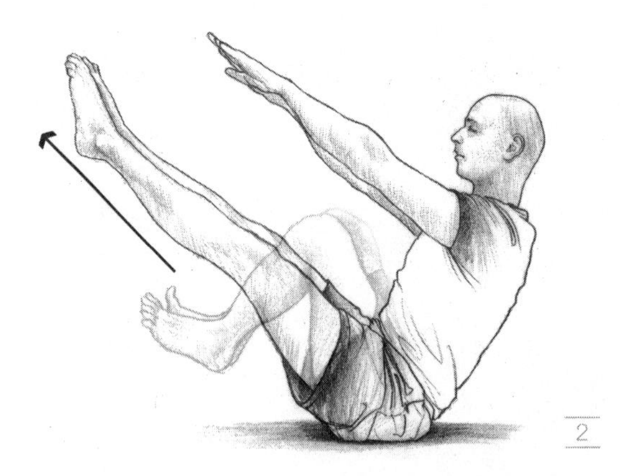

2

Using your powerhouse, extend your legs straight in the air as you inhale.

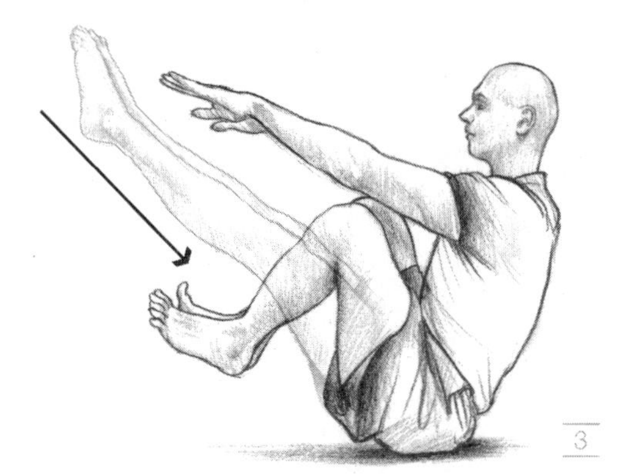

Keeping your heels high, draw your knees and your thighs to your chest as you exhale.

Perform 4 times.

THE BEAST WITHIN

BODY POSITION Keep your shoulders down and back as you reach forward. Don't arch your back. Keep your powerhouse pulled in and up throughout the exercise. Bring your thighs close to your chest in this starting position.

THE MIND IN MOTION Extend your legs at a height that causes no discomfort and that you can control. The illustrations in this section demonstrate a fairly high leg height, which you should be familiar with, after mastering the Teaser from the traditional mat workout (see page 89). To simulate the height of the reformer's foot bar more accurately, and to make the exercise more difficult, you may raise your legs to only about two-thirds of the illustrated height. Keep your toes pointed even when you bring your legs in. Do not lean back as you extend your legs.

CAUTIONS The challenge for men is to integrate leg and powerhouse strength by contracting their powerhouses throughout the movement. Don't simply default to your strong legs and release your powerhouse. This exercise can easily strain your hip flexors, be sure to stop if they begin to cramp. If you begin to feel discomfort in your back, lie down and hug your shins with your knees to your chest. Proceed slowly or leave this exercise out if you have shoulder, back, hip, knee, or leg problems.

STOMACH MASSAGE TWIST

BENEFITS: DEVELOPS BALANCE, COORDINATION, AND SPINAL ROTATION; STRENGTHENS THE WAISTLINE, POWERHOUSE, AND LEGS; WORKS THE LUNGS

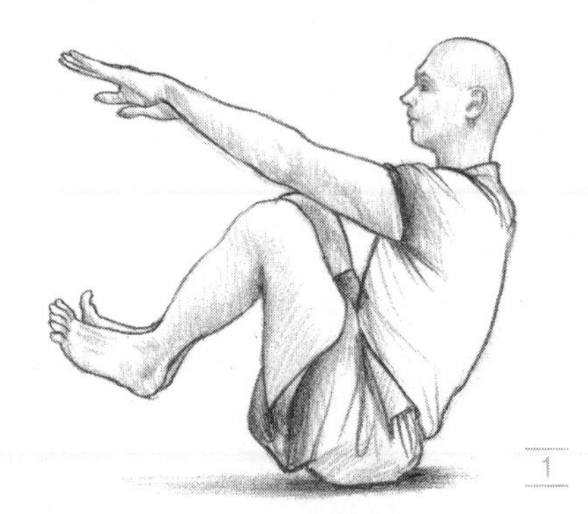

After the Stomach Massage Reach Up, remain in the same starting/finishing position. Inhale.

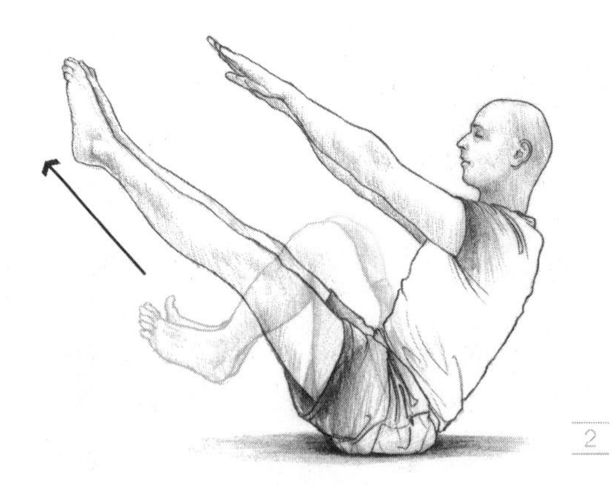

Extend your legs up.

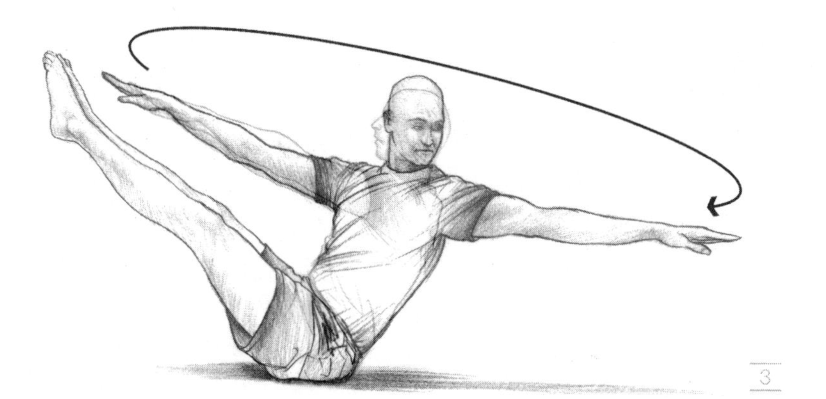

3

Twist from your waist and, keeping your right arm still, reach your left arm behind you as you exhale.

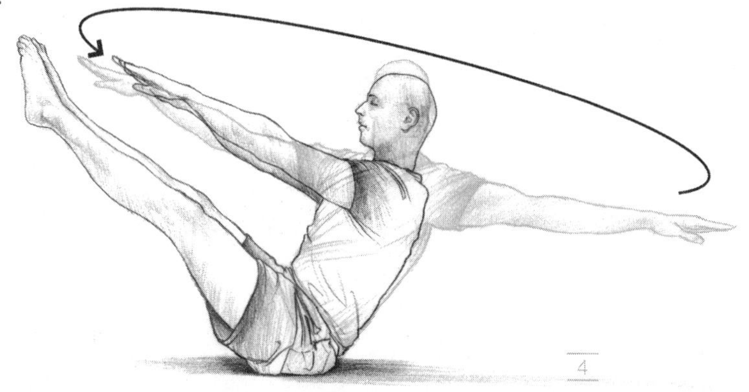

4

Untwist and reach your left arm forward as you inhale.

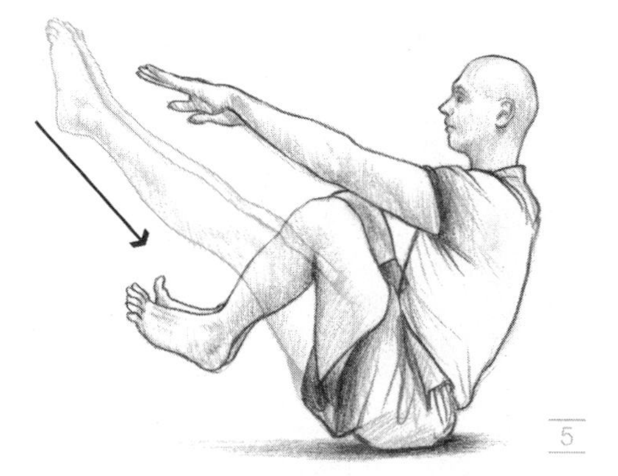

5

Bring your legs in. Repeat the whole sequence on the right side.

Perform twice, 2 times on each side.

THE BEAST WITHIN

BODY POSITION Keep your shoulders down and back as you reach forward. Don't arch your back. Keep your powerhouse pulled in and up throughout the exercise. When you pull your legs in, bring your thighs close to your chest.

THE MIND IN MOTION Twist from your waist up. Keep your heels together. Maintain a tall spine and anchor your sit bones to the floor. Don't arch your spine as you twist. Control this twisting movement; don't throw your body around. Keep your shoulders down and away from your ears. Keep your neck long and straight; don't tilt it to any one side. Keep your powerhouse engaged. For control purposes, steps 2 and 3 are shown as two separate moves. In typical practice you straighten your legs *as* you twist, in a single motion, but this often results in a sloppy execution. In the illustrated version, you must demonstrate more control by first extending your legs, holding them, and then twisting from your waist. This requires you to hold your legs out longer, which is difficult at first, but helps you develop greater strength and control. Once you can control the movement this way, you may try extending your legs at the same time that you twist.

CAUTIONS Due to tightness in the legs and back, men tend to have a small range of motion when they twist. Don't throw your body around to increase your range of motion; let your spinal rotation develop gradually with practice. This exercise can easily strain your hip flexors; be sure to cease the exercise if they begin to cramp. If you begin to feel discomfort in your back, lie down and hug your shins with your knees to your chest. Proceed cautiously or leave this exercise out if you have shoulder, back, hip, knee, or leg problems.

THE TENDON STRETCH

BENEFITS: STRENGTHENS THE ARMS, UPPER BODY, POWERHOUSE, HIPS, AND LEGS

After the Stomach Massage Twist, sit up tall with your legs straight. Place your palms on the floor alongside your hips. Pull your powerhouse in and up. Inhale and straighten your arms to lift your buttocks in the air.

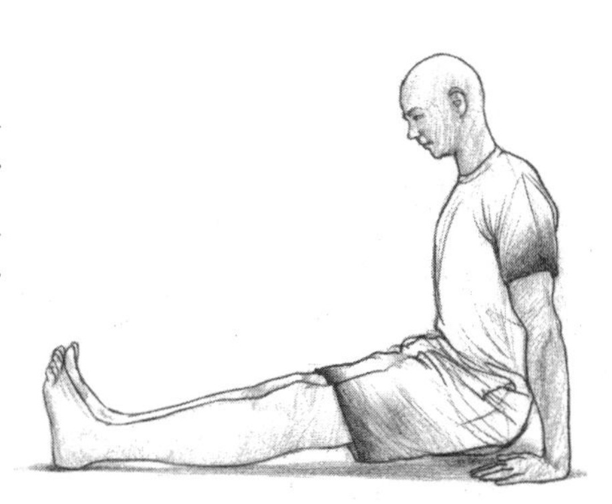

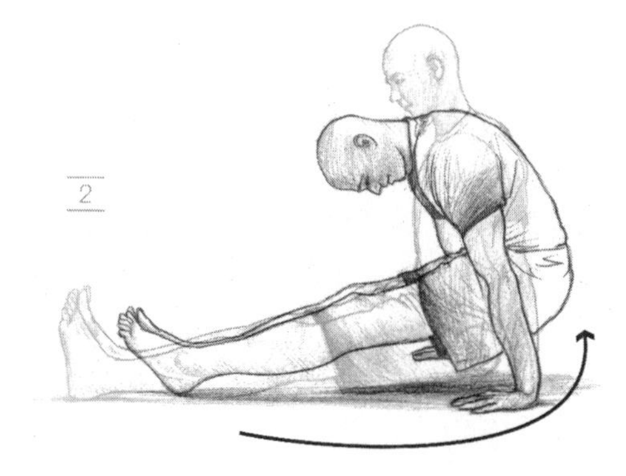

Exhale. Pull your powerhouse behind your arms and lift your buttocks higher off the floor. Let your feet slide back along the floor. Look down to your navel.

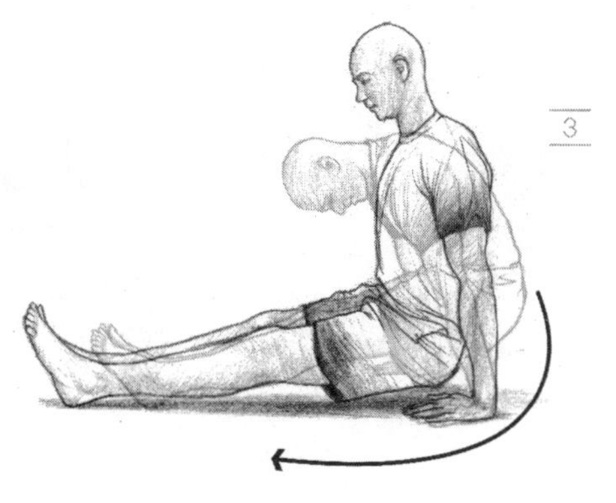

Inhale and return to the starting position. Look toward your toes.

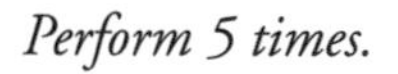

Perform 5 times.

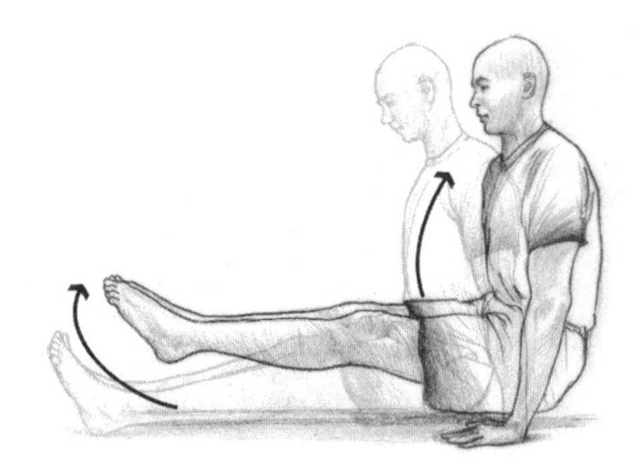

For an optional challenge, pull your powerhouse in and lift both your legs and buttocks into the air, hold this position for a few breaths. Perform this last step only once.

THE BEAST WITHIN

BODY POSITION Wear socks to help you slide. Lock your elbows and knees. You may perform this exercise on either fists or flat palms.

THE MIND IN MOTION Look at your navel when you lift your hips up and back off the floor. Use your powerhouse to control the movement; men have a tendency to muscle through the exercise with just their arms and shoulder strength. To move evenly and with control, you must pull in your powerhouse while engaging your arm and upper body strength. You may also perform this exercise with one leg out to the side, while your arms frame the single forward leg (not illustrated). When you lift your hips up and back, keep your side leg in the air. (On the reformer your feet would make contact with the reformer at your arch, with your heels dropping over the edge. This would stretch the Achilles' tendons as you perform the movement. This effect is difficult to reproduce on the mat, although the powerhouse and upper body work is easily duplicated.)

CAUTIONS Leave this exercise out if you have neck, shoulder, wrist, elbow, back, knee, or foot problems.

THE SHORT SPINE MASSAGE

BENEFITS: MASSAGES AND LENGTHENS THE SPINE; STRENGTHENS THE POWERHOUSE AND UPPER BODY

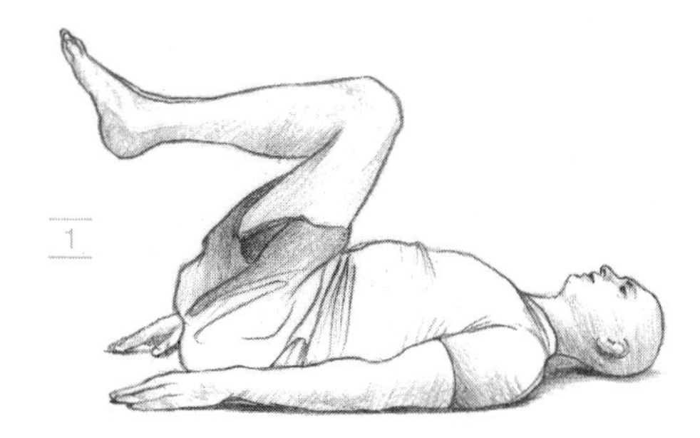

After the Tendon Stretch, lie on your back with your knees to your chest and your arms alongside your body. Keep your shoulders down and away from your ears and your spine anchored to the floor. Exhale and pull your powerhouse in.

Inhale and extend your legs out and up. Squeeze your buttocks. Keep your powerhouse in.

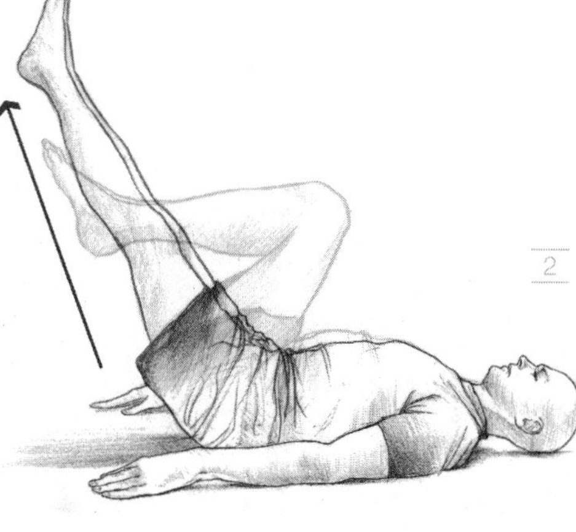

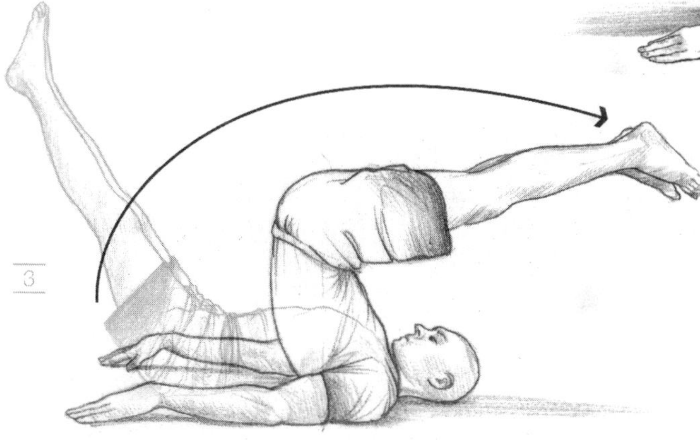

Press your arms into the floor as you begin exhaling, peel your hips and then your spine off the floor one vertebra at a time. Keep your powerhouse pulled in.

Continue exhaling as you lower your knees to your ears.

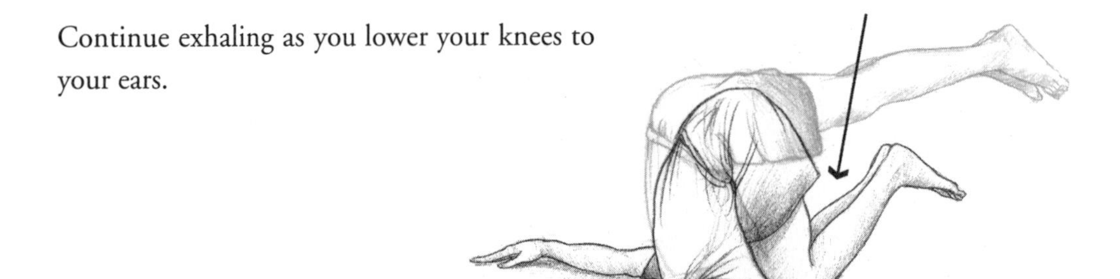

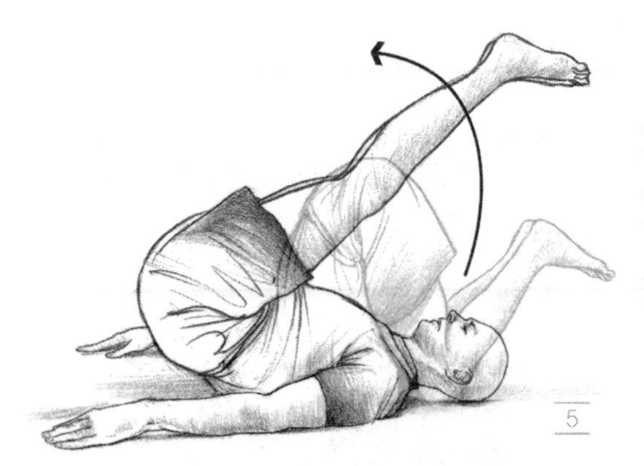

Inhale as you roll your spine back down one vertebra at a time. Keep your feet back, and allow your legs to straighten as you roll down.

When you can not roll down any farther with your feet behind you, bend your knees and lower your heels to your bottom; roll the remainder of your spine down to the floor as you exhale.

Perform 5 times.

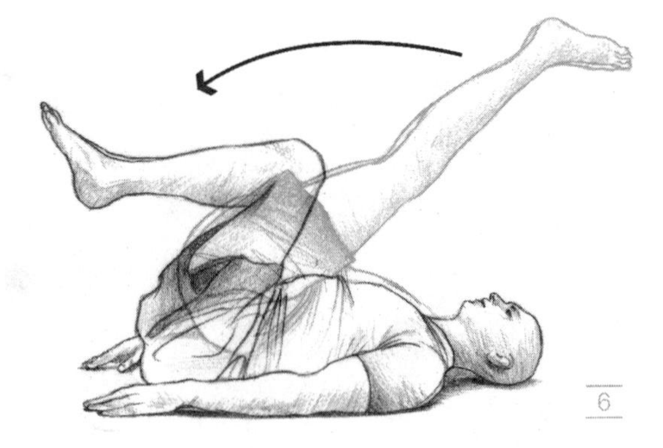

THE BEAST WITHIN

BODY POSITION Stabilize your body throughout the movement by pressing your arms into the mat. Keep your shoulders on the mat and away from your ears. To help keep your shoulders anchored and your chest open, it helps to imagine your collar bones reaching away from the center line of your body.

THE MIND IN MOTION Don't throw your legs up and over your head with momentum. Peel your hips and spine up one vertebra at a time by using your powerhouse. Keep your spine lifted, when you lower your knees to your ears during step 4; don't let your hips collapse. Although illustration 4 shows my knees reaching for the floor, most people shouldn't lower their knees that low. You risk putting too much pressure on your neck and losing control of your powerhouse by collapsing your spine and hips. As you roll down in step 5, don't allow your spine to fall to the mat; control the descent by using your powerhouse to lay your spine down on the mat one vertebra at a time. Keeping your feet back as you descend helps you to stretch the backs of your legs and maintain control. For a more difficult version, keep your heels glued to your backside and roll your spine down with control. (On the reformer, this is a more basic version.) Try both variations to determine which one challenges your strength more.

CAUTIONS Men with heavy hips and legs tend to rely on upper body strength combined with momentum to bring their legs overhead. This is dangerous for the neck. Proceed slowly or leave this exercise out if you have neck, shoulder, elbow, back, hip, or weight problems.

HEADSTAND I

BENEFITS: STRENGTHENS THE UPPER SPINE, POWERHOUSE, HIPS, AND SHOULDERS

Note about the Headstand: Many of Joseph Pilates's early clients were boxers and wrestlers. The headstands helped them to develop the necessary upper spine strength and flexibility required for these taxing sports. If your lifestyle or fitness goals don't require much upper spine or neck strength, then skip this exercise.

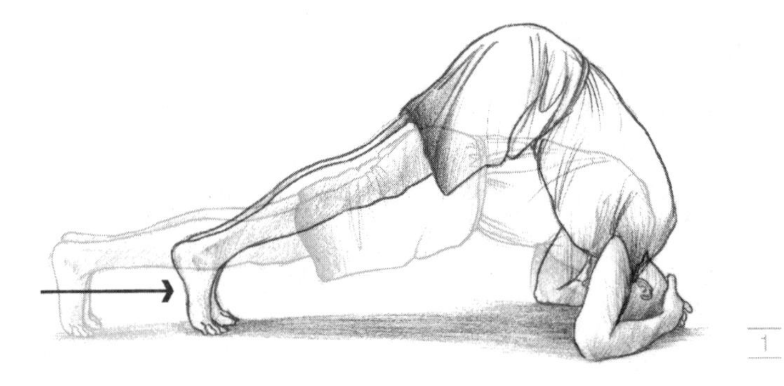

After the Short Spine Massage, turn over and place your forearms on the mat with your elbows one forearm's distance away from each other; keep your fingers interlaced. Your elbows and hands should form a triangle in which you will distribute your body weight. Secure your head in your hands (you may place a small towel or pillow beneath your head as a cushion). Straighten the rest of your body and lift your powerhouse in and up. Exhale and slide your feet in toward your head as you pull your hips up in the air.

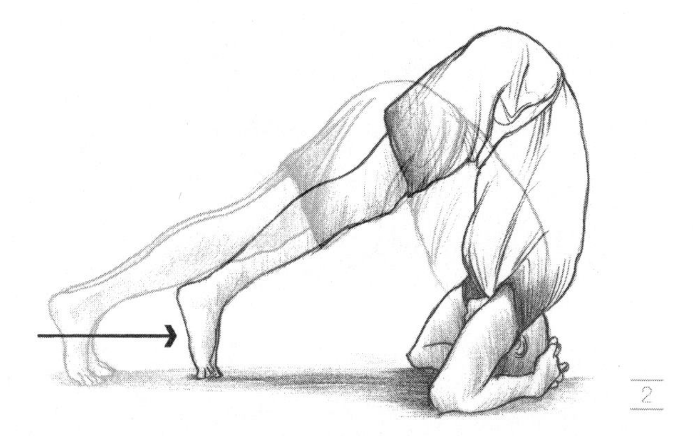

Continue exhaling as you slide your feet in as far as possible, with your hips reaching toward the ceiling.

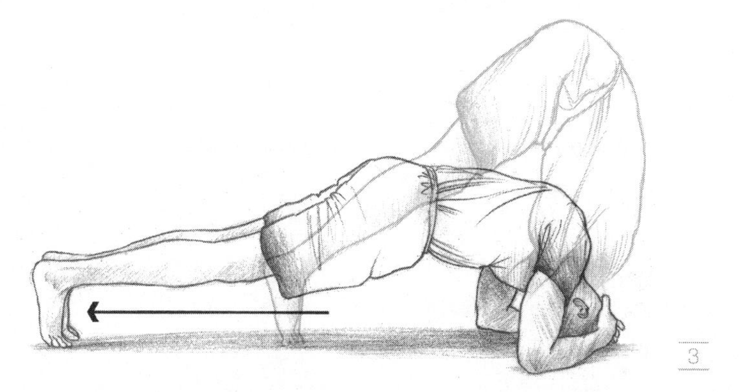

Inhale and slide your feet back out, away from your hands and head. Keep your powerhouse pulled in.

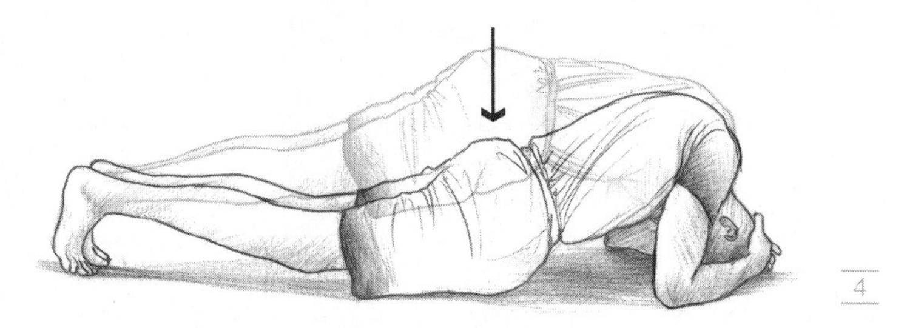

Lower your hips, but not all the way to the floor (clothing may sag toward floor).

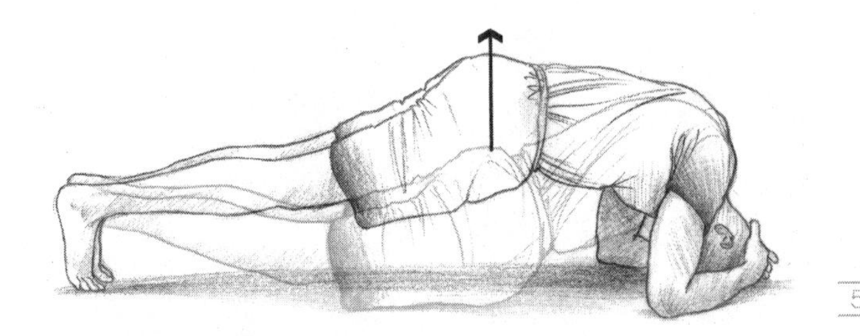

Lift your hips to the starting position.

Perform 3 times.

THE BEAST WITHIN

BODY POSITION Support your head against interlaced hands, with the top of your head on a cushioned floor. In the studio on the reformers, we typically use a pad and a small towel. Distribute your body weight onto your forearms. Do not arch your lower back.

THE MIND IN MOTION Wear socks if you perform the foot slides, as illustrated in steps 1 to 3. If you prefer not to slide, you may walk your feet one at a time toward and away from your hands instead (not illustrated). Keep your powerhouse active even as you lower your body. Your level of control will dictate how far you can move your feet back in step 3. *You should only lower and lift your hips in steps 4 and 5 if you can slide or walk your feet out as far as illustrated. If you can not slide or walk out that far, just perform steps 1 through 3.* Keep your neck long; don't arch your back!

CAUTIONS This is a precarious body position. Again, if your fitness goals and/or life-style don't require this level of neck strength and flexibility, leave the Headstand out. Proceed slowly or leave this out if you have, neck, shoulder, elbow, back, hip, knee, or foot problems.

HEADSTAND II

BENEFITS: STRENGTHENS YOUR LEGS, BACK, SHOULDERS, BUTTOCKS, NECK, AND ARMS; OPENS THE HIP FLEXORS

After Headstand I, turn over onto your back. Bend your knees and place your feet hip-width apart near your bottom. Bend your arms back by your head and place your palms flat under your shoulders. Exhale and pull your powerhouse in.

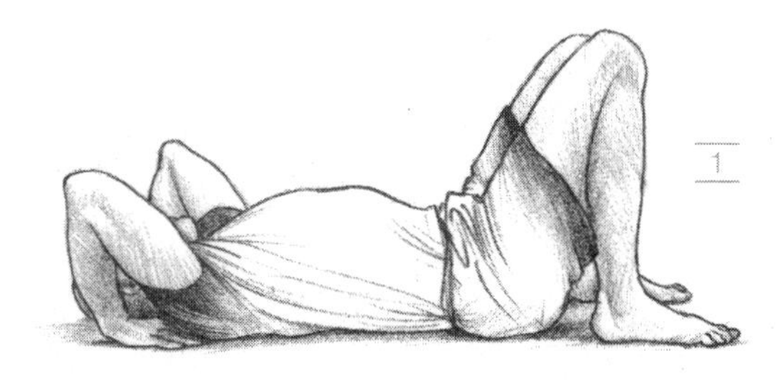

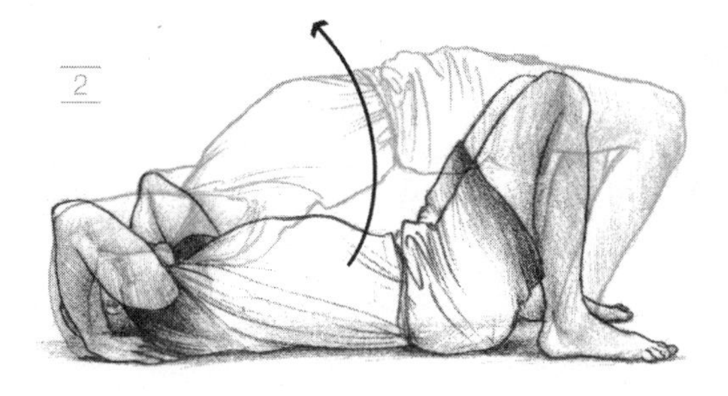

Inhale and squeeze your buttocks. Simultaneously press your hands and feet into the floor and lift your body up into a Backbend—only as high as necessary for you to place the top of your head on the floor.

Keep your neck long. Squeeze your buttocks and hold the position for a breath or two.

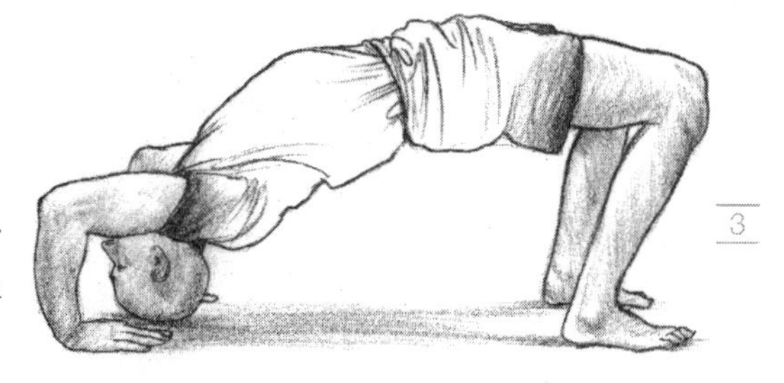

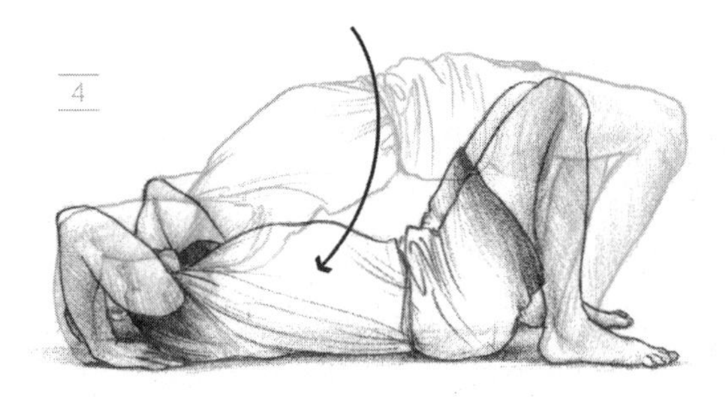

Bring your chin to your chest and lower your body to the starting position.

Perform this exercise only 1 time.

THE BEAST WITHIN

BODY POSITION Approach this exercise with caution. Use a pillow under your head, if necessary, and make certain your feet won't slip (i.e. create traction with bare feet, a sticky mat, a non-slip floor, etc.). Keep your neck long. Distribute your weight onto your hands as well, not just on your head. Squeeze your buttocks. Keep your elbows in.

THE MIND IN MOTION Take it easy when you place the top of your head on the floor or pillow. Simply hold the position (see illustration 3). There are other variations of this exercise, but they are superfluous for all but a small percentage of the population. (If you've ever wrestled or done grappling style martial arts, you've probably done neck bridges or something that resembles this exercise.)

CAUTIONS Get a spotter who has experience spotting backbends and bridges to watch you when you attempt this exercise. Do not roll onto your forehead or the back of your head; be sure that just the top of your head makes contact with the floor. Leave the Headstand II out if you have neck, shoulder, wrist, elbow, back, hip, knee, or foot problems.

SEMI-CIRCLE

BENEFITS: STRETCHES YOUR THIGHS, HIP FLEXORS, AND CHEST; STRENGTHENS THE BUTTOCKS, BACK, POWERHOUSE, AND LEGS

After the Headstand II, lie down on your back. Bend your knees and place your heels hip-width apart near your buttocks. Clasp your ankles with your hands. Pull your powerhouse in and up. Exhale.

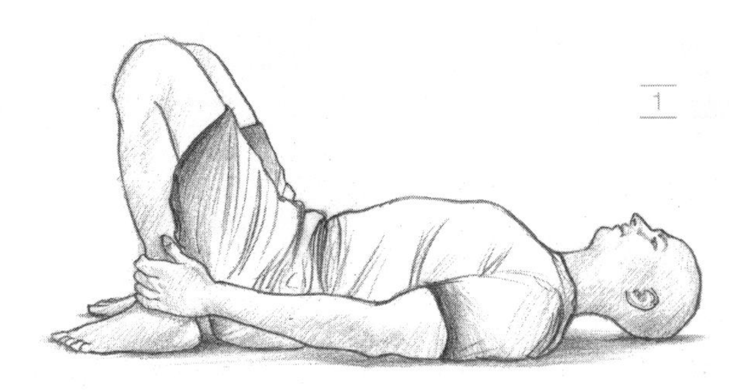
1

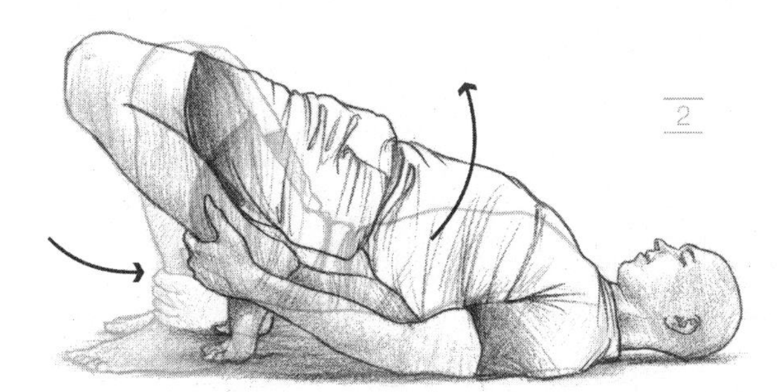
2

Begin inhaling as you roll forward onto the balls of your feet, with your heels lifted. Your buttocks will simultaneously lift up. Your knees will extend past your feet and your body will slide toward your heels.

Simultaneously slide your shoulders and upper body back, lift your buttocks as high as you can, and lower your heels to the floor. Your shins should be about vertical to the floor.

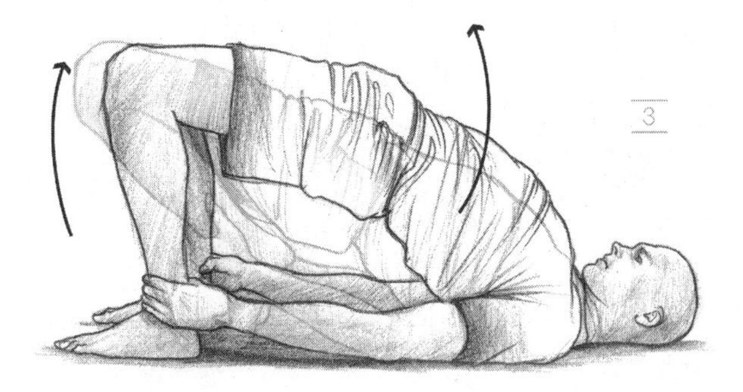
3

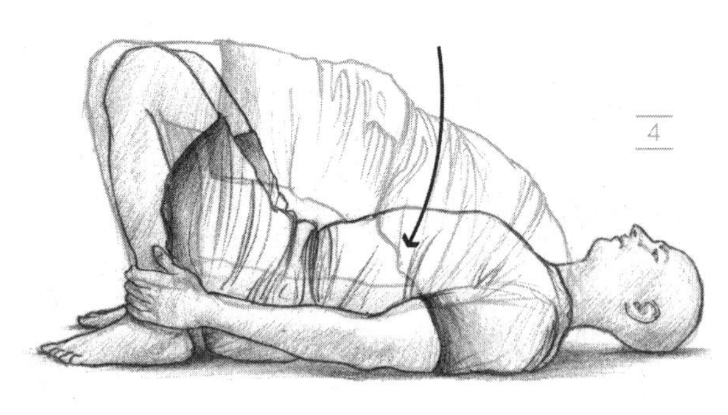

Exhale as you lower your body down to the floor.

Perform 3 times, then perform the exercise in reverse 3 more times. The reverse movement follows as such: Lift your bottom up high as in step 4, roll onto the balls of your feet as in step 3, lower your bottom and slide your body back as in step 2, and you will arrive in the starting position.

THE BEAST WITHIN

BODY POSITION Your heels need to be close to your bottom to make pivoting onto the balls of your feet easier on your knees. Your shoulders and upper back bear your weight when you slide backward. You should feel no tension in your neck.

THE MIND IN MOTION Don't push into the back of your head as you move. Keep your shoulders down. After you finish the exercise, you may work on heightening your bridge by simply holding the position in step 3. This will serve as a progressive step toward the High Bridge, which comes later in the reformer on the mat (see page 312). If you can grasp your ankles comfortably with your feet flat on the floor, you'll find that your chest and hips will be quite lifted. Concentrate on lifting your chest on the inhale and driving your hips toward the ceiling on the exhale. Hold this position for a breath or two and then lower your spine one vertebra at a time down onto the mat. While there are other variations and stretches that accompany this exercise, this is the safest version.

CAUTIONS This exercise can be tough on the knees because there is a lot of flexion (bend) in the knees throughout the exercise. Don't even consider this exercise if your knees are "tricky" or bad. Proceed slowly or leave this one out if you have any neck, shoulder, back, hip, *knee,* ankle, or foot problems. You must wear clothes that allow you to slide, otherwise your movement will be stop-and-go. Your feet, however, need good traction.

CHEST EXPANSION

BENEFITS: CORRECTS POSTURE; EXPANDS LUNG CAPACITY; RELEASES TENSION IN THE NECK; OPENS THE CHEST; STRENGTHENS THE UPPER BACK; LENGTHENS THE NECK (THIS IS A FANTASTIC EXERCISE!)

After the Semi-Circle, bring yourself upright onto your knees keeping them shoulder-width apart; place your feet together behind you and your arms straight out in front of you. Keep your shoulders down. Inhale and bring your straight arms down past your hips.

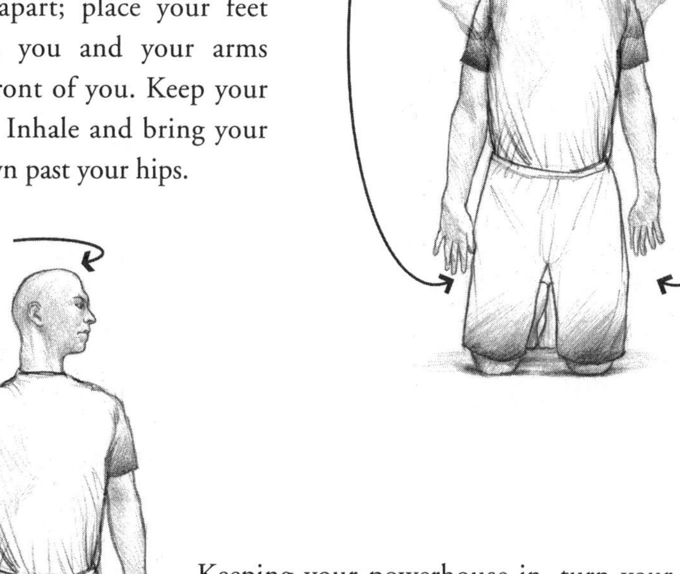

1

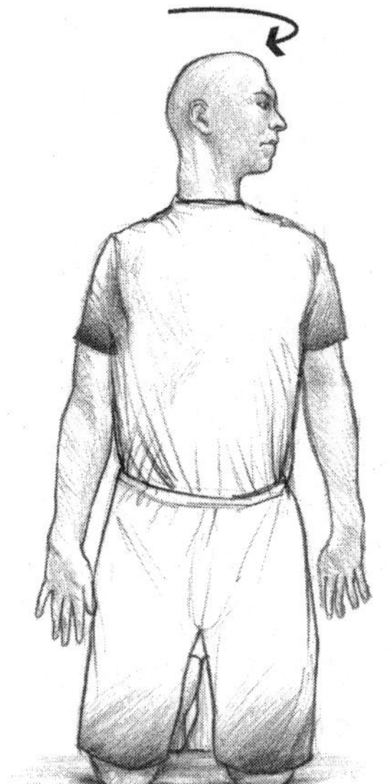

2

Keeping your powerhouse in, turn your head to your left. Hold your breath.

Maintaining a firm powerhouse, turn your head to your right. Hold your breath.

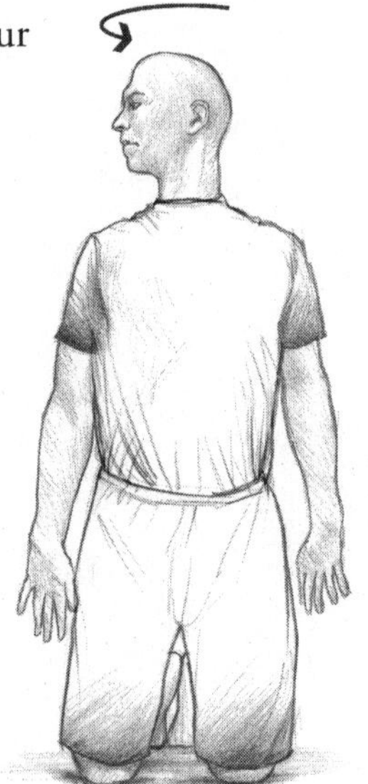

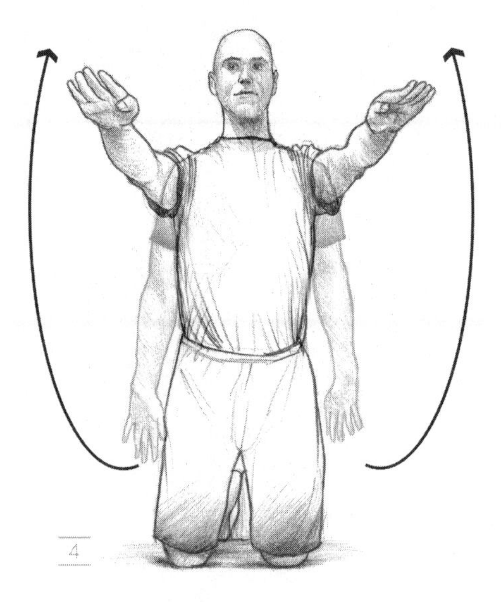

Look forward and exhale as you lift your arms to the starting position. Keep your shoulders down as you raise your arms up. Repeat the whole sequence, but this time look to your right first. This is considered 1 set.

Perform for a total of 2 sets.

THE BEAST WITHIN

BODY POSITION Keep your spine long and your buttocks engaged. Hold your powerhouse firmly. Don't sit back; maintain one vertical line from your knees to the crown of your head. Keep your shoulders down and away from your ears. You may be either on the tops of your feet or on the balls and toes of your feet. You may also place your feet apart, lined up with your separated knees. You may perform this exercise with your hands open or with fists.

THE MIND IN MOTION If you choose the first option, begin with loose fists and clench your fists when they are behind you. If you have bad knees, you may perform this exercise standing on your feet, in Pilates stance. There is a seldom used device, found in some Pilates studios, called a neck tensameter. Attached to either leg springs or a "guillotine," its function is to strengthen the neck. After having a client use the neck tensameter, Joseph Pilates would have him perform either a Chest Expansion or a Reverse Chest Expansion (not illustrated) to release tension in the neck. This is also the reason why the Chest Expansion follows soon after the Headstands.

CAUTIONS Leave this exercise out if you have neck, shoulder, knee, or foot problems.

THE THIGH STRETCH

BENEFITS: STRETCHES THE LEGS; STRENGTHENS THE LEGS AND BUTTOCKS; DEVELOPS CONTROL OF THE HIPS AND SPINE

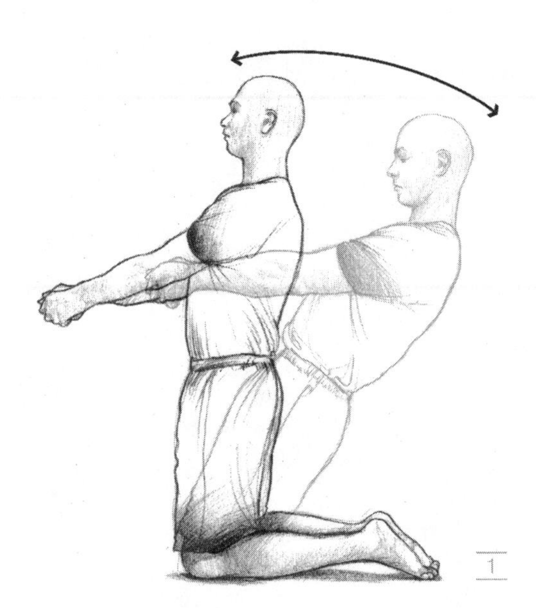

After the Chest Expansion, take the same starting position except bring your hands together and slightly lower than your shoulders. Pull your powerhouse in and up. Bring your chin to your chest. Squeeze your buttocks and inhale as you hinge backward from your knees, keeping your body rigid and strong. Squeeze your buttocks and return to the upright starting position as you exhale slowly.

Perform 3 times.

THE BEAST WITHIN

BODY POSITION Your feet may be together or apart in line with your knees. Your hands may be shoulder-width apart as well. Maintain a tall, straight line from your knees to the crown of your head throughout the movement.

THE MIND IN MOTION It's very important that you squeeze your buttocks firmly throughout the exercise. It will help you control the descent. It will also help prevent your hip flexors from contracting and consequently breaking the straight line of your body as you return to the starting position. Your forward-reaching hands will act as a minor counterweight to help you return to the upright position. Don't arch or hinge anywhere on your spine. Contract your powerhouse hard. The farther back you lean, the more intense the stretch in your thighs will feel. If you need assistance coming up, simply lift your straight arms a bit as if you were holding the horses' reins on a stagecoach. If you fall back too far and need to bail out, sit down on your heels first and, once you are stable, round your back with your forehead to your knees.

CAUTIONS Don't even consider this exercise if you have problematic knees. Leave this exercise out if you have neck, back, hip, knee, ankle, or foot problems.

THE BACKBEND

BENEFITS: STRENGTHENS THE LEGS BUTTOCKS, BACK, SHOULDERS, AND SPINE; OPENS THE HIP FLEXORS AND CHEST; DEVELOPS FLEXIBILITY IN THE SPINE

After the Thigh Stretch, remain in the same starting position, except hold your hands together against your chest as if you're praying. Pull your powerhouse in and squeeze your buttocks. Inhale and pivot backward from your knees as you reach your arms straight overhead and behind you.

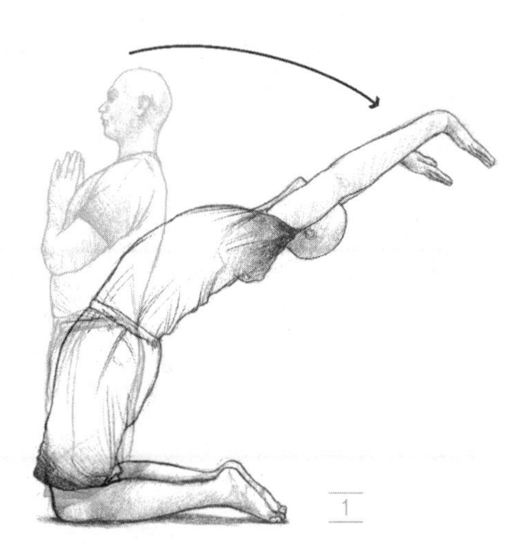
1

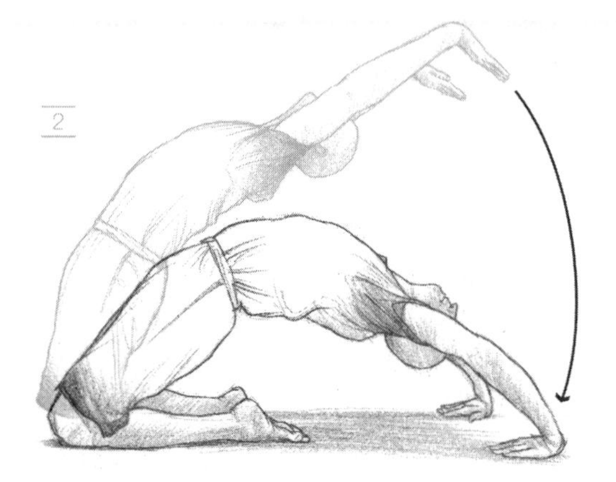
2

Find the floor with your hands, and keep your spine arched. Hold this position for a moment.

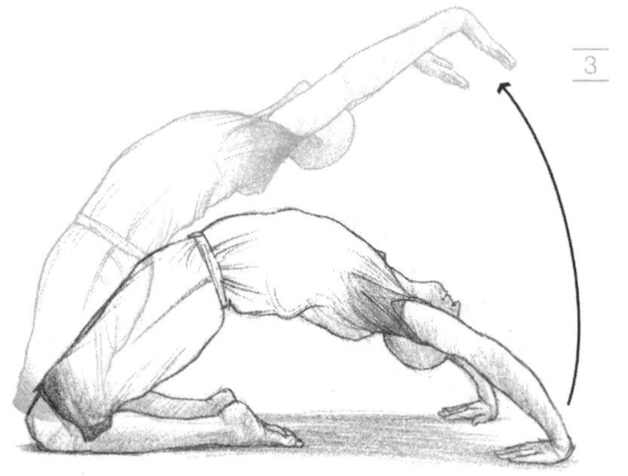
3

Squeeze your buttocks and bend your elbows slightly. Push off the floor with your hands and straighten your arms back up to reverse the Backbend. Begin exhaling slowly as you push off the floor.

Sit back on your heels with your head to your knees to release your back.

Perform only 1 time.

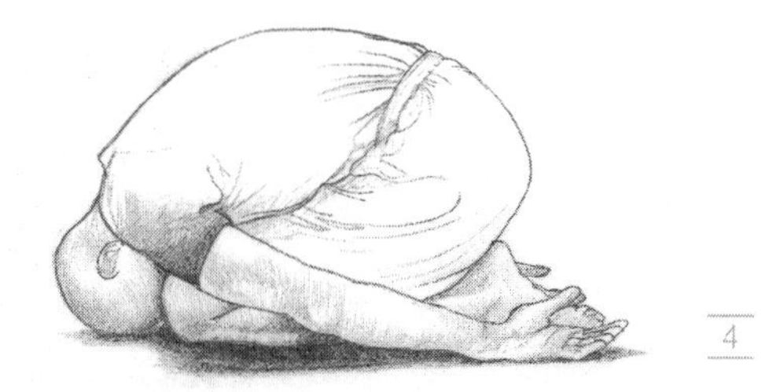

THE BEAST WITHIN

BODY POSITION Place your feet apart. Keep your spine long.

THE MIND IN MOTION Men typically find the Backbend difficult, as they tend to be stiff in the spine, hips, and shoulders. Squeeze your buttocks to protect your back and control the movement. Lift your powerhouse in and up. Imagine arching your back over a barrel so that the entire spine would be supported by the barrel. You may simply hold the Backbend position (see illustration 2), or you may bend and straighten your arms three times (not illustrated) before lifting yourself back up.

CAUTIONS You will need abundant leg, buttock, and powerhouse strength combined with a flexible spine and shoulder girdle to perform this exercise. If you are lacking in any of these areas, then leave the Backbend out. Have someone familiar with Backbends spot you. It isn't a fun day when your head hits the floor! Leave this out if you have neck, shoulder, wrist, elbow, back, hip, knee, or ankle problems.

THE SWAKATE SERIES
SWAKATE, UMPA, PROFILE, LOTUS

SWAKATE

BENEFITS: STRENGTHENS THE ARMS, SHOULDERS, BACK, BUTTOCKS, AND POWERHOUSE

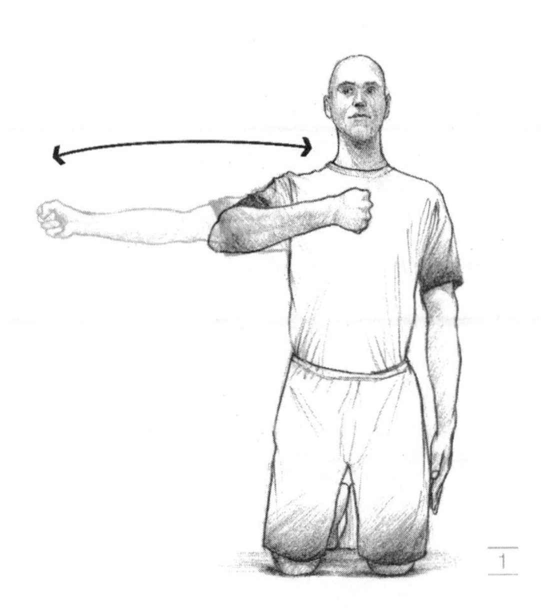

After the Backbend, come up into a kneeling position. Place your knees slightly apart, and hold your body upright in one straight line from your knees to the crown of your head. Keep your left arm down at your side. Lift your right arm to chest height and lightly touch your chest with a loose right fist. Keep your shoulders down. Inhale and straighten your right arm out to the side. Tighten your right fist, arms, powerhouse, back, and buttocks. Exhale and return to the starting position.

Repeat 3 times with your right arm, then 3 times with your left arm.

THE BEAST WITHIN

BODY POSITION Keep your buttocks engaged. Keep your powerhouse pulled in and up. Your shoulder should remain down. The front of your body should be flat, as if it were against a wall.

THE MIND IN MOTION Create tension in your arm and back when you extend your arm. On a reformer the springs would perform this function. The arm movement is very much the same as a back fist strike in martial arts. The nonworking hand is either firmly flat against the side of your body or closed forming a fist. The Swakate Series of exercise is considered a men's series. It is seldom taught to women, though it should be.

CAUTIONS Leave this out if you have knee, elbow, or foot problems. If this exercise bothers your shoulder, then leave it out as well.

NOTE Of all the questions I've asked my mentor, there are two that seem to have no clear answers. The first question is "What was the story behind Joseph Pilates's tattoos?" The second is "What does 'Swakate' [pronounced swa-ka-tee] mean?" I've heard some interesting explanations, but no clear definition. The names for all the exercises in the following Swakate Series are a bit odd: Swakate, Umpa, Hoopla, Profile, and Lotus. (We will not be doing Hoopla, which is a combination of Swakate and Umpa, and an arm-circling variation of the Profile. Both lose their effect without spring resistance.)

THE SWAKATE SERIES
SWAKATE, UMPA, PROFILE, LOTUS

UMPA

BENEFITS: STRENGTHENS THE ARMS, SHOULDERS, BACK, BUTTOCKS, AND POWERHOUSE

After the Swakate, remain on your knees in the same position. Keep your right arm bent at your side. Pull your powerhouse in and up. Inhale and lift your right arm toward the ceiling, keeping your right shoulder down. Exhale and pull your arm back down to the starting position.

Perform 3 times with your right arm, then perform 3 times with your left arm.

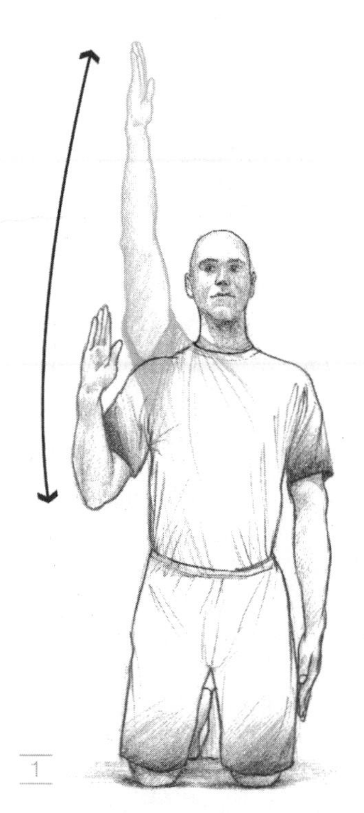

THE BEAST WITHIN

BODY POSITION Squeeze your buttocks. Keep your powerhouse engaged and your spine tall. Keep the front of your body flat and firm, as if it were pressed against a wall. Keep your nonmoving hand either flat against your side or in a clenched fist.

THE MIND IN MOTION When you extend your arm toward the ceiling, keep your corresponding shoulder down. When your arm is fully raised, tense your arm, stomach, and buttocks. Hold this position for a second or two. When you lower your arm down, engage your back muscles and concentrate on pulling your elbow down with tension.

CAUTIONS Leave this exercise out if you have shoulder, elbow, knee, or foot problems.

THE SWAKATE SERIES
SWAKATE, UMPA, PROFILE, LOTUS

PROFILE

BENEFITS: STRENGTHENS THE ARMS, BACK, SHOULDERS, POWERHOUSE, AND BUTTOCKS; LENGTHENS THE WAIST

After the Umpa, lower your left fist to the floor with a straight arm. Reach your right elbow toward the ceiling with your right fist loosely clenched above your head. Keep your knees and hips squarely facing forward. Look at the floor toward your left fist. Bend only at your side; don't bend forward. Pull your powerhouse in and squeeze your buttocks. Inhale and reach your right fist toward the ceiling. When your right arm is straight, tighten your right fist. Exhale and bend your right elbow to return to the starting position.

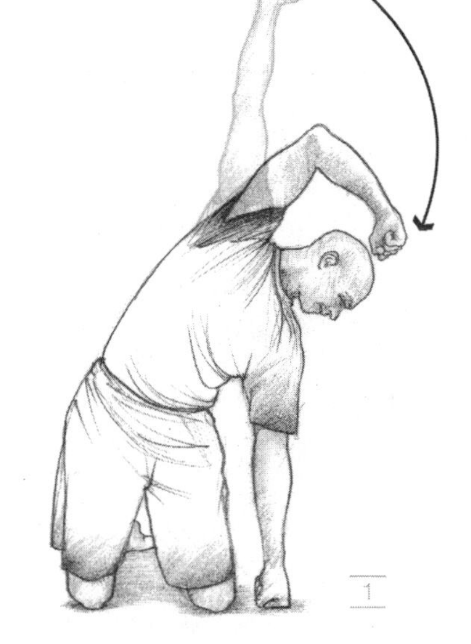

Perform 3 times to your left side, then 3 times to your right side.

THE BEAST WITHIN

BODY POSITION Squeeze your buttocks. Lift your powerhouse in and up. Keep the front of your body firm and flat. Lock your stationary arm on the floor and keep your supporting shoulder down.

THE MIND IN MOTION When your active arm is extended, contract the muscles of your powerhouse, arm, and back. As you raise your arm toward the ceiling, pull that shoulder down and contract your back muscles down as well.

CAUTIONS Placing your fist on the floor will strengthen your wrist, especially if its weak. Make certain that any weight or pressure that you transfer to your fist—which should be minimal, since the bulk of your mass and powerhouse is stabilizing you—is directed into the knuckles of your pointer and middle fingers. Leave this exercise out if you have neck, shoulder, elbow, back, or knee problems.

THE SWAKATE SERIES
SWAKATE, UMPA, PROFILE, LOTUS

LOTUS

BENEFITS: STRENGTHENS THE ARMS, BACK, SHOULDERS, POWERHOUSE, AND BUTTOCKS

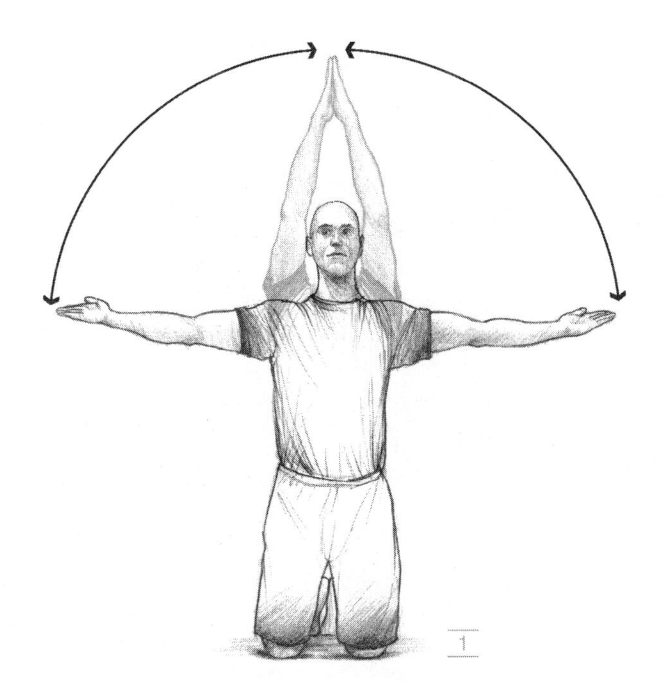

After the Profile, face forward and come up into a kneeling position as you did for the Swakate and Umpa. Place your knees slightly apart, and hold your body upright in one straight line from your knees to the crown of your head. Straighten your arms out to the sides. Keep your shoulders down. Inhale and lift your arms up overhead. Tighten your arms, powerhouse, back, and buttocks. Exhale and return to the starting position.

Perform 3 repetitions

THE BEAST WITHIN

BODY POSITION Squeeze your buttocks and tighten your powerhouse. Keep your neck and spine long. Don't break the straight line of your body at the hips. Don't lean back.

THE MIND IN MOTION Keep your shoulders down as you lift your arms up. If you choose to keep your palms open, push them together momentarily when they are overhead to create tension. If you use fists, clench them momentarily when they are overhead. If you need to bend your elbows slightly to help keep your shoulders down, then maintain the same slight bend throughout the movement.

CAUTIONS Leave this exercise out if you have shoulder or knee problems.

SNAKE/TWIST

BENEFITS: DEVELOPS FLEXIBILITY IN THE SPINE AND HIPS; IMPROVES BALANCE AND COORDINATION; STRENGTHENS THE POWERHOUSE AND UPPER BODY

Sit onto your left buttock and hip with your knees slightly bent. Place your hands flat on the floor to your left, with your right hand slightly closer to your body than your left. Rest your right heel on the arch of your left foot.

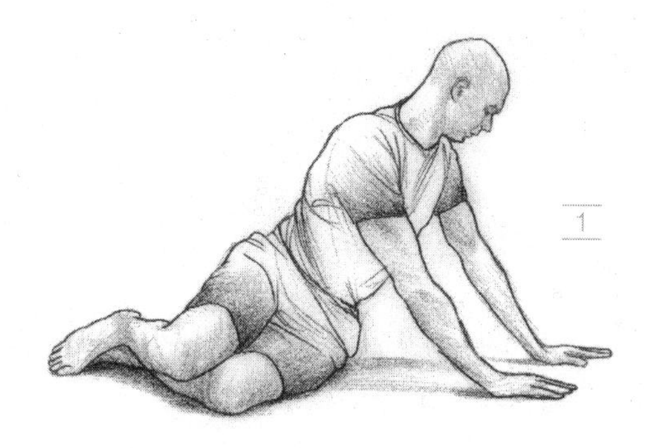

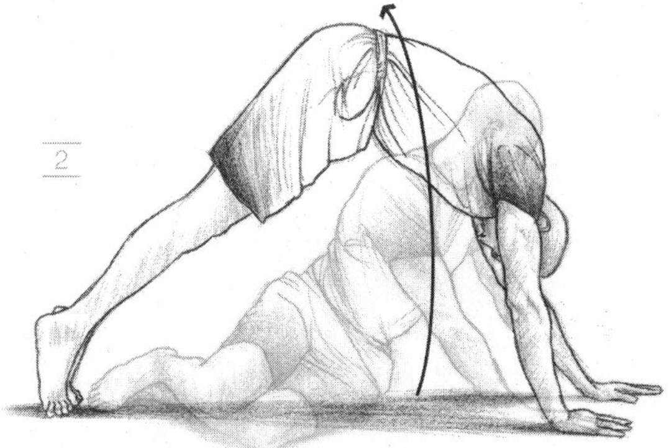

Exhale as you lift your hips and powerhouse into the air while straightening your legs. Look at your navel.

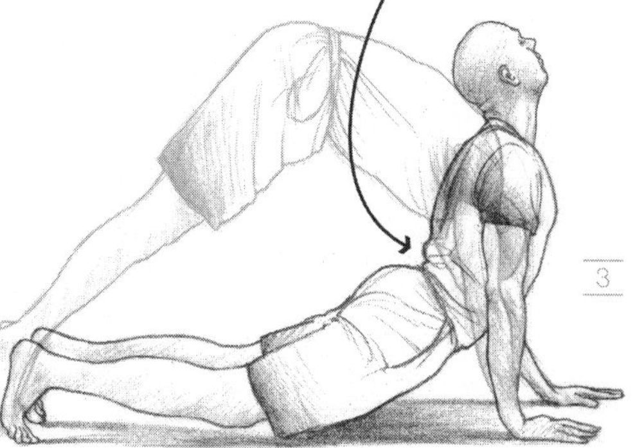

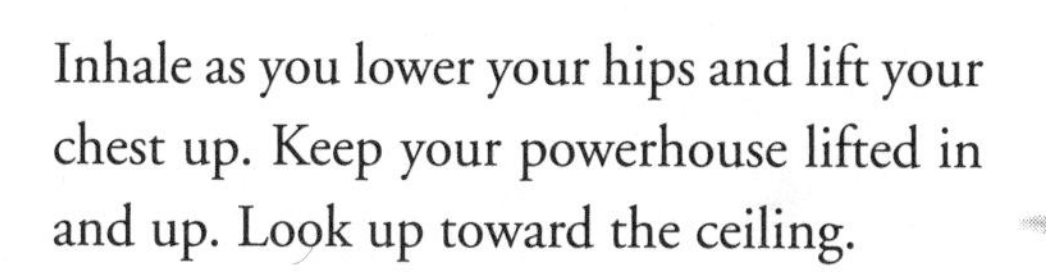

Inhale as you lower your hips and lift your chest up. Keep your powerhouse lifted in and up. Look up toward the ceiling.

Exhale and look back to your navel as you lift your hips and powerhouse into the air.

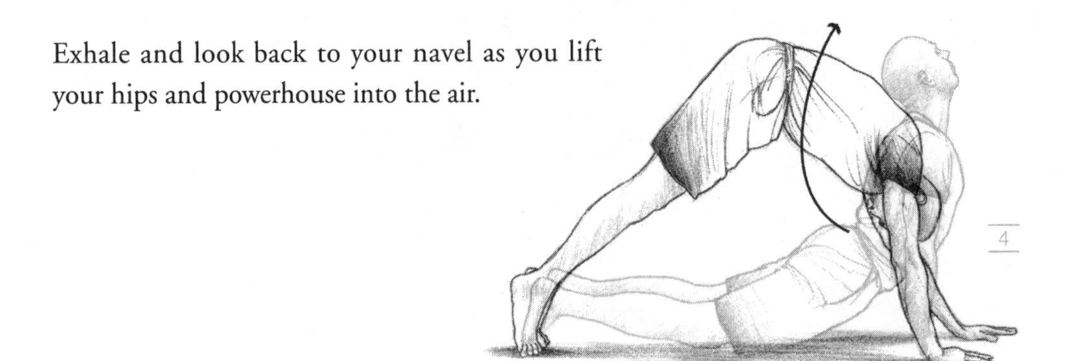

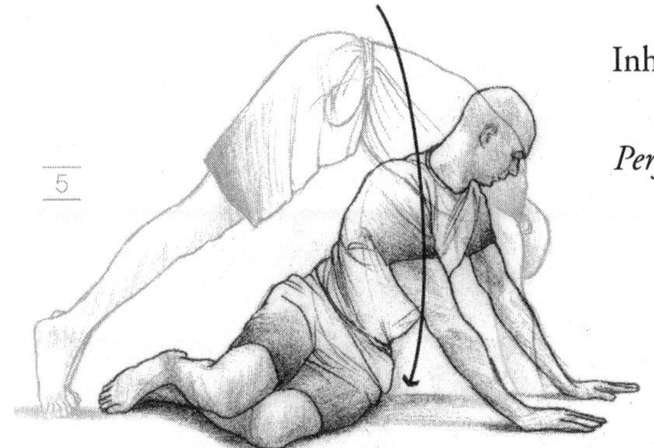

Inhale and lower your left hip to the mat.

Perform steps 2 through 5 twice.

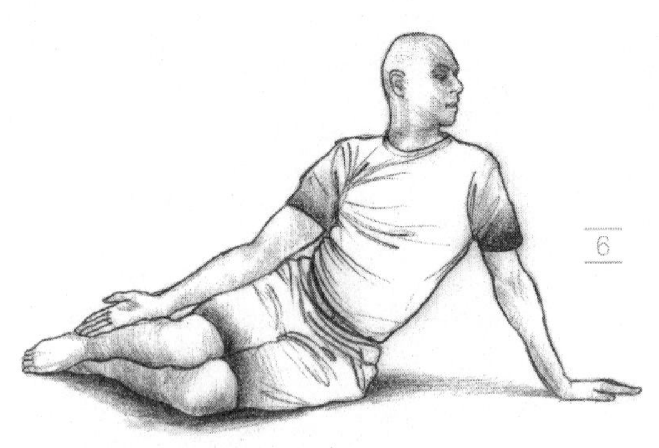

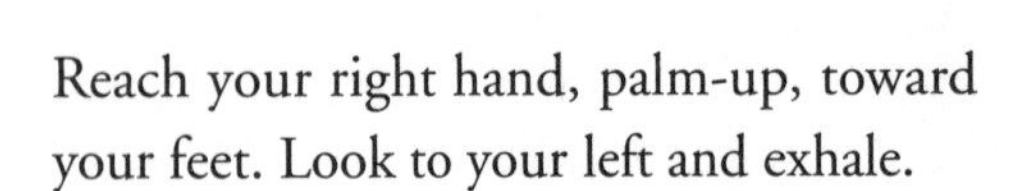
Reach your right hand, palm-up, toward your feet. Look to your left and exhale.

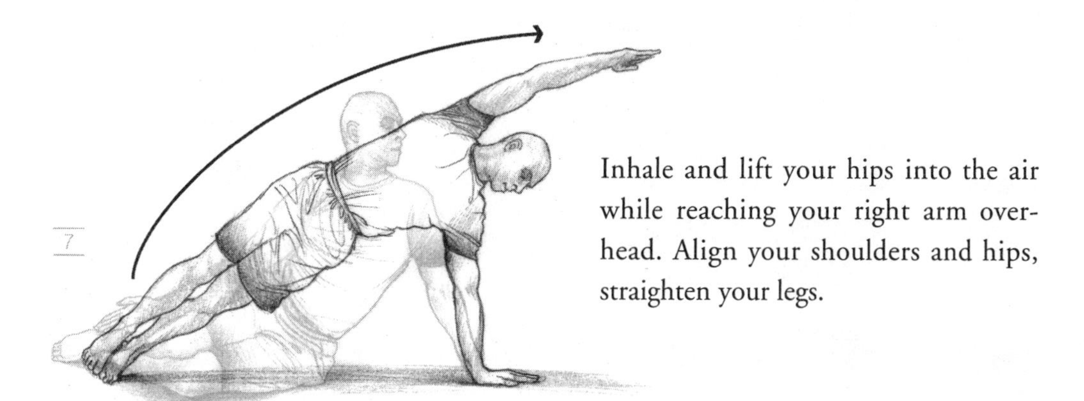

Inhale and lift your hips into the air while reaching your right arm overhead. Align your shoulders and hips, straighten your legs.

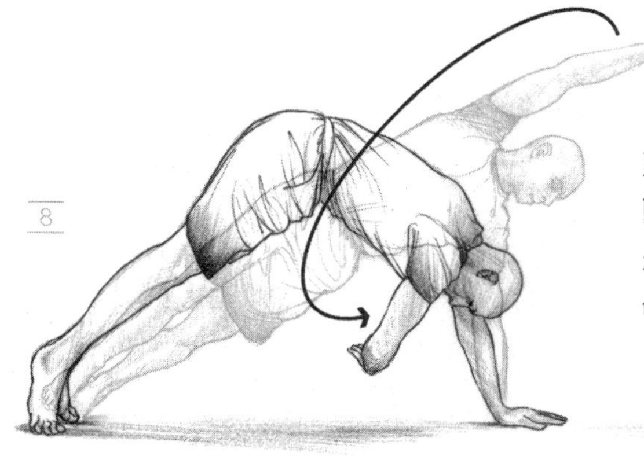

Exhale and rotate your body, anchoring both sets of toes on the floor. Feed your right arm under your torso to twist your torso slightly.

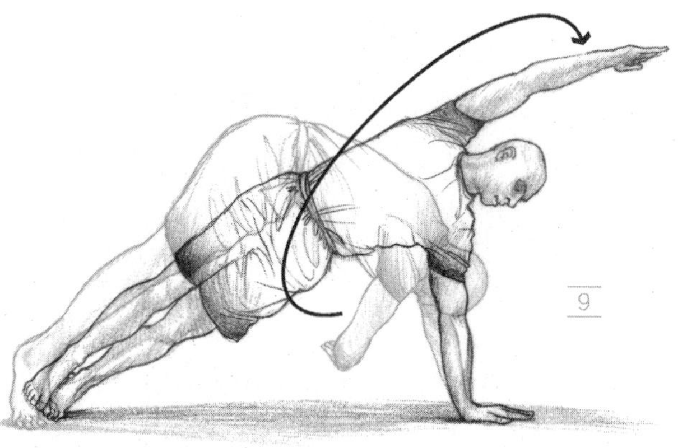

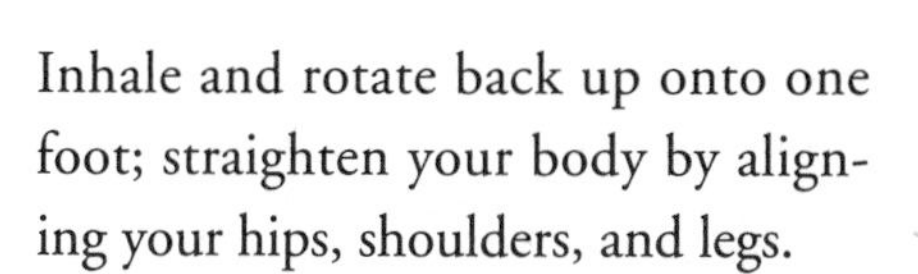

Inhale and rotate back up onto one foot; straighten your body by aligning your hips, shoulders, and legs.

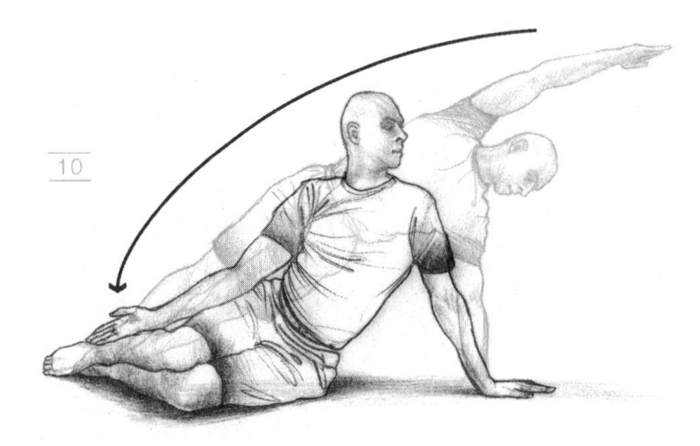

Exhale and lower your left hip to the floor, with your right hand reaching palm-up toward your feet in the starting position.

Repeat steps 7 through 10 once. Then repeat the entire sequence, steps 1 through 10, on your right side.

THE BEAST WITHIN

BODY POSITION Focus on maintaining a long spine throughout this exercise.

THE MIND IN MOTION Your position when you bring your hips into the air (see illustration 2), should resemble that of the Elephant—except that you're on your toes and balls of your feet, with your heels lifted. Your hips and sit bones should *not* be reaching away from your hands with your back flat. When you lift your hips up from the starting position, your back will be rounded. When you arch up (see illustration 3), lift your sternum to the ceiling. Keep your arms and legs straight. Keep your shoulders down and back when you are arched; don't allow your head to sink into your shoulders. Keep your neck long. Pull your powerhouse firmly in and up when you raise your hips and bottom into the air. The Twist (steps 6 to 10) is typically added to the Snake (steps 1 to 5) to demand more strength, balance, and coordination. You may either square your hips above the floor when you rotate onto both feet (see illustration 8)—or for a more challenging Twist, leave your hips in the initial lifted position on only one foot (see illustration 7) as you twist your arm under your torso.

CAUTIONS Men tend to be less flexible in the spine than women. Don't sink into any one spot in your spine. Lengthen your entire body. Proceed slowly or leave the Snake/Twist out if you have neck, shoulder, wrist, elbow, back, hip, knee, or foot problems. If you are overweight, be extra careful not to release your powerhouse or let your girth pull on your lower back.

HEADSTAND PULLING STRAPS

BENEFITS: STRENGTHENS THE NECK, SHOULDERS, LEGS, BUTTOCKS, BACK, AND HIPS

Note: This exercise is almost exclusively reserved for men in Pilates. But even for men it is rarely recommended because it requires significant strength and control to be performed safely and properly. If you are not sure whether you're strong enough or flexible enough, or whether this exercise is necessary for your lifestyle or fitness goals, skip it. If you do attempt the Headstand Pulling Straps, ask someone who's familiar with Neck Bridges to spot you.

After the Snake/Twist, turn over onto your back. Place your feet flat on the floor near your buttocks, hip-width apart. Reach your arms overhead and place your palms flat under your shoulders. Exhale and pull your powerhouse in. Inhale and lift your body up until you are resting on just your hands, feet, and the top of your head.

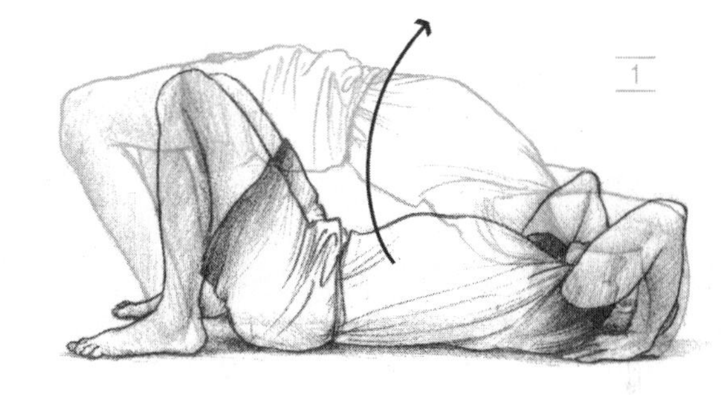

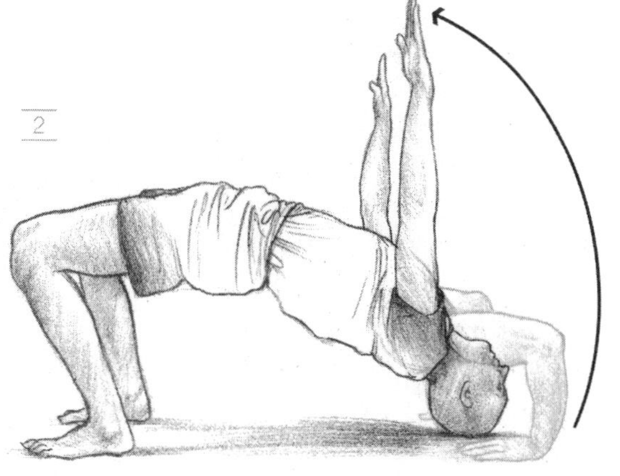

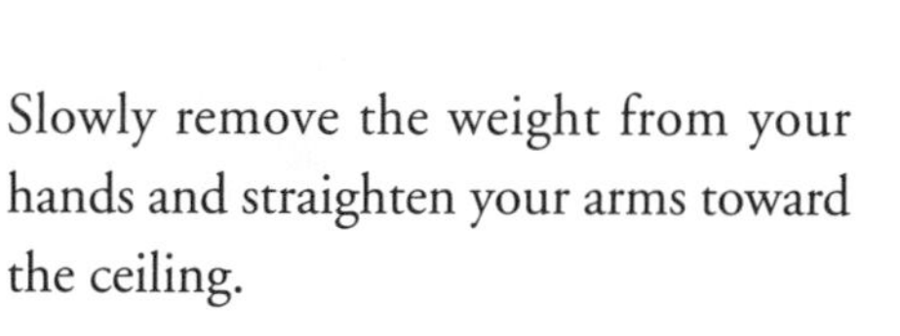

Slowly remove the weight from your hands and straighten your arms toward the ceiling.

Exhale and lower your straight arms. Keep your buttocks and powerhouse engaged.

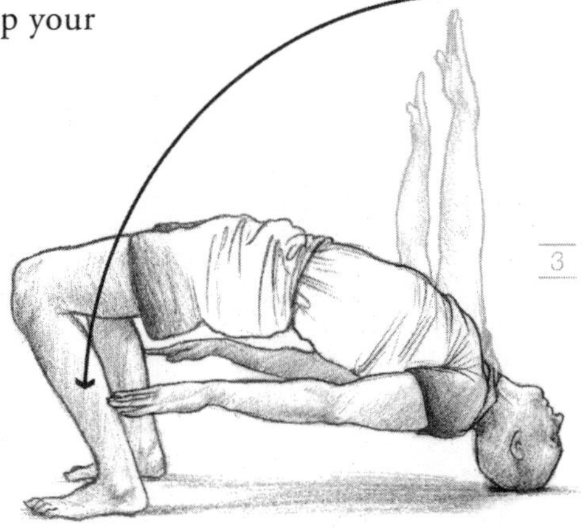

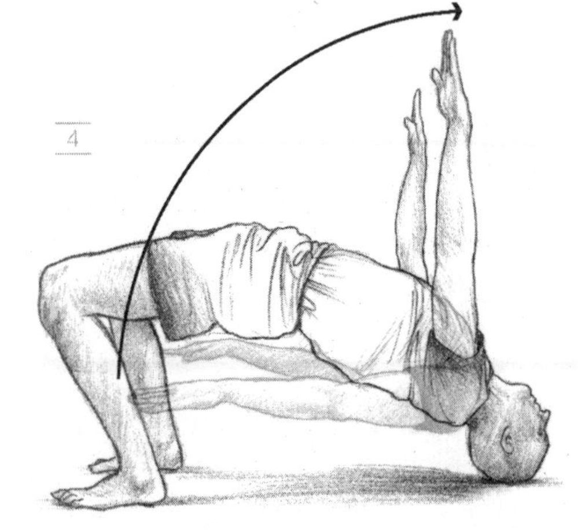

Inhale and return your straight arms toward the ceiling.

Lower and lift your arms 3 times, (see illustrations 3 and 4).

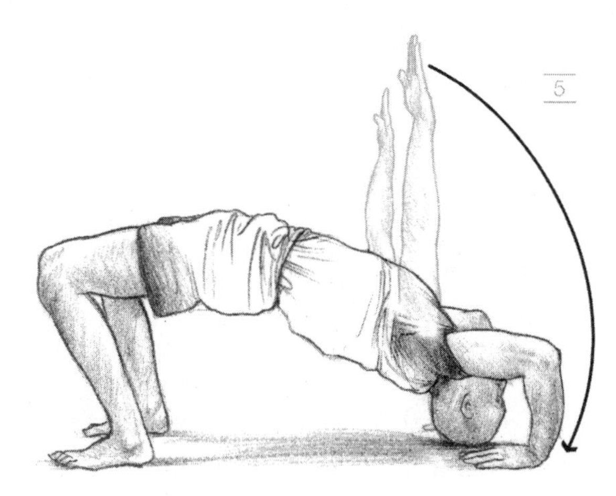

Return your hands to the floor below your shoulders.

Exhale and bring your chin to your chest.
Lower your body to the floor.

Perform this exercise only 1 time.

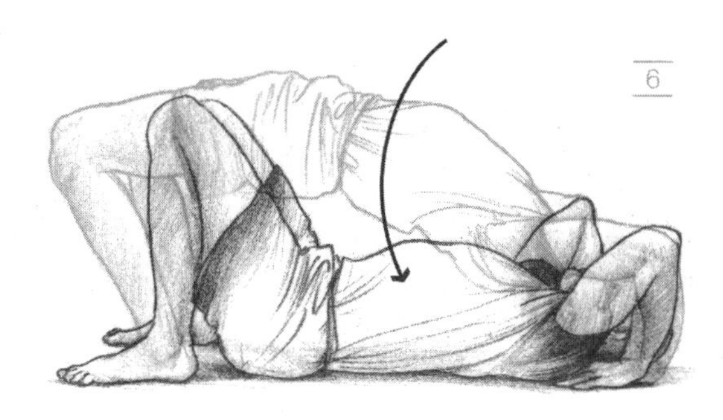

THE BEAST WITHIN

BODY POSITION Approach this exercise with caution. Secure a cushion or small pillow that will *not move* under your head if necessary, and be sure that your feet have very good traction. Keep your neck long. Squeeze your buttocks.

THE MIND IN MOTION Squeeze your buttocks firmly throughout the movement. Be certain your neck is safe and secure before you extend your hands to the ceiling. You shouldn't feel any pain. Don't roll onto either your forehead or the back of your head while positions 2 through 5. Focus on keeping your neck long. Keep your powerhouse drawn in. Your fingertips may touch the floor as you lower your straight arms in step 3. The range of motion for your arms depends on your balance and control. If you feel any discomfort, place your hands back under your shoulders, bring your chin to your chest, and lower your back to the floor with control.

CAUTIONS Leave this exercise out if you have neck, shoulder, wrist, elbow, back, hip, knee, or foot problems.

THE CORKSCREW

BENEFITS: STRENGTHENS THE POWERHOUSE, BUTTOCKS, SHOULDERS, ARMS, WAIST, AND SIDES; IMPROVES FLEXIBILITY OF THE SPINE AND BODY

Note: This is exactly the same as the Corkscrew from the traditional mat exercises *(see page 57)**. The following illustrations depict the advanced variation of the Corkscrew, which is appropriate for reformer on the mat.*

After the Headstand Pulling Straps, lie fully extended on your back. Place your arms along your sides with your shoulders down and away from your ears. Pull your powerhouse in, exhale, and bring your straight legs up to a vertical 90-degree angle to the floor, keep your entire spine on the floor during this movement.

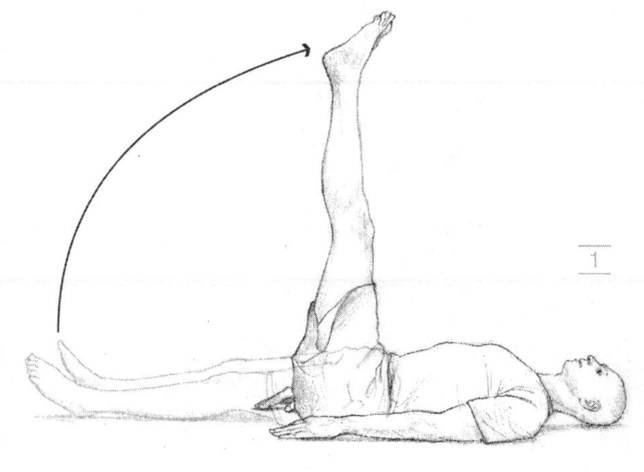

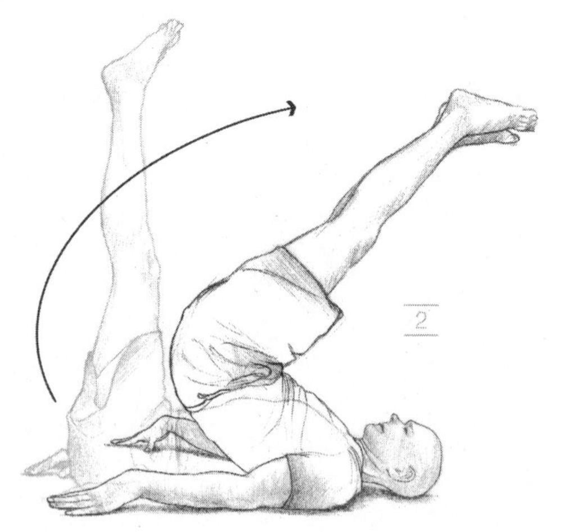

Inhale as you press your hands and arms into the floor. Using your powerhouse, peel your hips and spine—off the floor—one vertebra at a time until your knees are approximately above the mouth/chin region of your face. When your knees are above your face, you will be rolled up to about your mid to upper back.

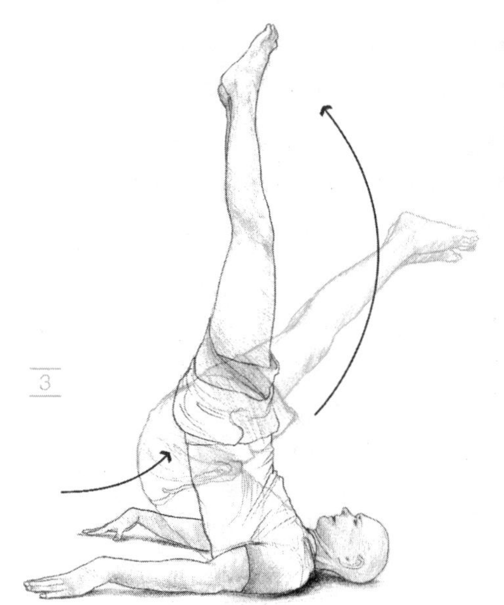

Continuing to press your arms into the floor, drive your hips forward and squeeze your buttocks as you reach your legs straight up toward the ceiling. Keep your stomach pulled in.

Lower both legs together to an angle slightly above parallel to the floor, while keeping your spine and hips lifted.

4

5

Exhale and lower the right side of your body down to the floor as you begin to circle your legs around in a clockwise direction (circle down the right side).

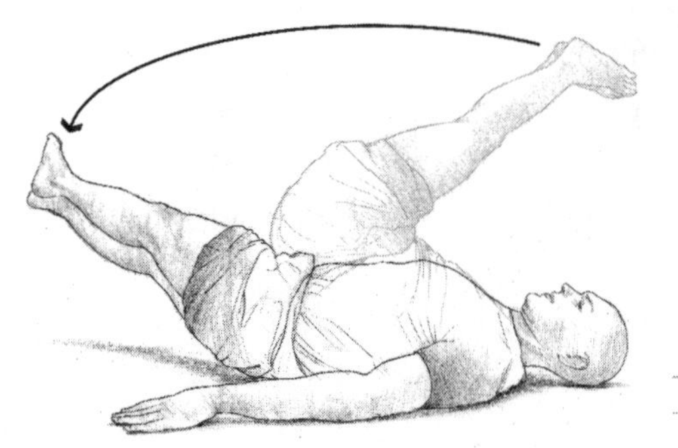

Once your tailbone and spine are down, continue to circle your legs around clockwise.

Inhale as you begin to lift up onto the left side of your body. Keep the powerhouse pulled in.

7

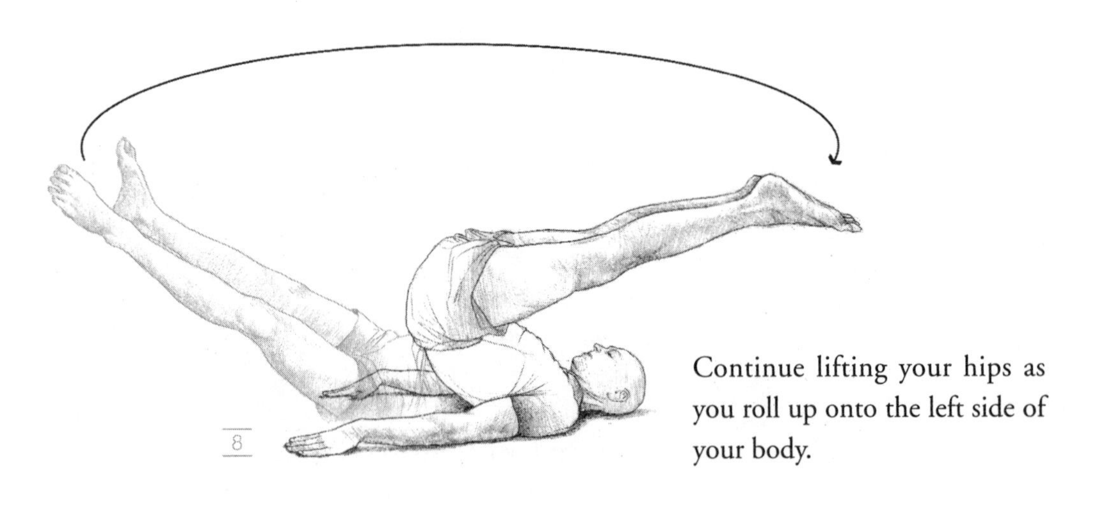

Continue lifting your hips as you roll up onto the left side of your body.

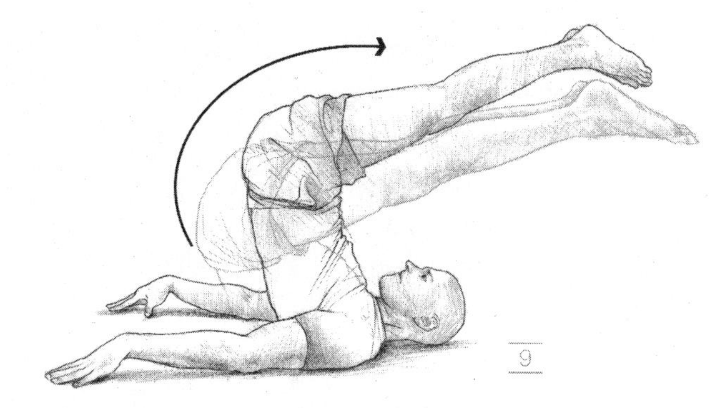

Arrive with your legs overhead at an angle just above parallel to the floor; your weight should be evenly distributed across your upper back, shoulders, and arms.

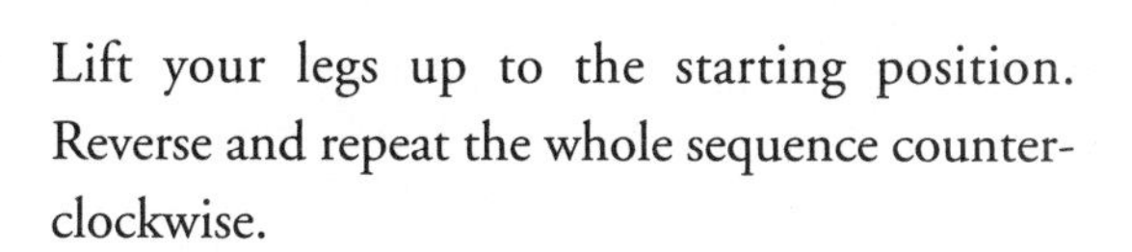

Lift your legs up to the starting position. Reverse and repeat the whole sequence counterclockwise.

Perform 3 times in each direction.

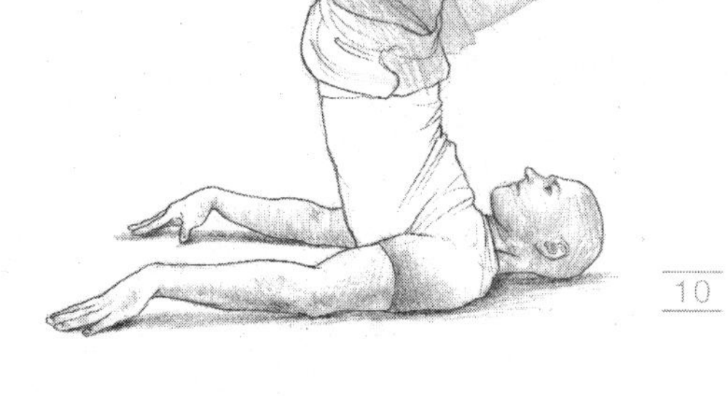

THE BEAST WITHIN

BODY POSITION At all times keep your shoulders away from your ears. Anchor your shoulders and arms down onto the mat. Reach your arms long toward your feet. Try to keep your elbows and knees straight throughout the exercise.

THE MIND IN MOTION By now, you should be adept at this exercise, but I'll reiterate the same modifications that applied to the traditional mat Corkscrew, just in case you need them. The easiest way to learn this exercise is to begin by not lifting your bottom in the air. Lie on your back with only your legs in the air (see illustration 1). Circle your legs around clockwise, then circle them counterclockwise. Exhale during the first half and inhale during the second half of each circle. Control the entire movement. Don't allow momentum to take away your control. Keep the circle small. If tightness in your back or legs makes it difficult, try this exercise with bent knees. If you have a problematic lower back, keep your hands under your buttocks when circling your legs in a small circle and don't lift your hips and spine—or simply leave this exercise out. You mustn't allow your lower back to arch up off the mat when your buttocks, spine, and torso are on the floor. When you have mastered this "spine down" version, you may then progress to lifting your hips only slightly at the end of each circle—as per the hip lift in step 2, but not as high off the ground. Finally, you may attempt the complete Corkscrew sequence as illustrated.

For more of a challenge, lower your feet as low as possible (see illustration 5) with your hips lifted as you begin to circle your legs around. Keep your powerhouse pulled in throughout the movement.

CAUTIONS Proceed slowly or leave this exercise out if you have neck, shoulder, elbow, back, or hip problems.

CONTROL BALANCE/ARABESQUE

BENEFITS: STRENGTHENS THE POWERHOUSE AND UPPER BODY; DEVELOPS BALANCE, FLEXIBILITY, AND CONTROL

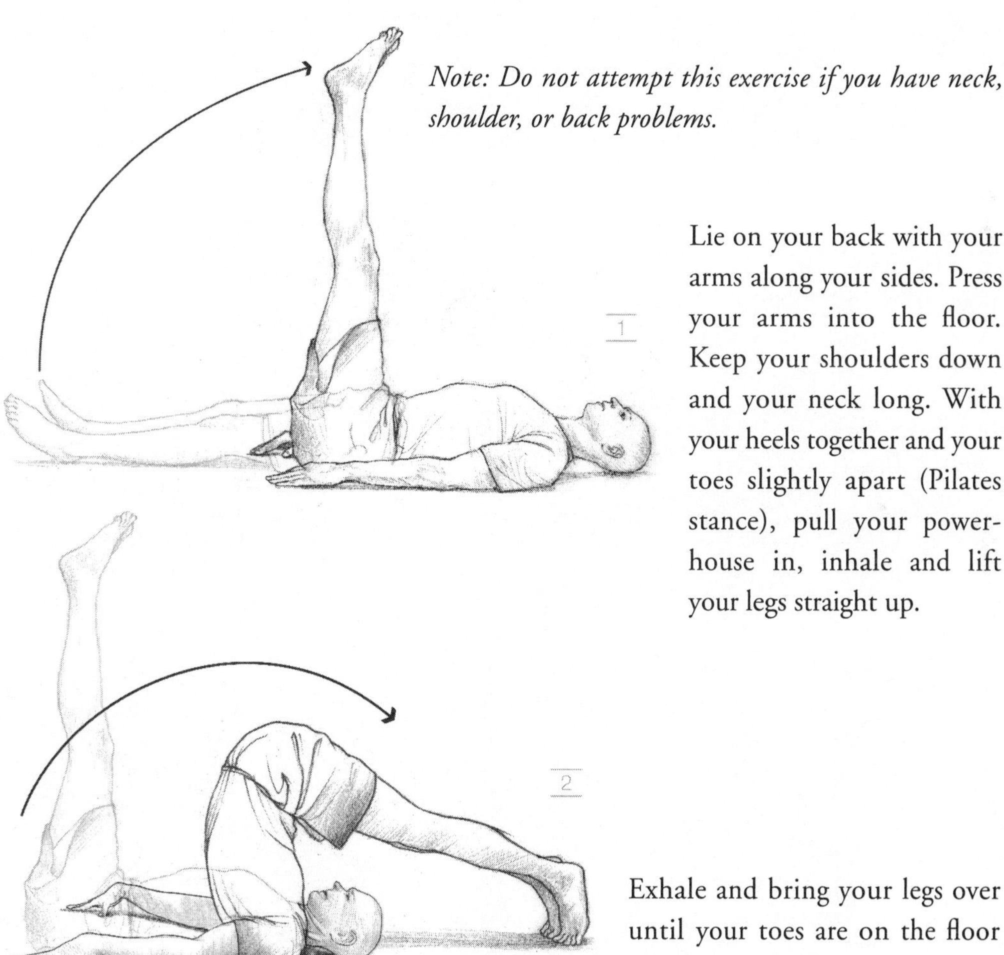

Note: Do not attempt this exercise if you have neck, shoulder, or back problems.

Lie on your back with your arms along your sides. Press your arms into the floor. Keep your shoulders down and your neck long. With your heels together and your toes slightly apart (Pilates stance), pull your powerhouse in, inhale and lift your legs straight up.

Exhale and bring your legs over until your toes are on the floor behind your head.

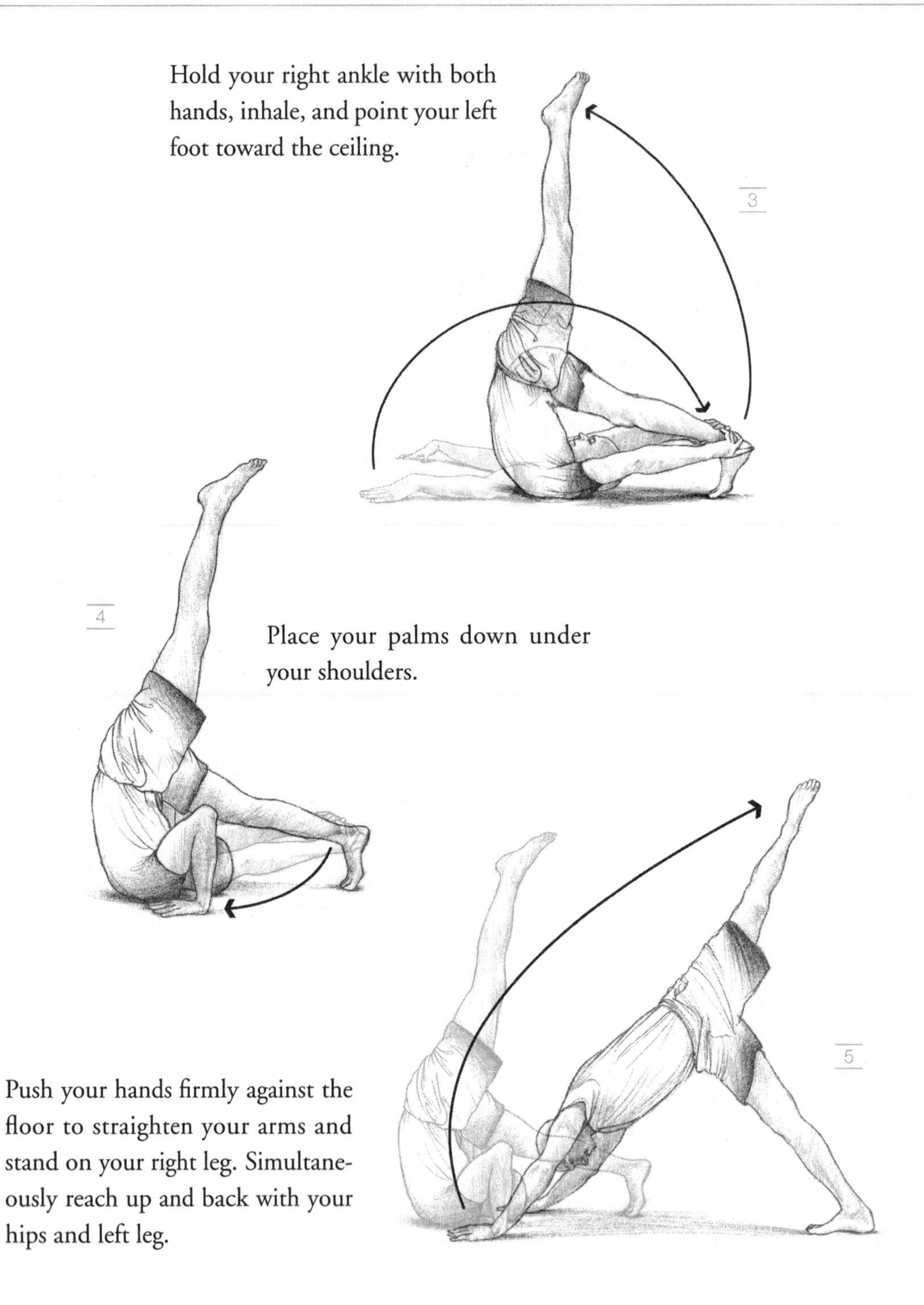

Hold your right ankle with both hands, inhale, and point your left foot toward the ceiling.

Place your palms down under your shoulders.

Push your hands firmly against the floor to straighten your arms and stand on your right leg. Simultaneously reach up and back with your hips and left leg.

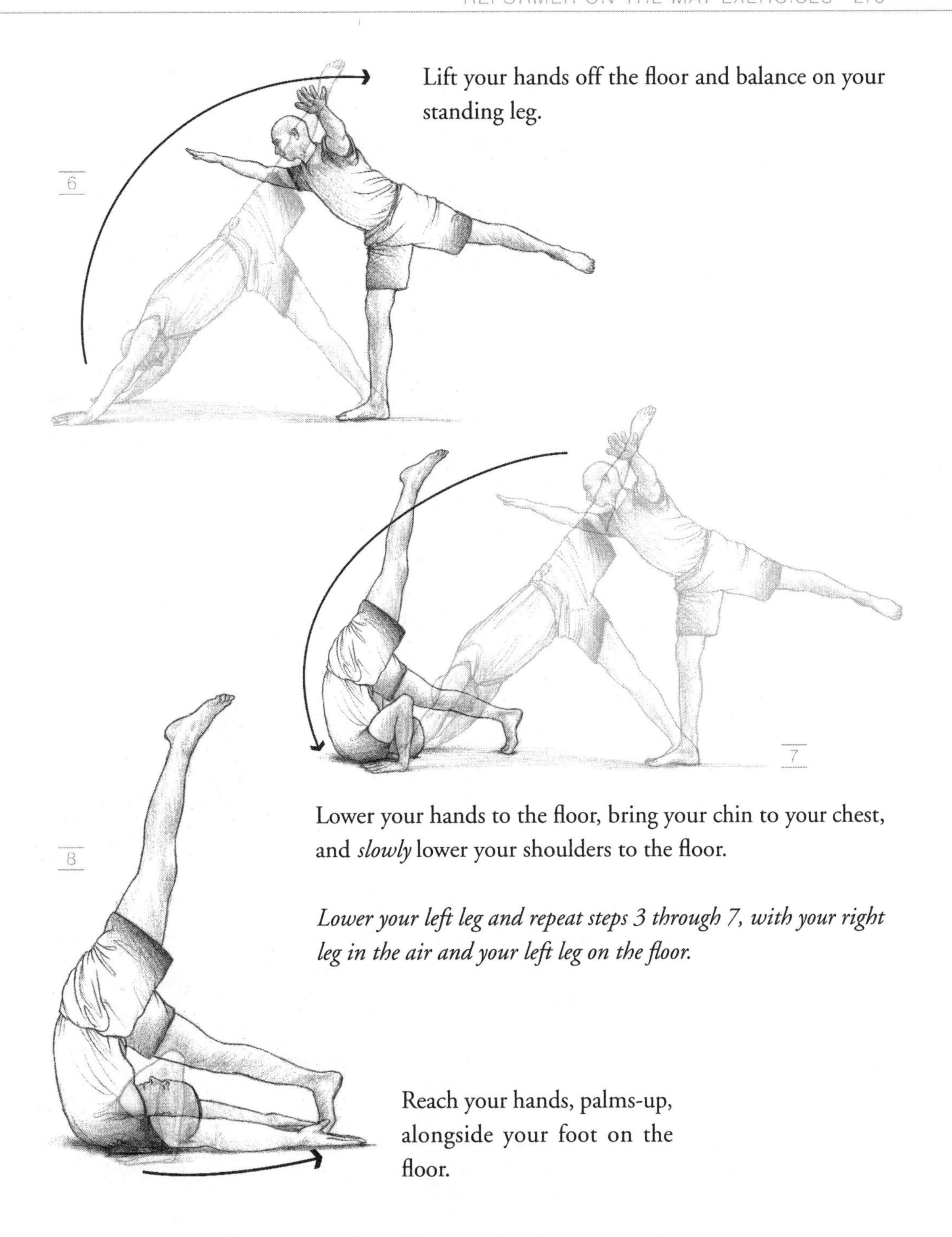

Lift your hands off the floor and balance on your standing leg.

Lower your hands to the floor, bring your chin to your chest, and *slowly* lower your shoulders to the floor.

Lower your left leg and repeat steps 3 through 7, with your right leg in the air and your left leg on the floor.

Reach your hands, palms-up, alongside your foot on the floor.

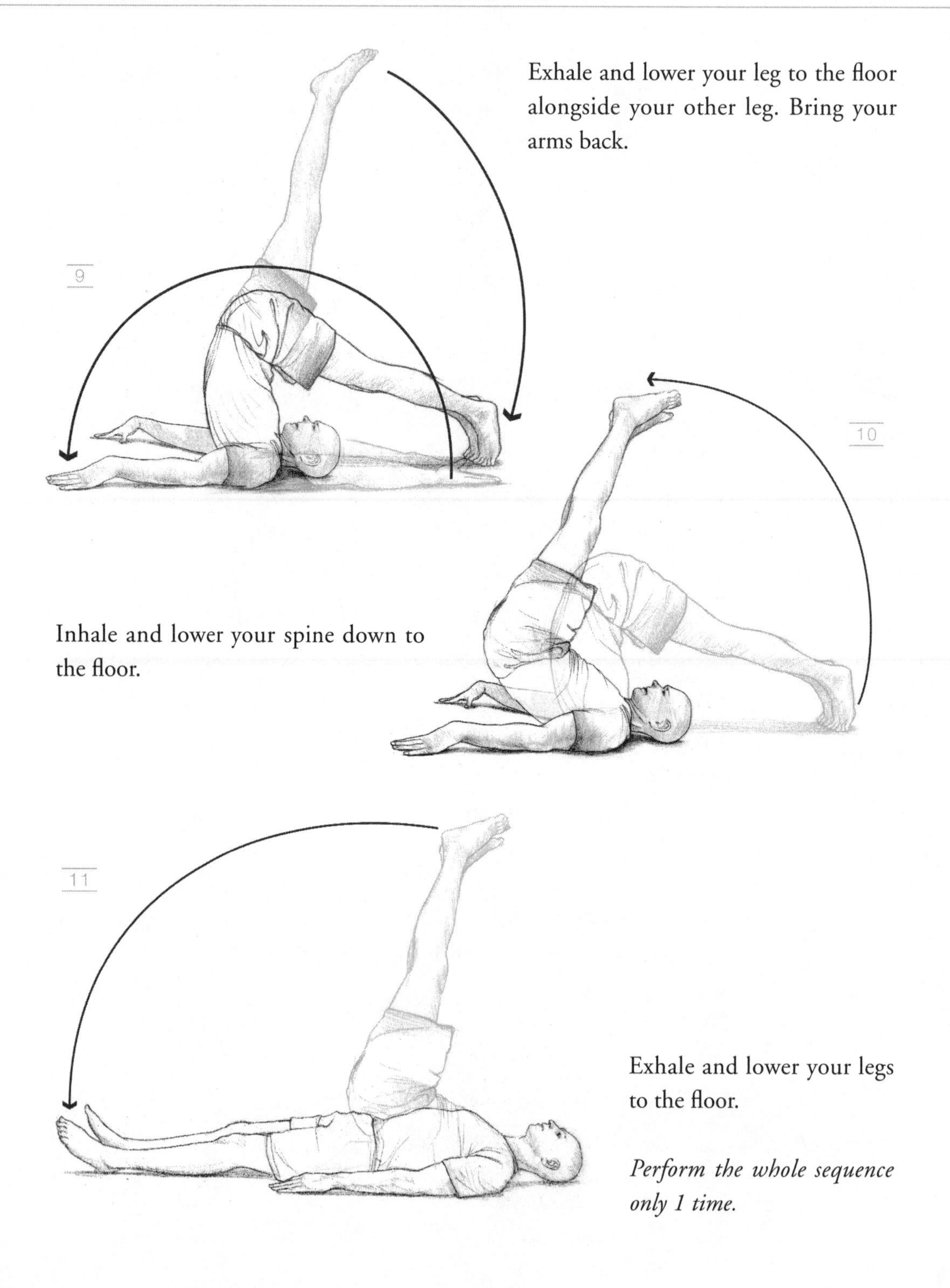

Exhale and lower your leg to the floor alongside your other leg. Bring your arms back.

Inhale and lower your spine down to the floor.

Exhale and lower your legs to the floor.

Perform the whole sequence only 1 time.

THE BEAST WITHIN

BODY POSITION Your entire spine should be on floor when you begin.

THE MIND IN MOTION If you don't have the upper body strength and spinal flexibility (especially in the neck) that you need to push off the mat, then leave out the back roll into Arabesque (see illustrations 4, 5, 6, and 7) and perform only the balance control portion of the exercise (see illustrations 1, 2, and 3). Hold your powerhouse in throughout.

Here is a detailed breakdown of what happens when you push off the floor in steps 5 and 6. Keep pressing your hands firmly into the floor and allow your head to come up without any pressure on your head or neck. Your standing foot may slide back a bit, which is fine. Let your elevated leg reach up and away. The hand push should be enough to allow you to lift your shoulders and head off the floor without impediment. If you don't immediately come off the floor smoothly and easily, then end the exercise. When standing while balancing on one leg, bend your supporting knee if you start to lose your balance.

When you lower yourself back down to the floor in step 7, place your hands on the floor where they originally were and bring your chin to your chest. Or, you may first bring your hands to the floor—closer to your body—and then walk your hands out to their original push-off spot. You may also bend your supporting knee to make it easier to reach your hands out that far. Bend your elbows and let your shoulders and upper back meet the mat softly. Don't place yourself onto your upper neck. Men tend to have the upper body strength but lack the flexibility in the upper spine to execute this move smoothly.

CAUTIONS This exercise is both difficult to execute and precarious for your neck. Proceed slowly and carefully. Leave this out if you have wrist, elbow, knee, or foot problems. Again, don't even attempt the Control Balance/Arabesque if you have neck, shoulder, balance, or back problems.

THE GRASSHOPPER

BENEFITS: STRENGTHENS THE LEGS, BUTTOCKS, HIPS, BACK, AND POWERHOUSE

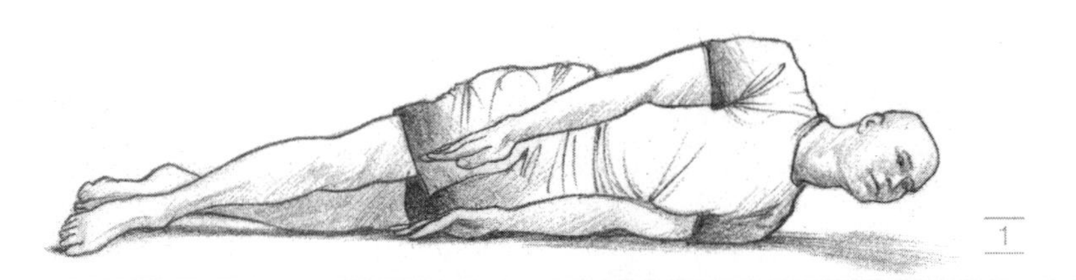

Start by lying on your left side, with your arms extended and your palms facing the floor. Your right leg is momentarily crossed over your left.

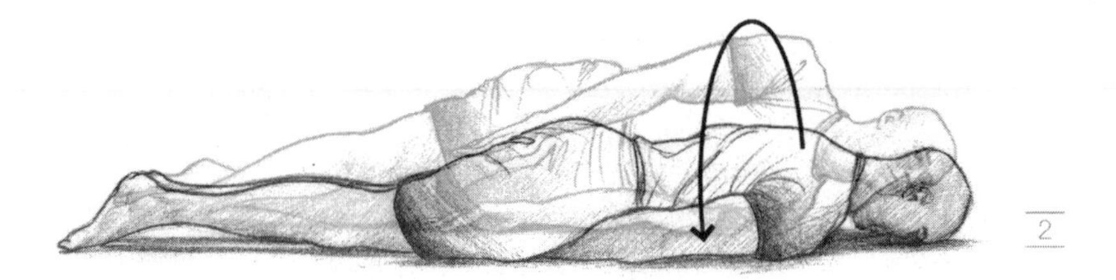

Roll onto your stomach and place your palms flat on the floor underneath your thighs. Rest your forehead on the cushioned floor. Pull your shoulders down and away from your ears.

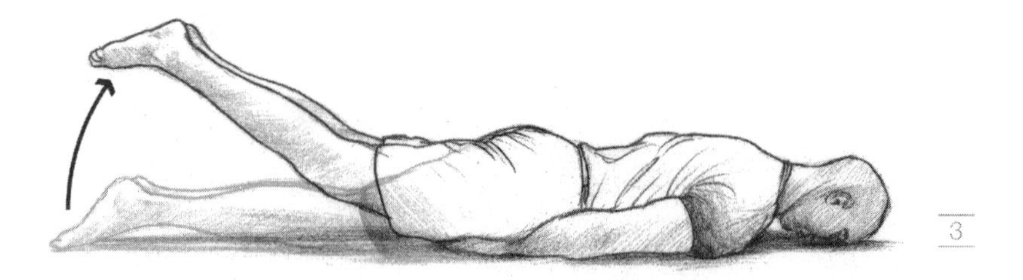

Pull your powerhouse in and up. Press your legs together and lift them up to the ceiling as you contract your buttocks firmly and begin to inhale.

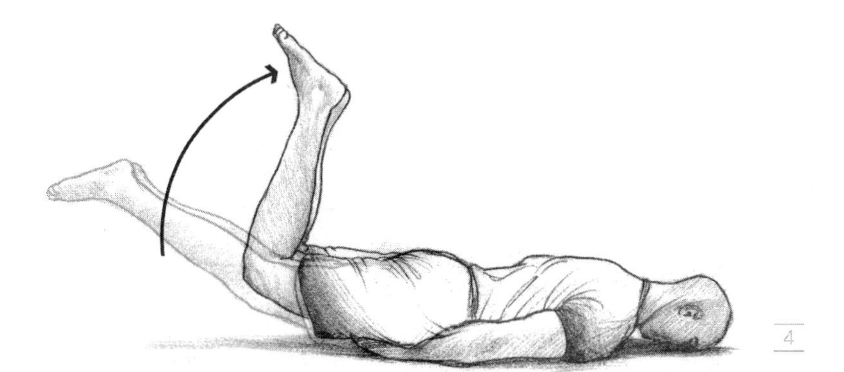

Bend your knees and lift your legs higher.

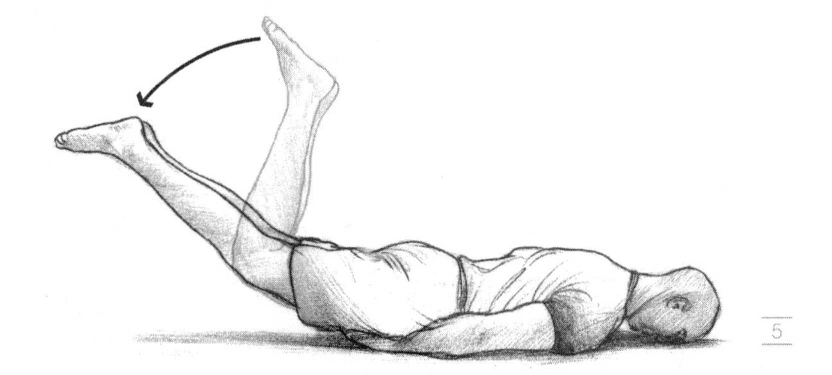

Straighten your legs in the air.

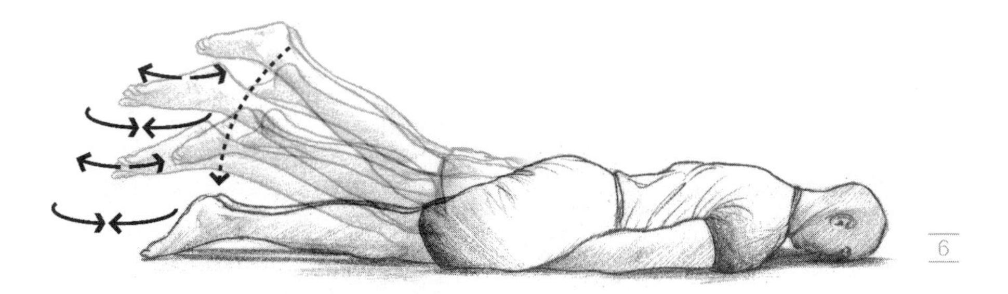

Begin exhaling as you clap your heels together while simultaneously lowering your legs to the floor.

Perform 3 times.

THE BEAST WITHIN

BODY POSITION When you're on your stomach, you may have your palms up against your thighs or against the floor (as instructed). It's more difficult with your palms down. Keep your forehead on the mat to avoid hurting your neck.

THE MIND IN MOTION Squeeze your buttocks and pull your powerhouse in and up to initiate the leg lifts, keep them engaged throughout the movement. Do not initiate the leg lift from your lower back. Think of lengthening your legs as you lift them. Lower your legs with control; do not succumb to gravity.

CAUTIONS If you feel strain in your lower back, stop the exercise and sit back on your heels (as at the end of the Swan) to release your back muscles. Men typically have a small range of leg motion in the Grasshopper. Proceed slowly or leave this out if you have neck, shoulder, wrist, elbow, rib, back, hip, or knee problems.

ROCKING PULL

BENEFITS: STRENGTHENS THE BACK, ARMS, LEGS, POWERHOUSE AND BUTTOCKS; STRETCHES THE CHEST AND SHOULDERS

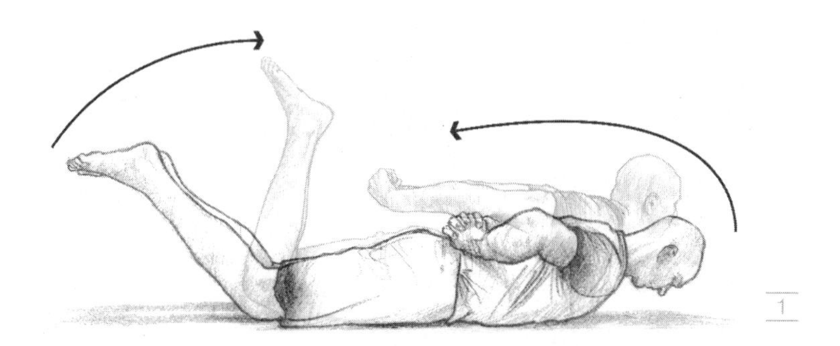

After the Grasshopper, stay on your stomach. Bend your knees until your lower legs are roughly at a 45-degree angle off the floor. Lift your forehead off the floor while maintaining a long neck. Interlace your hands on your lower back with your elbows bent. Pull your powerhouse in and squeeze your buttocks. Inhale, straighten your arms, lift your chest, and bring your feet toward your buttocks.

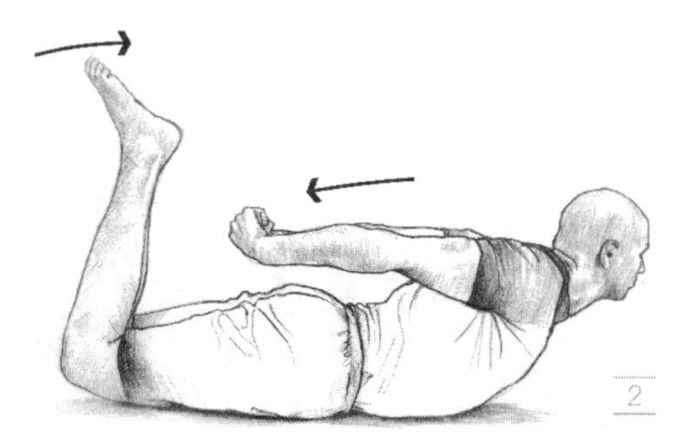

Hold this position for two seconds, and then exhale as you return to the starting position.

Perform 5 times.

THE BEAST OF WITHIN

Nowadays, people usually perform the traditional mat Rocking exercise and leave this version out. Both versions should be performed in the reformer on the mat workout. After the Rocking Pull, you may add the Rocking from the traditional mat workout (see page 120). When this exercise is performed on the reformer, it is often referred to as Hamstring Curls. They are two different exercises with the same leg movement.

BODY POSITION You begin with your legs bent. On the reformer, your legs would have to be slightly bent to create the necessary tension to keep the straps from falling off on your feet. In the reformer on the mat, the initial leg bend engages the hamstring muscles from the outset.

THE MIND IN MOTION When your arms are straight, keep them as high as you can off your back. Press your hips down. Squeeze your buttocks hard and pull your powerhouse in as you lift your chest off the floor; don't hinge in any one spot on your spine. Tight shoulders and a broad back may inhibit your from straightening your arms. If this is the case for you, simply separate your hands and reach your fingers back with your palms up when you're in the raised position.

CAUTIONS Leave this exercise out if you have neck, shoulder, rib, back, hip, or knee problems.

SWIMMING

BENEFITS: STRENGTHENS THE ARMS, SHOULDERS, BACK, BUTTOCKS, AND LEGS; LENGTHENS THE SPINE

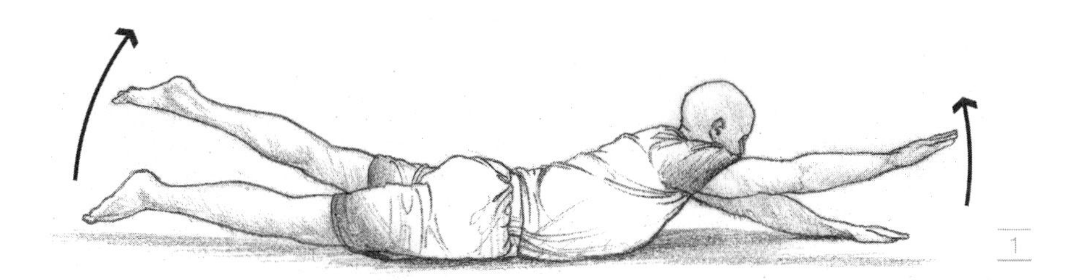

After the Rocking Pull or Rocking, if you added it in as instructed, remain on your stomach and extend your arms and legs out. Exhale and pull your powerhouse in. Squeeze your buttocks and lift your right arm and left leg into the air. This is 1 stroke.

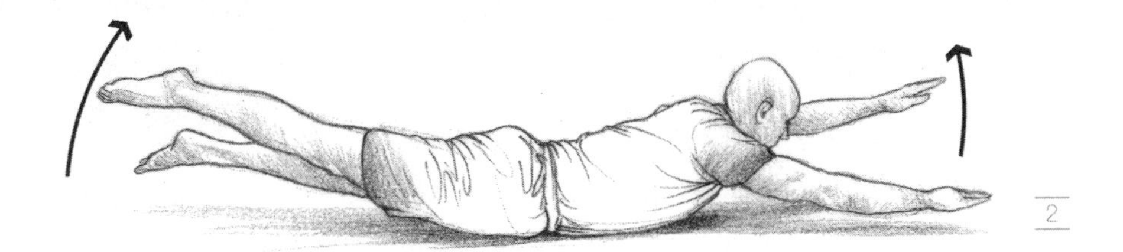

Then lift your left arm and right leg while lowering your alternate limbs just off the floor. Continue alternating raising your right arm and left leg, then your left arm and right leg, while keeping all four limbs off the floor at all times. Move continuously as if you're swimming, inhaling for 5 strokes and exhaling for 5 strokes. This is 1 set.

Perform for 3 to 4 sets.

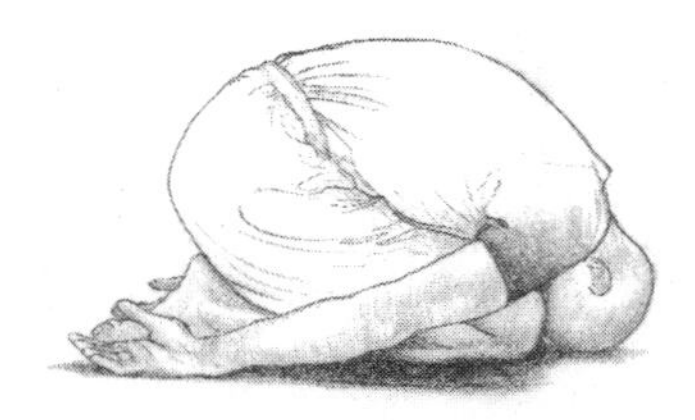
3

Sit back on your heels with your forehead on your knees.

THE BEAST WITHIN

This is the exact same exercise as in the traditional mat work.

BODY POSITION Keep your body lifted as high off the floor as possible. Try to keep your elbows and knees locked straight. Don't let your arms or legs touch the floor. Keep your shoulders down and away from your ears.

THE MIND IN MOTION A stroke is defined as the single lifting motion of an arm and the opposite leg. Lift the entire length of your body up, with particular focus on lengthening your spine. Do not hinge in any one spot on your back. Squeeze your bottom, hold your powerhouse in, and keep your sternum lifted off the floor. If you cannot straighten your arms and legs, then keep the most minimal bend in your elbows and knees throughout the exercise. If you begin to feel discomfort in your lower back, stop the exercise and sit back on your heels (see illustration 3).

CAUTIONS Men tend to have tightness in the back, which can make it difficult to lift and lengthen the spine in this exercise. Leave this out if you have neck, shoulder, rib, back, or knee problems.

LONG SPINE MASSAGE

BENEFITS: STRENGTHENS YOUR POWERHOUSE, BUTTOCKS, AND UPPER BODY

1

After Swimming, turn over onto your back, fully extended. Hold onto a sturdy object, such as an I-beam, a staircase beam, or anything stable and secure that you can firmly grip. Pull your powerhouse in and inhale. Exhale as you lift your legs together into the air.

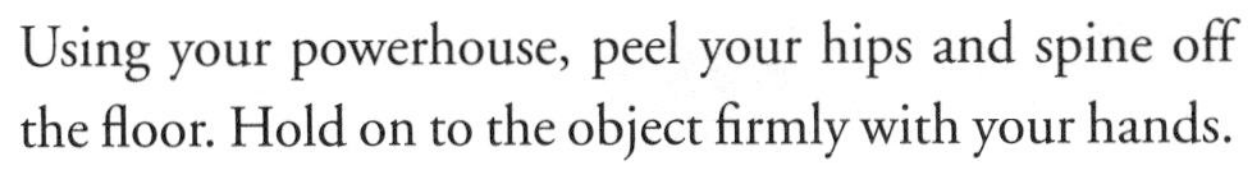

Using your powerhouse, peel your hips and spine off the floor. Hold on to the object firmly with your hands.

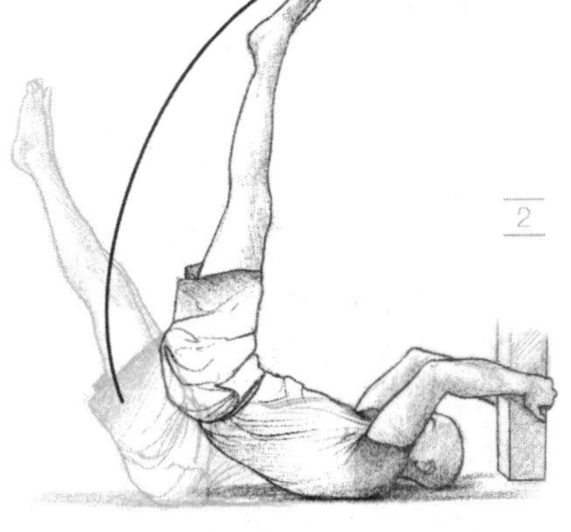

2

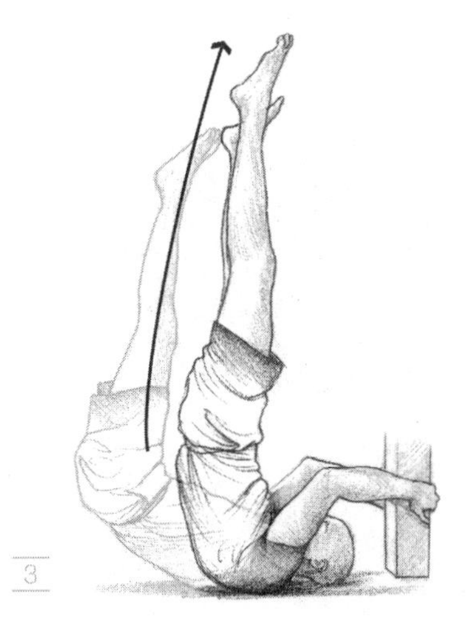

3

Inhale and open your legs shoulder-width apart. Lengthen your spine straight up and reach your toes to the ceiling. Keep your tailbone tucked under and your buttocks firmly engaged. Your weight should be on your upper back—not on your neck.

Lower your body with control while maintaining the straight line of your body. Keep your powerhouse, buttocks, and hands strongly engaged.

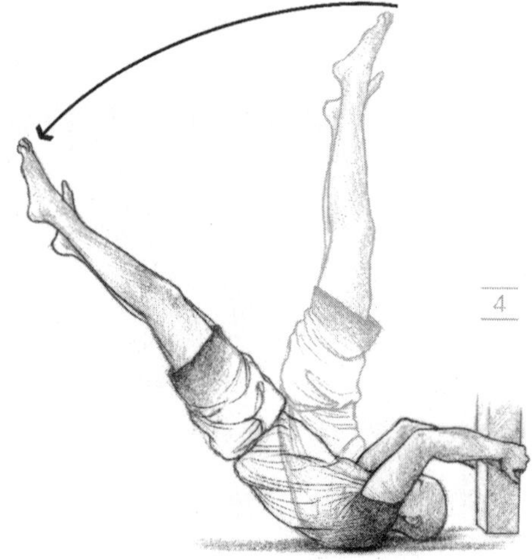

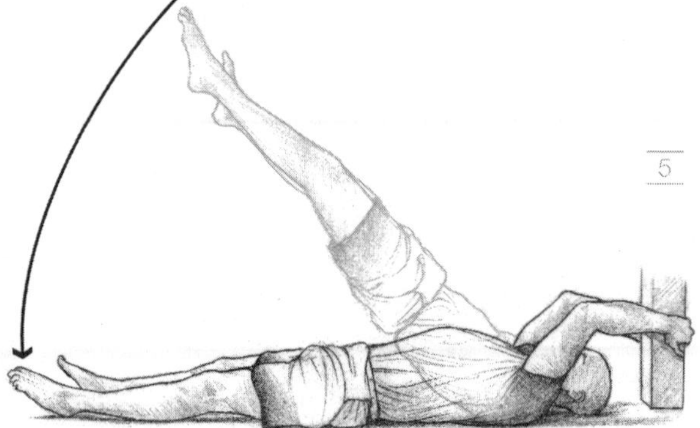

Continue lowering your body all the way to the floor and then exhale.

Perform steps 1 through 5 for a total of 3 repetitions.

After the 3 repetitions, begin again in the starting position, keeping your legs shoulder-width apart. Peel your hips and spine off the floor using your powerhouse. Hold onto the object firmly with your hands.

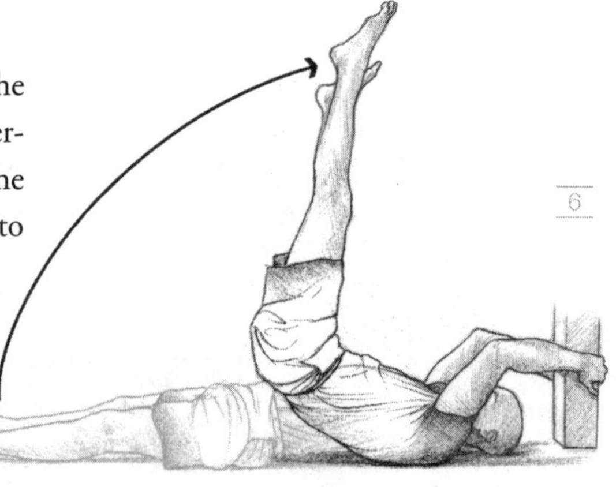

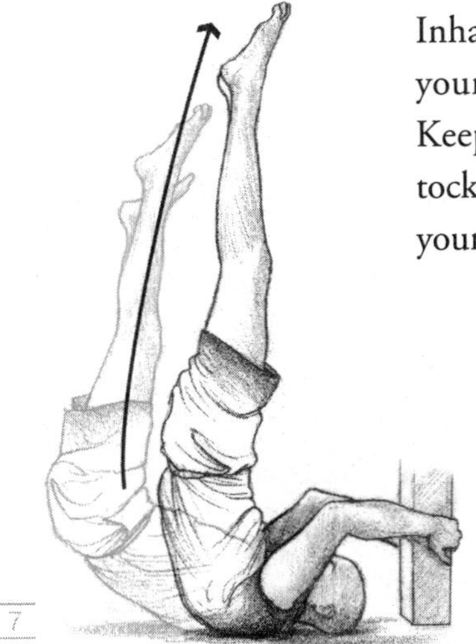

Inhale and bring your legs together. Lengthen your spine and reach your toes to the ceiling. Keep your tailbone tucked in and your buttocks firmly engaged. The weight should be on your upper back—not on your neck.

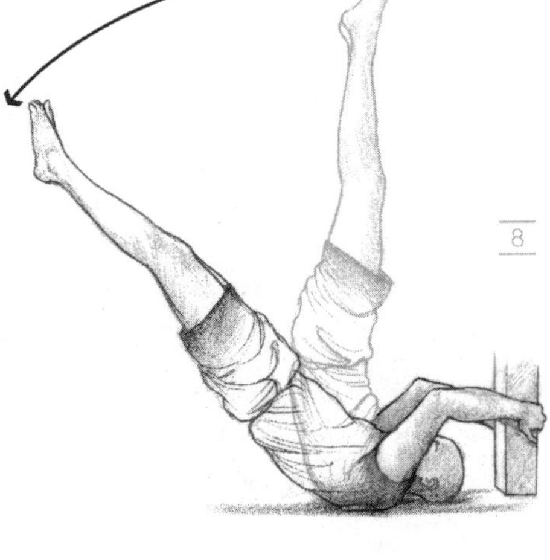

Lower your body slowly with control. Keep your powerhouse, buttocks, and hands strongly engaged. Squeeze your legs together.

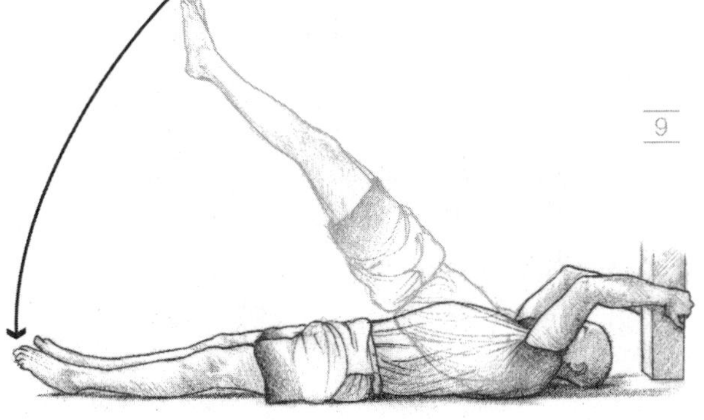

Continue lowering your body all the way to the floor, and then exhale.

Perform steps 6 through 9 for a total of 3 repetitions.

THE BEAST WITHIN

If you ordered a reformer for home delivery in Joseph Pilates's day, you would have received a sheet of photos showing a robust sixty-five-year-old Joseph Pilates performing the reformer exercises. The exercise called Long Spine Massage looked exactly like Short Spine Massage, except that you held your legs straight with your feet over your face throughout the roll down movement. You never bent your knees. On the reformer, both exercises are performed with straps on the feet to help control the roll down movement of the spine. This exercise, as illustrated here, was originally called Control Stretch. It was performed with neither straps on the feet nor rolling the spine down. In the modern day it tends to go by the name Long Spine Massage Without Straps. Sometime in the past, the two exercises morphed together, and it is now performed with straps on the feet—probably to help control the movement because this illustrated version is outright tough.

BODY POSITION From your head to your toes, keep your body long.

THE MIND IN MOTION Bend at your hips only as much as necessary to your lift hips and spine off the floor. Don't bend so much at your waist that the weight of your legs pulls you up and you disengage your powerhouse. Use your powerhouse strength to lift yourself up as well as to as to control your descent. When your spine is off the floor and your feet are extended toward the ceiling, you should feel the weight on your upper back and shoulders—not in your neck. Tuck your tailbone. You must squeeze your bottom hard and pull your powerhouse in. If during the descent you feel that you're about to lose control, don't let your body fall. Instead lower yourself to the floor by bending at the hips and begin to roll your spine down one vertebra at a time. It will resemble the Jackknife exercise from the traditional mat work. If you do "jackknife" down, you will be safer but will also have lost most of the working benefit of the exercise. With practice, you'll eventually be able to hold your body rigid throughout the movement.

CAUTIONS Proceed slowly or leave this exercise out if you have neck, shoulder, hand, back, or hip problems.

KNEE STRETCHES I

BENEFITS: STRENGTHENS THE UPPER BODY AND THE POWERHOUSE

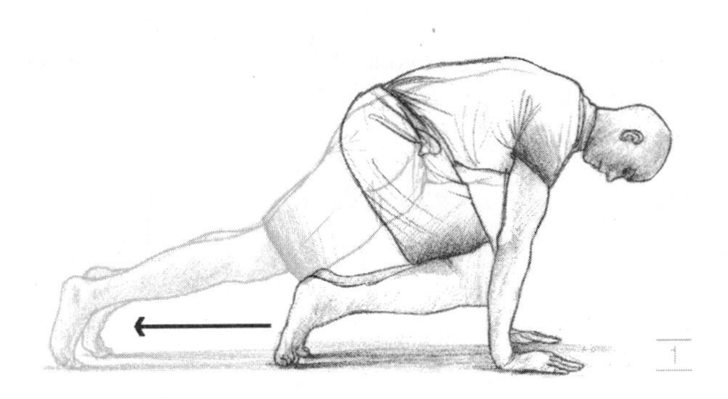

After the Long Spine Massage, turn over onto your hands and knees. Round your back and look at either your navel or between your wrists. Pull your powerhouse in and up. Lift your knees about two to four inches off the floor. Exhale and bring your knees in toward your chest. Now you are in the starting position. Inhale and slide your feet out until your legs are nearly straight. Wear socks to facilitate sliding.

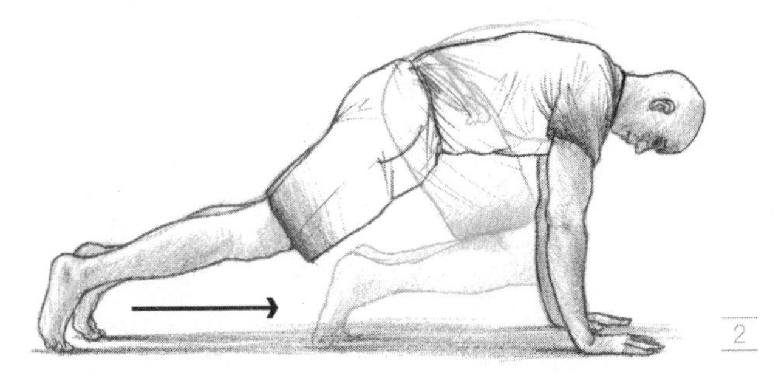

Exhale and slide your feet forward, bring your knees to your chest, until you're back in the starting position.

Perform a total of 8 repetitions.

THE BEAST WITHIN

BODY POSITION In this version of the Knee Stretches, you must keep your back rounded and your powerhouse pulled in and up. Don't arch your back. Keep your shoulders pulled down into your body and away from your ears.

THE MIND IN MOTION In this exercise, support your body weight with your hands. Don't jam into your knees when you extend your legs out and behind you. Your knees should be slightly bent. Don't hold the extended leg position; bring your legs back into the starting position immediately. Sustain continuous movement.

CAUTIONS Proceed slowly or leave this exercise out if you have neck, shoulder, wrist, elbow, back, hip, knee, ankle, or foot problems.

KNEE STRETCHES II

BENEFITS: STRENGTHENS THE POWERHOUSE AND UPPER BODY; IMPROVES AGILITY AND SPEED

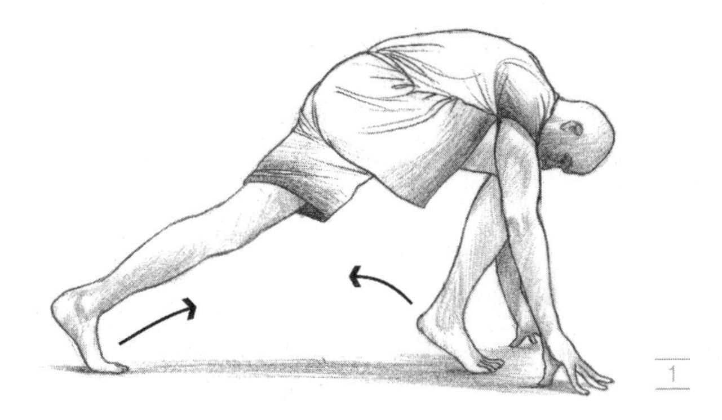

After the Knee Stretches I, assume the starting position of a professional sprinter. Place your fingertips on the floor, with one leg tucked in and the other leg extended behind you. Lift your powerhouse in and up.

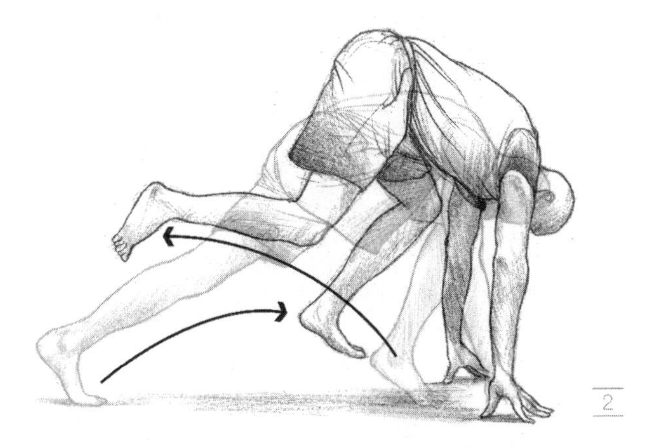

Inhale and, in a running motion, switch the position of your legs.

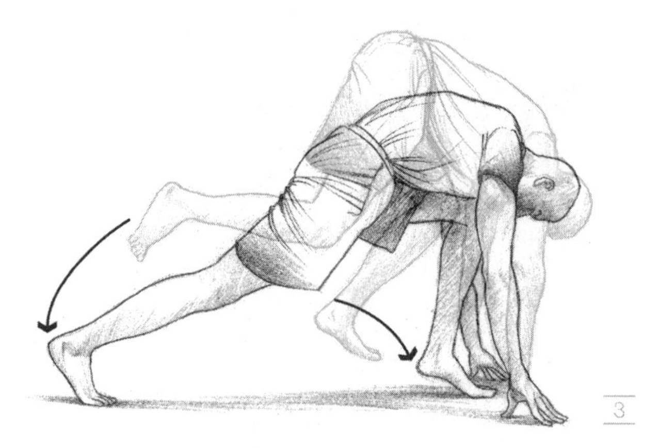

Exhale and switch your legs back.

Perform 8 repetitions.

THE BEAST WITHIN

BODY POSITION Don't arch your back; keep it rounded. You may perform this exercise on your palms instead of on your fingertips, but it might feel more natural on your fingertips.

THE MIND IN MOTION Land softly on the balls and toes of your feet with each leg switch. You may keep your front foot in the air to allow you to switch legs faster; your hips will not lift as much. Move smoothly.

CAUTIONS Proceed slowly or leave this exercise out if you have neck, shoulder, wrist, back, hip, knee, ankle, or foot problems.

KNEE STRETCHES III

BENEFITS: STRENGTHENS THE POWERHOUSE, ARMS, AND BUTTOCKS; IMPROVES FLEXIBILITY OF THE SPINE

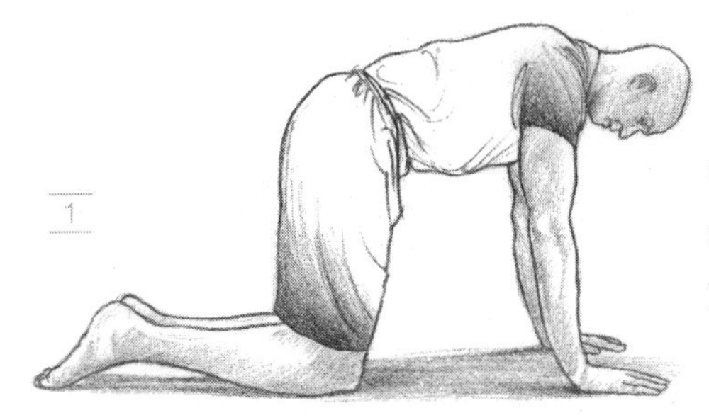

Get down on all fours, with your knees underneath your hips and your wrists underneath your shoulders.

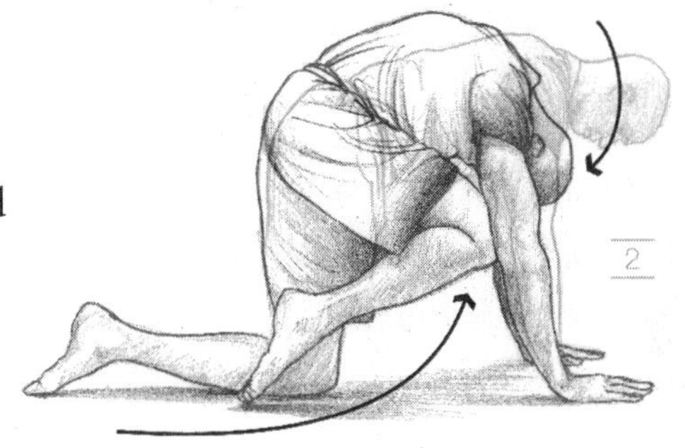

Exhale and bring your right knee and forehead together, as you pull your powerhouse in.

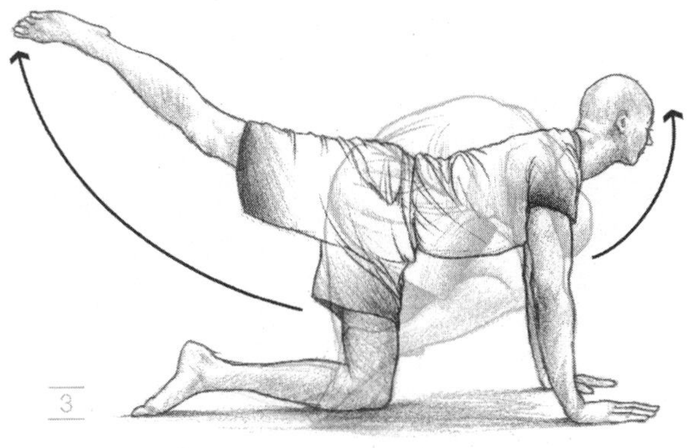

Inhale and extend your right leg back and up as you look forward and up. Keep your hips square and your powerhouse pulled in.

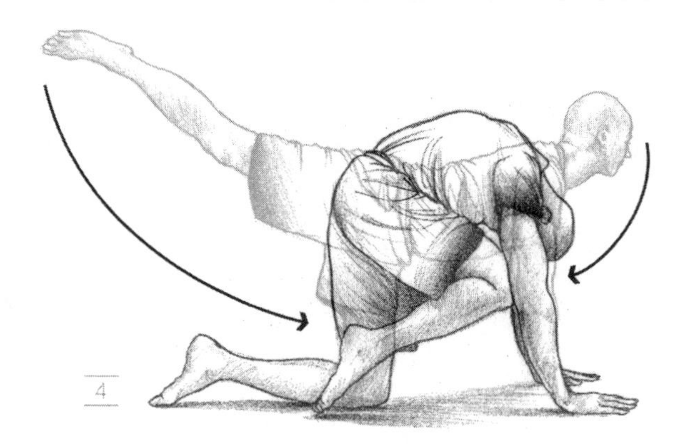

Exhale and bring your knee and forehead back together.

Perform 5 knee stretches with your right leg, then 5 with your left leg.

THE BEAST WITHIN

BODY POSITION Pad the floor if your knees are tender. If your wrists are weak, perform this exercise on the first two knuckles of your fists.

THE MIND IN MOTION Try to touch your knee to your forehead. You probably won't be able to do this at first, but this is the eventual goal. Keep your arms straight when you extend your leg back. Lengthen your entire spine when your leg is extended. Don't simply arch your lower back. Don't lean to the side of your supporting leg. Keep your powerhouse lifted into your spine throughout the movement. To make this exercise more challenging, begin in a Push-up position and keep your supporting leg straight throughout the exercise.

CAUTIONS Proceed slowly or leave this out if you have neck, shoulder, wrist, elbow, rib, back, hip, or knee problems.

RUNNING

BENEFITS: EXERCISES THE POWERHOUSE; STRETCHES THE BACKS OF THE LEGS

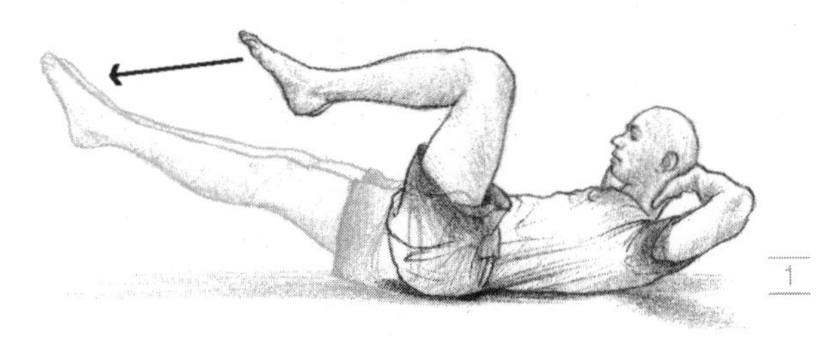

After the Knee Stretches, turn over and lie on your back. Pull your powerhouse in. Bend your knees to your chest as you exhale. Interlace your fingers behind your head and, using your powerhouse, lift your head off the floor. Inhale and extend your legs out.

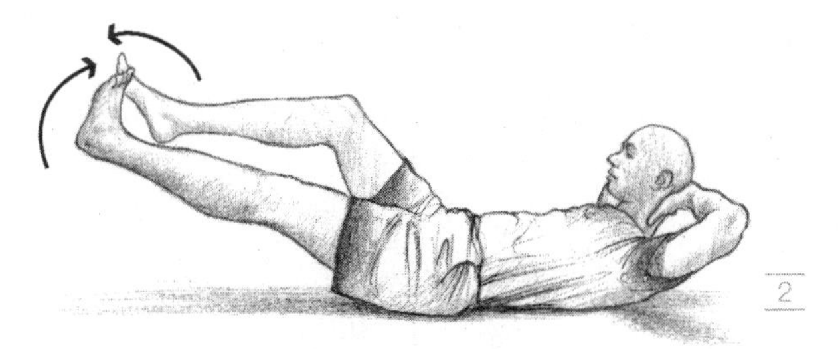

Keep the inside edges of your big toes touching each other. Bend your right knee and drop (or push) your left heel away from you.

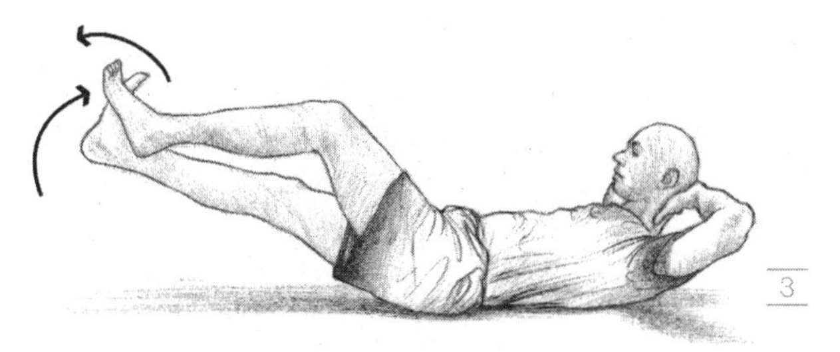

Switch by bending your left knee and dropping (or pushing) your right heel away from you. Inhale for 5 heel drops and exhale for 5 heel drops. This is 1 set.

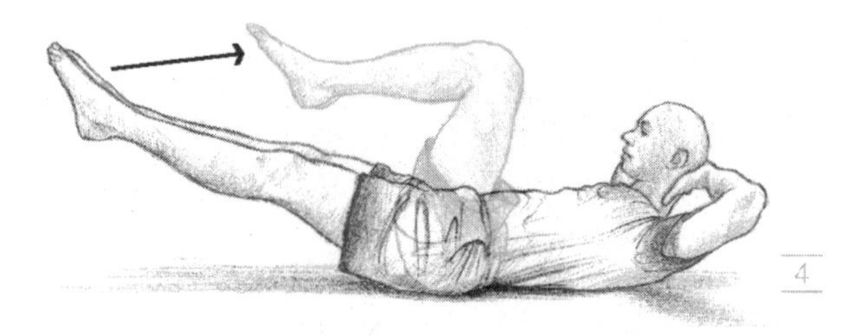

Finish your exhalation as you draw your knees to your chest.

Perform 2 sets.

THE BEAST WITHIN

BODY POSITION From your tailbone to the tips of your shoulder blades, keep your spine on the floor. Do not arch your lower back. Don't release your stomach. Keep your hands tightly interlaced or hand over hand. To lift your head, engage your powerhouse; do not pull it up with your hands. Keep your neck long.

THE MIND IN MOTION Keep your powerhouse in as you extend your legs out. Extend through the heel of your straight leg. If you have tightness in the legs and back—as many men do—you may find it difficult to extend your legs completely. Adjust the height of your legs to a position that you can maintain for the entire exercise. Ideally, you'd be able to extend them about fifteen to eighteen inches off the floor—approximately the height of a foot bar on a reformer. If you have heavy legs and/or your powerhouse is fatigued, you'll find it harder to hold your legs in the air for the duration of the exercise. If this is so, try fewer repetitions or discontinue the exercise.

CAUTIONS Leave this exercise out if you experience neck, back, knee, ankle, or foot problems.

PELVIC LIFT

BENEFITS: LENGTHENS THE SPINE; STRENGTHENS THE POWERHOUSE, LEGS, AND BUTTOCKS

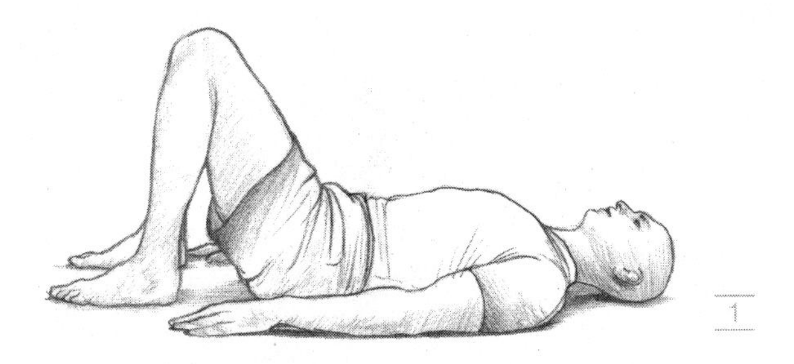

After Running, stay on your back. Bend your knees and place your feet flat on the floor, hip-width apart near your buttocks. Place your arms along your sides and draw your shoulders down and away from your ears. Pull your powerhouse in and exhale.

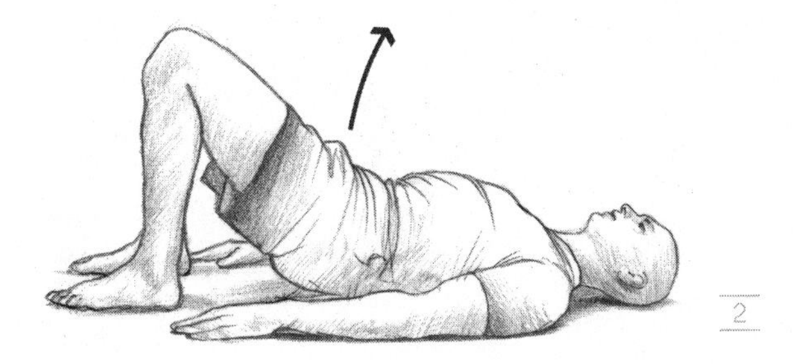

Inhale as you lift only your tailbone and hips in the air. Exhale and lower them down to the floor.

Perform up to 10 times.

THE BEAST WITHIN

BODY POSITION Anchor your body and feet to the mat.

THE MIND IN MOTION Pull your powerhouse in and up and lift only your pelvic girdle into the air. Don't come up too high. Lengthen your spine away from your ribs as you lift your hips. Keep your shoulders pulled down and away from your ears; keep your fingers reaching long toward your feet. As you lift and lower your tailbone, keep your hips squared.

CAUTIONS Leave this exercise out if it aggravates your lower back, feet, hips, or knees.

CONTROL PUSH-UP FRONT

BENEFITS: STRENGTHENS THE ENTIRE BODY

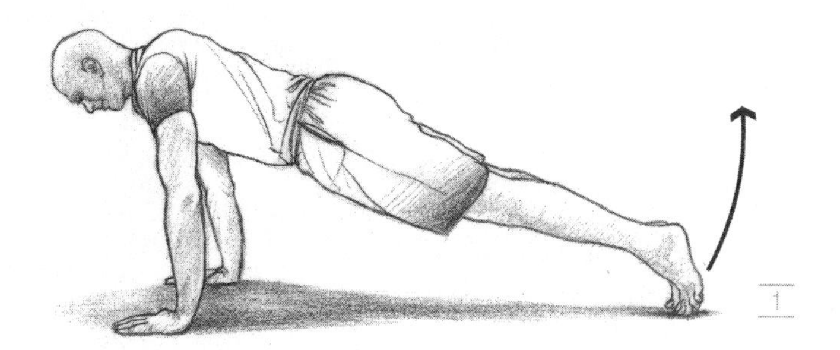

After the Pelvic Lift, turn over and assume a Push-up position. Inhale and lift your left leg high toward the ceiling.

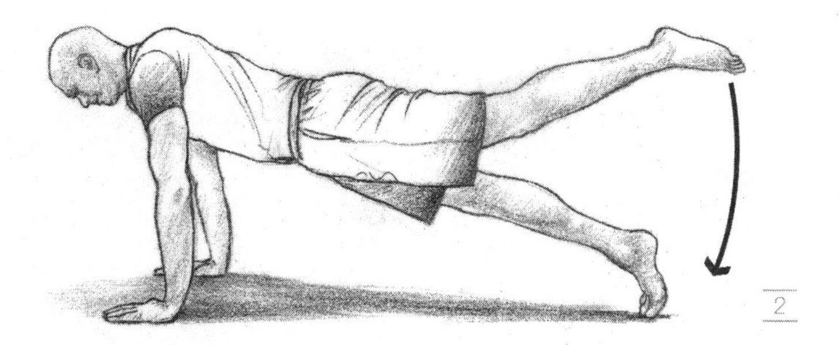

Exhale and lower it to back to the floor.

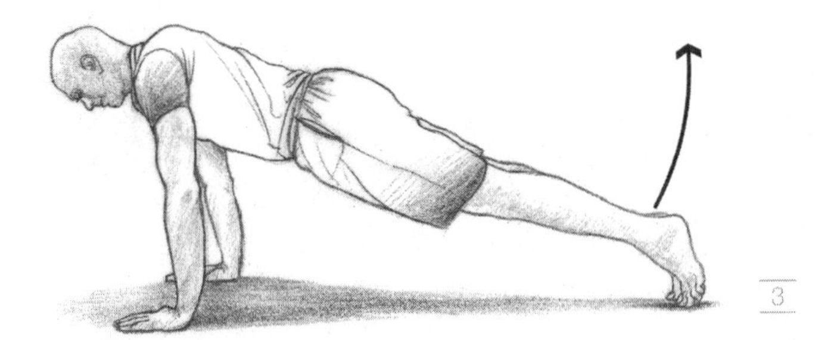

Inhale and lift your right leg high toward the ceiling.

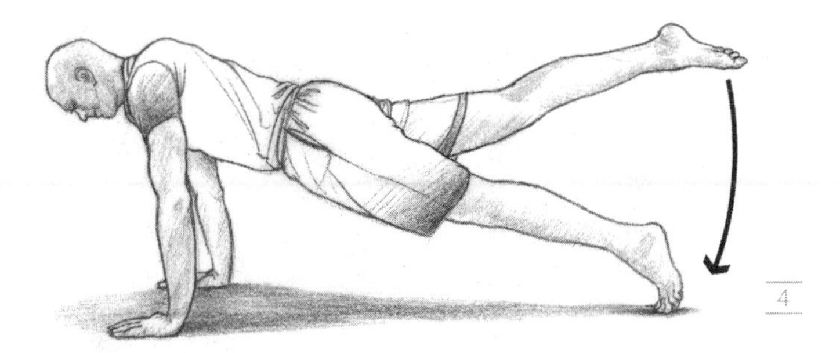

Exhale and lower it to the floor.

Repeat for a total of 3 times with each leg.

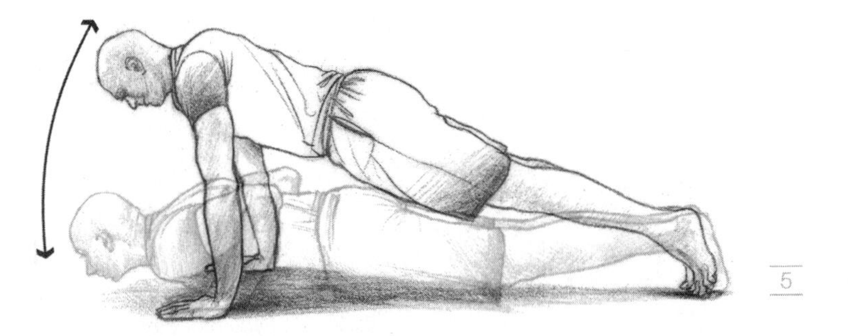

Inhale, look forward, and pull yourself into the floor. Exhale and rise up.

Perform 3 to 5 Push-ups as illustrated in step 5.

THE BEAST WITHIN

BODY POSITION When you take the Push-up position, place your wrists directly underneath your shoulders and lock your elbows. Secure your shoulders into their sockets. Keep your legs zipped together as in Pilates stance. Tuck your tailbone under and squeeze your buttocks. Keep your powerhouse firmly in.

THE MIND IN MOTION When you prepare for the Push-up in step 5, look slightly forward—not down. As you pull yourself down and push yourself back up, keep your entire body tight. Don't allow your head, hips, or lower back to sag. Don't allow your elbows to rotate out. Following these guidelines will make your Push-up more challenging and will strengthen your entire body. For an even greater challenge, try the Push-ups on only one leg at a time.

CAUTIONS If you are overweight, be extra sure to hold your navel to your spine to prevent your weight from pulling on your lower back. If you have wrist problems, try supporting yourself on the first two knuckles of your fists. If it still hurts, then skip the exercise. Leave this exercise out if you have neck, shoulder, elbow, or back problems.

CONTROL PUSH-UP BACK

BENEFITS: STRENGTHENS THE ARMS, NECK, SHOULDERS, BACK, POWERHOUSE, BUTTOCKS, HIPS, AND LEGS; OPENS THE CHEST; STRETCHES THE ARMS

After the Control Push-up Front, turn over and sit up with your legs straight and your hands flat on the floor behind you (not illustrated). Exhale and lift your hips and body up into a straight line as you engage your buttocks and powerhouse. Inhale and lift your left leg toward the ceiling.

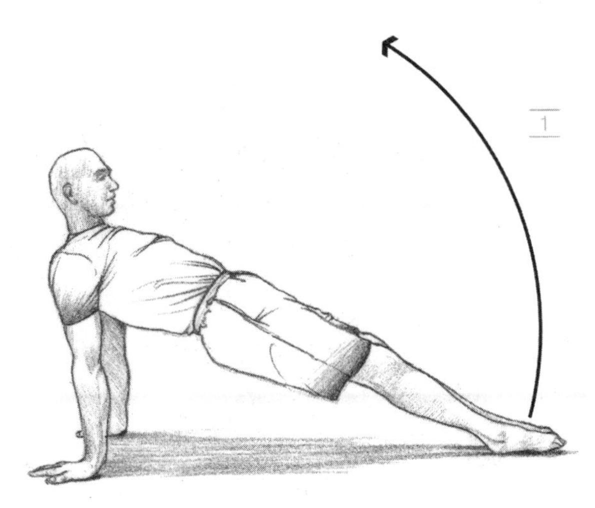

1

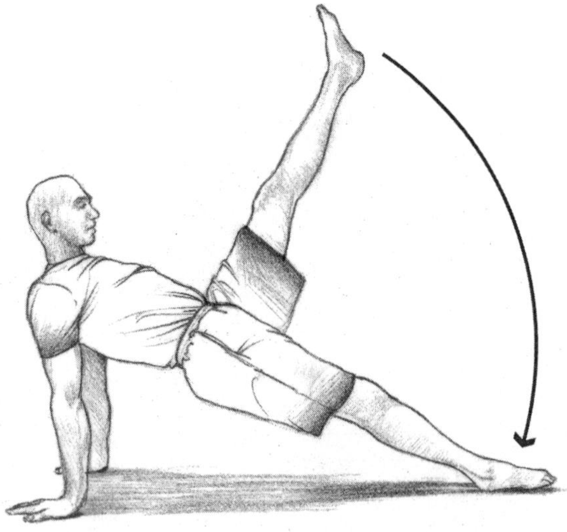

Exhale and lower your left leg to the floor.

2

Inhale and lift your right leg toward the ceiling.

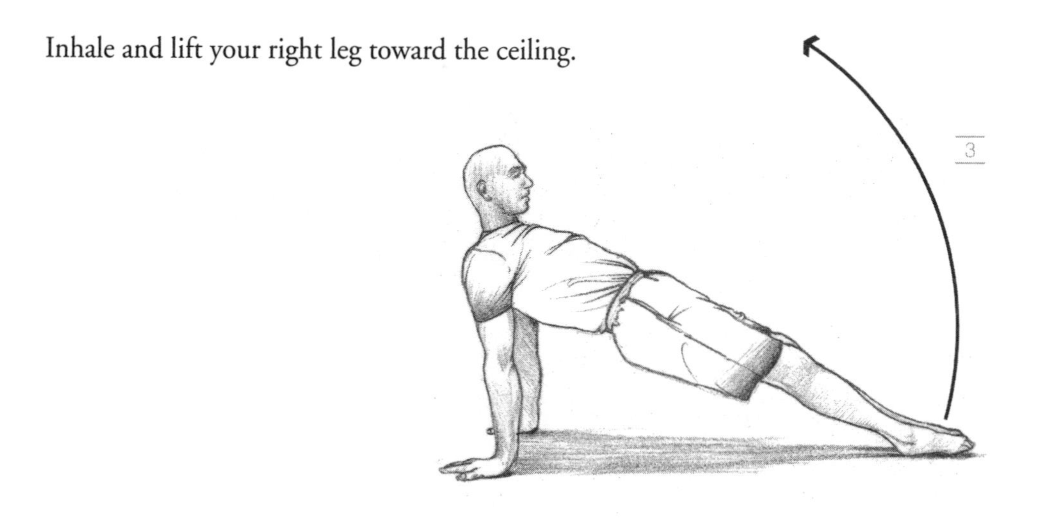

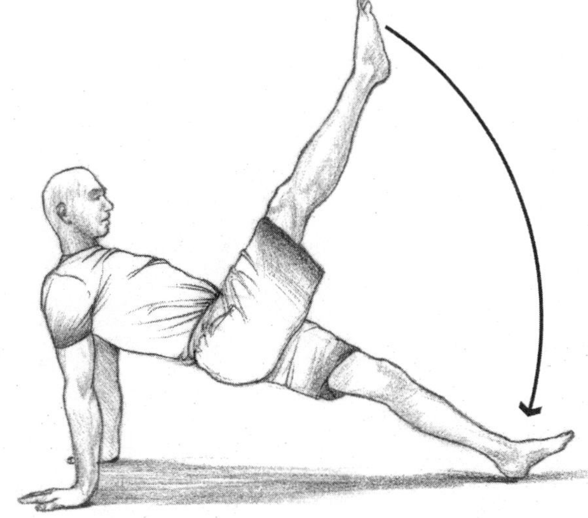

Exhale and lower your right leg down to the floor.

Perform 3 times.

THE BEAST WITHIN

This exercise is the Leg Pull Up from the traditional mat work.

BODY POSITION Keep your shoulders down and away from your ears. Keep your neck long; don't let your head sink down in to your shoulders. Lock your knees and elbows.

THE MIND IN MOTION: If you find it too difficult to lift your legs when you start out, simply hold the first position and breathe in and out a few times. It's okay to let your leg turn out when you lift it, but always lift with control. Don't kick haphazardly. Keep your bottom up and your hips square when you lift your leg. You may place your hands flat on the floor with your fingers turned in any direction that doesn't hurt your wrists—or, to strengthen your wrists, you may perform this exercise on your fists.

CAUTIONS Men tend to have a small range of motion when lifting their legs. As always, control is more important than range. Leave this exercise out if you have neck, shoulder, wrist, elbow, back, hip, knee, or ankle problems.

THE STAR

BENEFITS: STRENGTHENS AND LENGTHENS THE ENTIRE BODY; DEVELOPS BALANCE AND COORDINATION

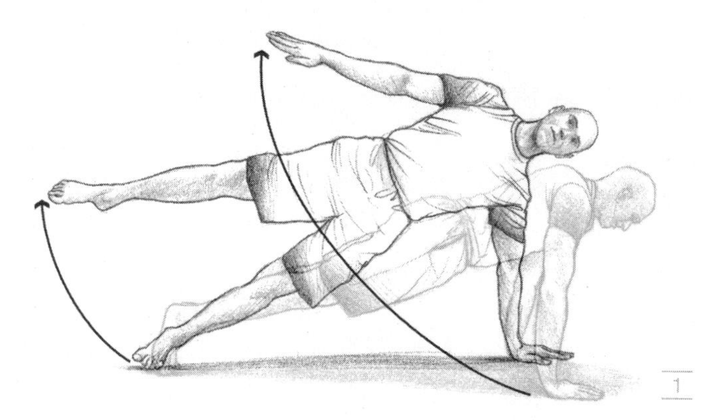

Assume a Push-up position. Turn onto your left hand and left leg. Lift your right leg 2 to 3 feet in the air above your left leg. Lift your right arm to just above parallel with the floor, keeping it in line with your body. This is the starting position.

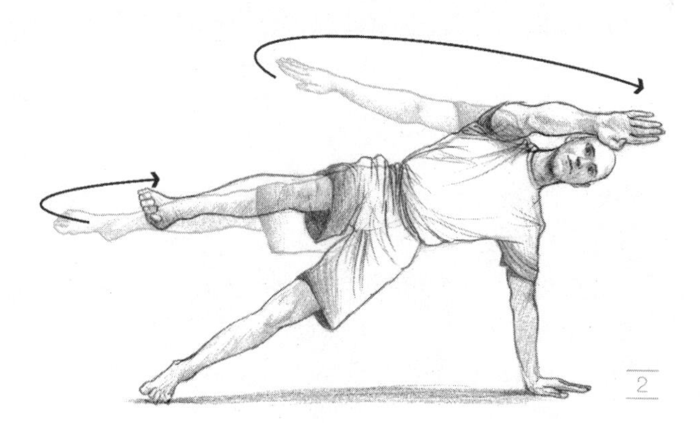

Inhale and bring your right arm and leg forward as far as you can, while maintaining control.

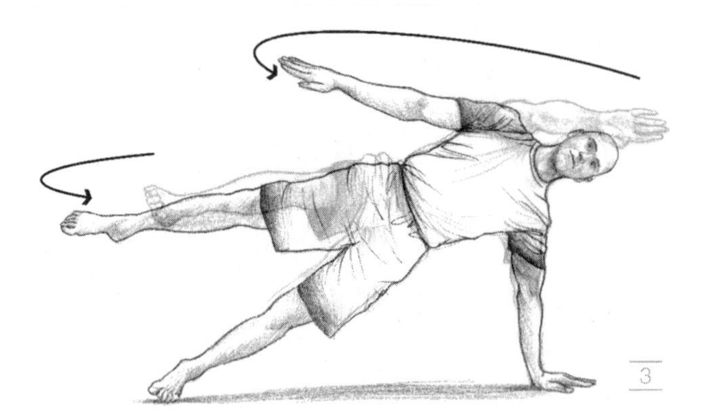

Bring your right arm and leg back to the starting position as you exhale.

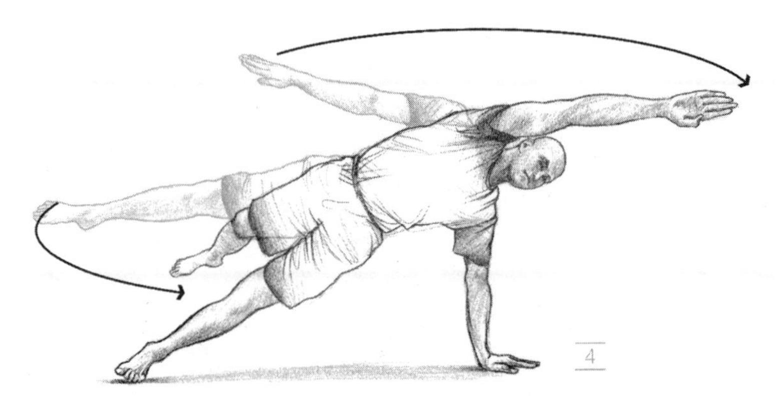

Inhale and extend your right leg back behind you as you bring your right arm forward again.

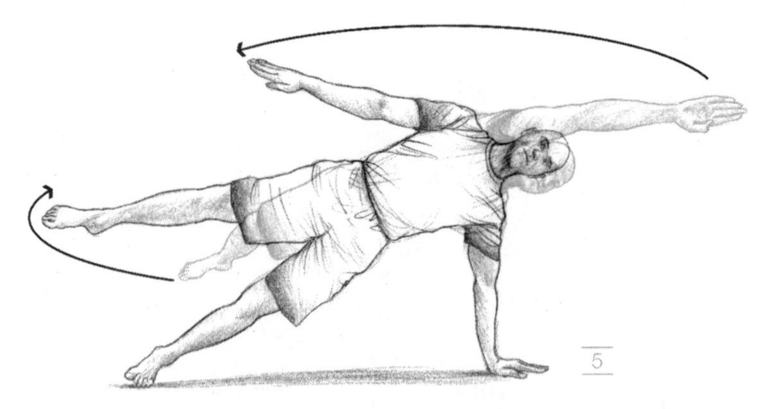

Exhale and bring your right leg forward and your right arm back to the starting position.

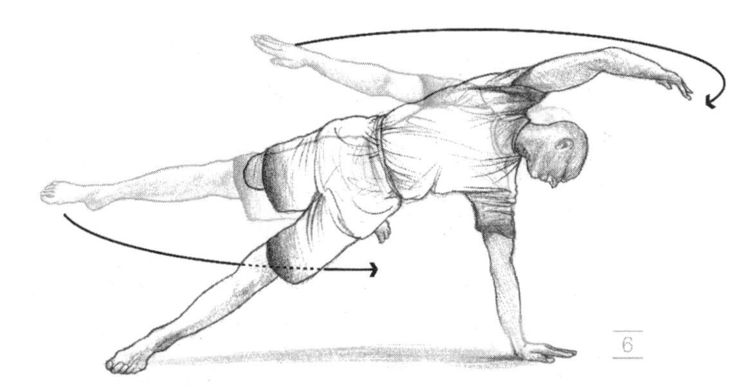

Inhale as you bend your leg behind you; reach your arm behind you with a bent elbow. Think of connecting your fingers to your toes to form a large circle. Look back toward your toes.

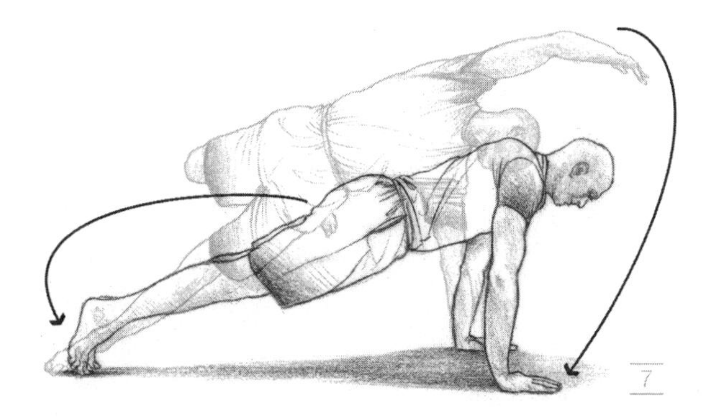

Exhale and come into a Push-up position.

Perform 1 repetition on each side.

THE BEAST WITHIN

BODY POSITION When you start out in the Push-up position, place your feet together so that when you turn onto one side you roll onto only the outside edge of your bottom foot. Keep your hips lifted. Keep your supporting shoulder away from your ear. Do not sink into your supporting arm. Lock your elbows and knees. Keep your hips and shoulders squared over one another. Don't allow them to roll. Keep your neck long.

THE MIND IN MOTION The Star is an exercise that accommodates all skill levels. If, for example, the Push-up position is a challenge, stop there. If just holding yourself up on one leg and one arm (see illustration 1) is testing your limits, then simply practice holding that position until it comes easily to you. Do not proceed further until you're able to do so with control.

Men tend to have the strength for this exercise but lack the flexibility to demonstrate much range of motion in the arms, legs, and spine. Remember, control is more important than range. A greater range of motion will come naturally with practice. Balance is typically a challenge as well; it too will come with strength and practice.

CAUTIONS Proceed slowly or leave this exercise out if you have neck, shoulder, wrist, elbow, back, hip, knee, or foot problems.

THE SIDE SPLITS

BENEFITS: STRENGTHENS THE INNER THIGHS; IMPROVES BALANCE AND POSTURE

Stand in Pilates stance with your arms open as if you were holding a large ball. Inhale and skim your right foot along the floor about 2 to 3 feet to the right.

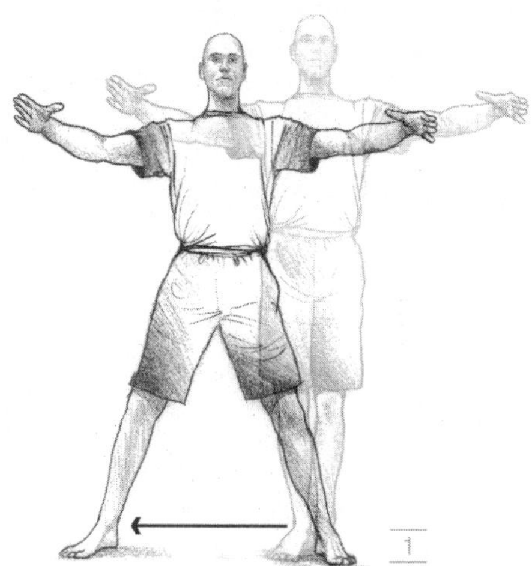
1

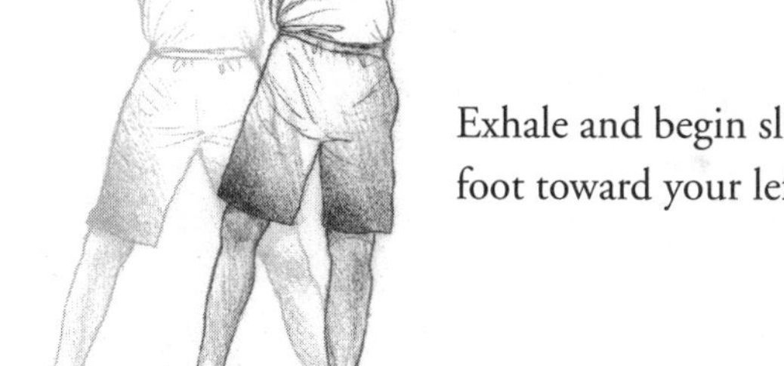
2

Exhale and begin sliding your right foot toward your left.

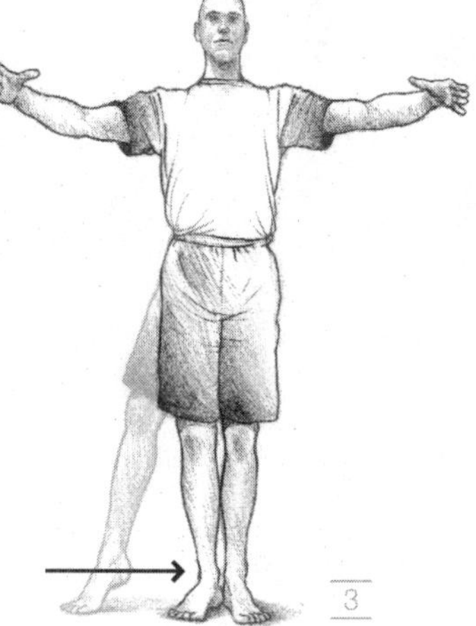
3

Finish exhaling as you return to Pilates stance.

Perform 3 times with your right leg, then 3 times with your left leg.

THE BEAST WITHIN

BODY POSITION You begin by standing in Pilates stance, except with your arms out to the sides and slightly bent elbows and wrists.

THE MIND IN MOTION Don't jump or step your foot out. Use your inner thighs to pull your leg back in. Keep your powerhouse engaged during the movement. (If you are able to perform full splits on the floor, this exercise won't be much of a challenge for you unless you slide your foot out farther when you begin.)

CAUTIONS Proceed slowly or leave this exercise out if it aggravates your hip, inner thighs, groin, ankles, or feet. Don't even attempt it if you have knee problems or injuries.

FRONT/RUSSIAN SPLIT COMBINATION

BENEFITS: STRENGTHENS AND LENGTHENS THE LEGS AND SPINE

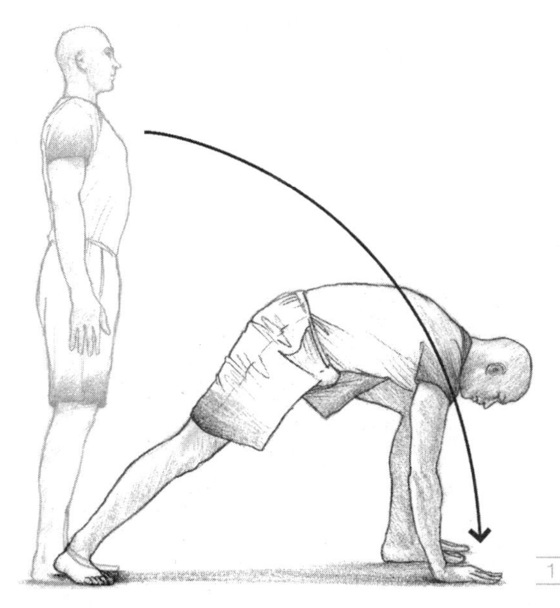

Standing in Pilates stance, exhale as you step forward with your left foot. Bend your left knee and place your palms shoulder-width apart on both sides of your foot, aligning your fingers and toes. Your knee should be directly above your ankle. Keep your rear foot flat and minimally turned out. Pull your powerhouse in and up.

Inhale and straighten your front leg as you pull your hips squarely up. Keep your palms on the floor and your powerhouse lifted.

Straighten and bend your front leg for a total of 5 repetitions.

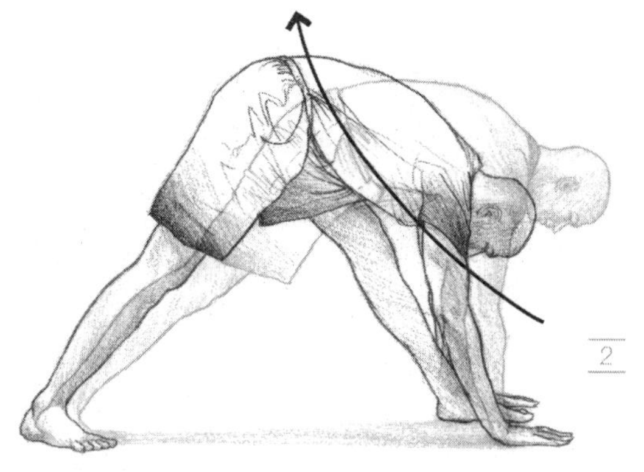

Inhale and lift your torso up. Bend your front knee, keep your hips square, and interlace your fingers behind your head. Keep your elbows wide.

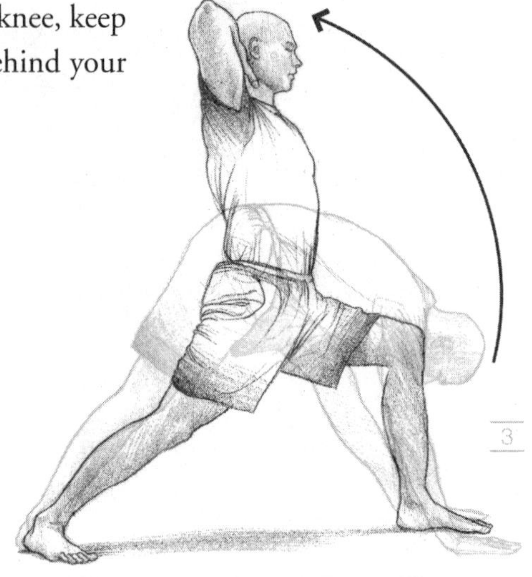

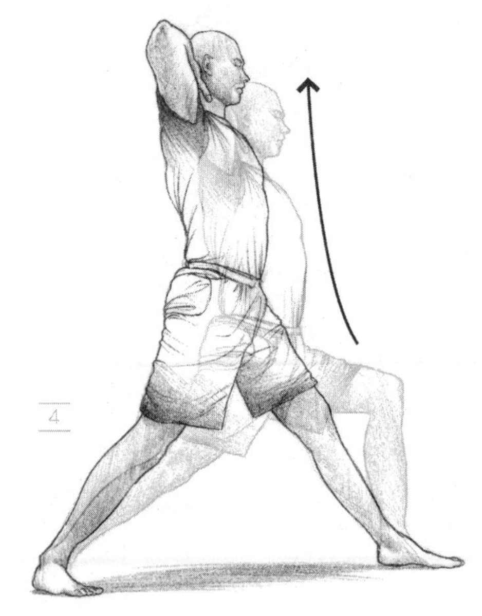

Exhale and straighten your front leg.

Bend and straighten your knee in this upright position for a total of 5 repetitions.

Lay your torso over your straight front leg. Place your palms on the floor on both sides of your front foot, keeping your shoulders and hips square. If you are flexible enough, lay your right cheek on your left shin. Hold this position for a few breaths.

Repeat the entire sequence (steps 1 through 5) with your right leg forward.

5

THE BEAST WITHIN

BODY POSITION This exercise is a partial combination of the Front Split and the Russian Split, which are performed on the reformer. Squeeze your buttocks to help maintain square hips. Lock your rear knee, and feel the weight on the outside edge of your rear foot. The farther apart your legs are, the more your rear foot will be turned out. Keep your powerhouse pulled in and up throughout the exercise.

THE MIND IN MOTION When you bend your front knee, don't let your knee overshoot your toes. This may be dangerous to your knee. When straightening your front leg with your hands on the floor, keep both feet grounded. Don't sacrifice square hips for better range of motion. When you come forward over your straight leg in step 5, keep both feet grounded. Keep your entire front foot grounded, but if you shift your weight slightly onto the inside edge of your front foot and lift your front kneecap by flexing your quadriceps, you'll help square your hips. If you have stiff legs, you will have a limited range of motion when your hands are on the floor. If you're not able to put your palms on the floor, try placing just your fingertips on the floor or hold onto your front calf or ankle.

CAUTIONS Proceed slowly or leave this exercise out if you have wrist, back, hip, knee, ankle, foot, or balancing problems.

THE HIGH BRIDGE

BENEFITS: OPENS THE CHEST AND HIP FLEXORS; STRENGTHENS THE SHOULDERS, ARMS, BACK, BUTTOCKS, AND LEGS; DEVELOPS FLEXIBILITY OF THE SPINE

After the Front/Russian Split Combination, lie on your back. Bend your knees and place your feet hip-width apart near your buttocks. Bend your arms back and place your palms on the floor underneath your shoulders. Exhale and pull your powerhouse in.

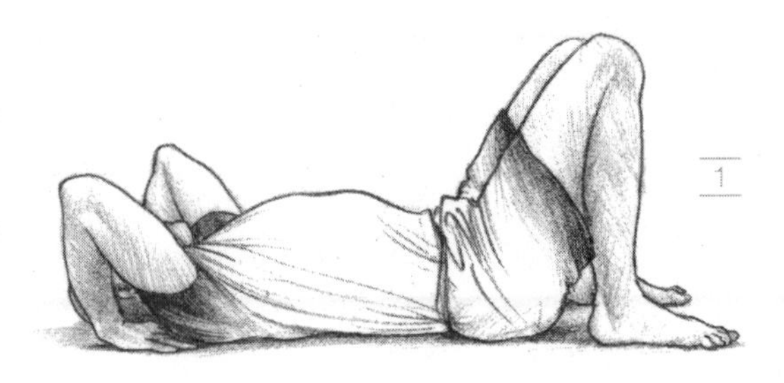

Step 2 is optional. It's helpful if you are new to Full Bridges or you need a transitional step to control the movement, but you may skip to Step 3 and bring your body straight up into a High Bridge. Inhale as you press your hands and feet into the floor, squeeze your buttocks, and lift your body up into a small backbend with the top of your head resting on the floor. Keep your weight distributed on your hands and feet.

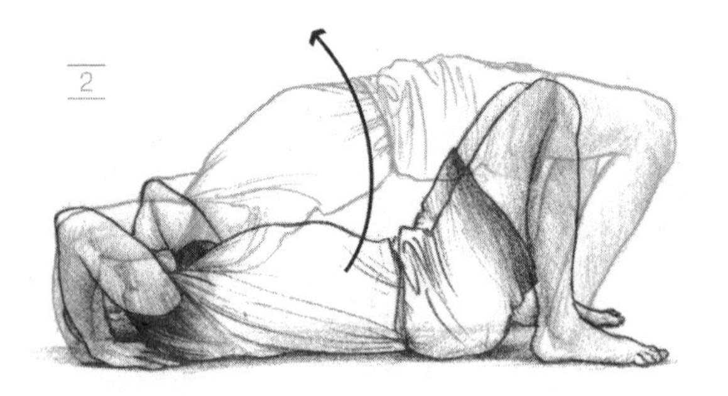

Lift your body all the way up by straightening your arms, squeezing your buttocks, and pressing into your feet. Hold the High Bridge for a few breaths.

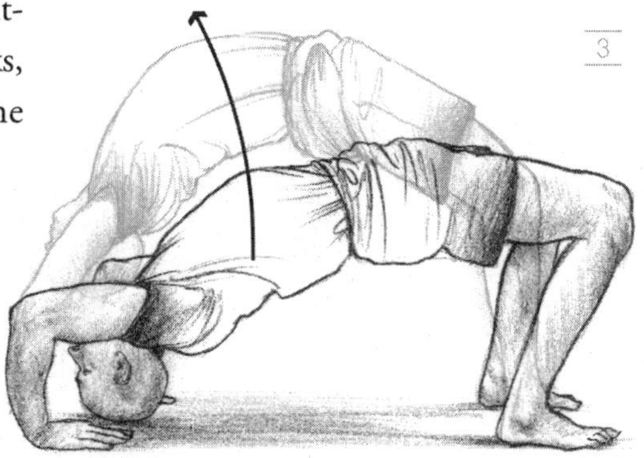
3

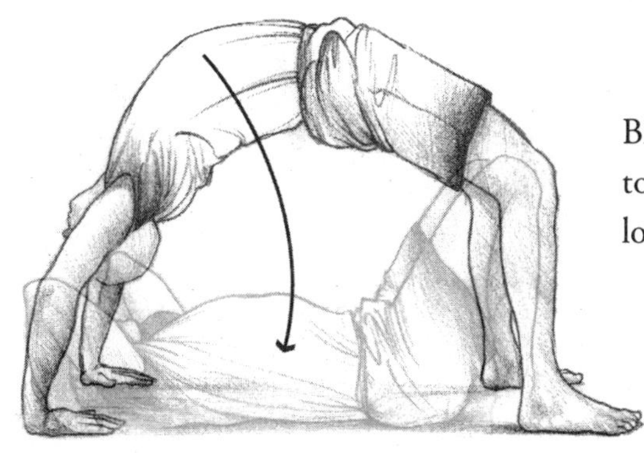
4

Bring your chin to your chest as you begin to exhale. Bend your elbows and slowly lower your body to the floor with control.

Settle into the starting position for a moment.

Perform steps 1 to 5 up to 3 times.

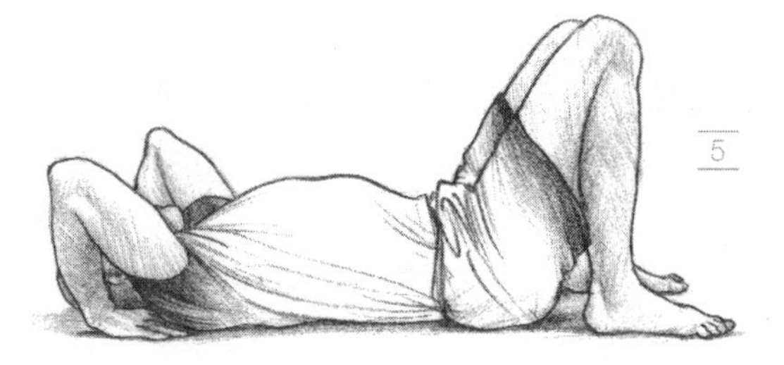
5

Stand up and perform a forward bend to release your back muscles.

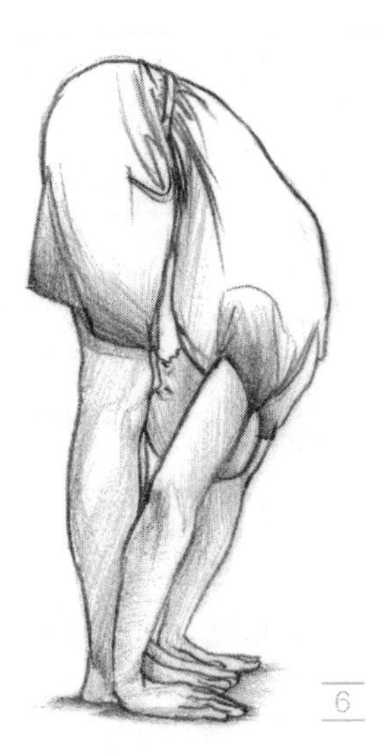

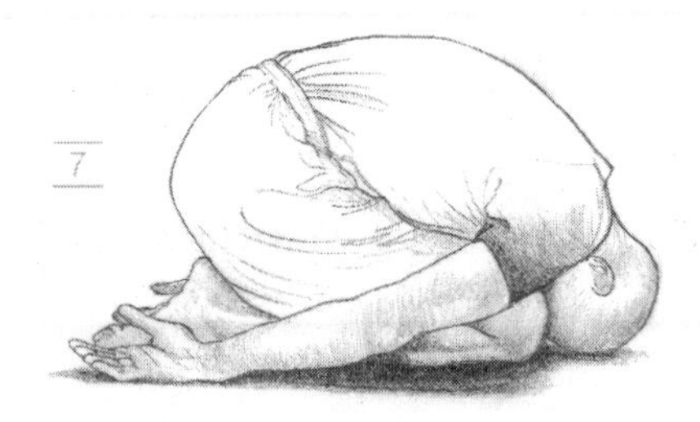

As an alternative to a standing forward bend, you may sit back on your heels and bring your forehead to your knees to release your back muscles.

THE BEAST WITHIN

BODY POSITION Be sure to place your hands and feet properly, as demonstrated in Step 1. Press firmly into your hands and feet.

THE MIND IN MOTION Don't perform the High Bridge on just the balls of your feet and toes; keep your feet flat on the floor. Squeeze your buttocks firmly to lengthen your hip flexors and help protect your back. If squeezing your buttocks causes any pain, leave this exercise out. When you're in the High Bridge position, try to keep your chest above your head. If you find that you're not ready for this exercise, simply bring your chin to your chest, bend your elbows, and lower yourself to the floor (see illustration 4). For men who come to Pilates with stiff bodies and no background in dance, martial arts, yoga, or gymnastics, performing the High Bridge is a satisfying accomplishment. Joseph Pilates put it this way: "If your spine is inflexibly stiff at 30, you are old; if it is completely flexible at 60, you are young."[8]

CAUTIONS I strongly recommend you perform this exercise with a spotter who has worked with inverted positions and back bending exercises. If being upside down makes you dizzy or light-headed, then you must have a spotter or skip this exercise completely. If you have tight hip flexors, upper back and/or shoulders, then don't risk the strain and potential injury. Leave the High Bridge out if you have neck, shoulder, wrist, elbow, back, hip, knee, or foot problems.

THE RUSSIAN SQUATS

BENEFITS: STRENGTHENS THE LEGS; INCREASES FLEXIBILITY OF THE SPINE, KNEES, AND HIPS

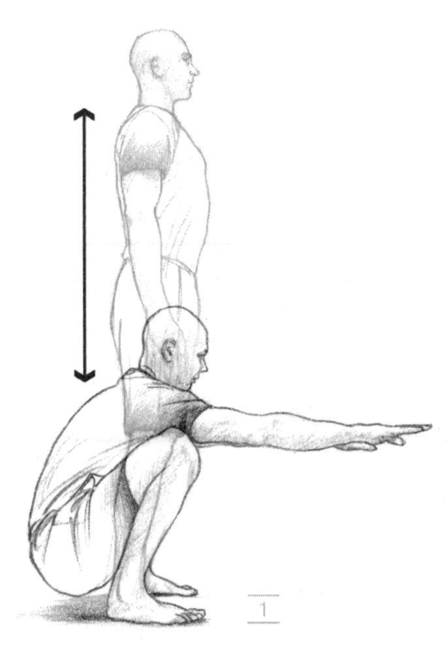

Stand up tall and then place your feet hip-width apart. Pull your powerhouse in and inhale. Keeping your shins vertical to the floor, reach your hands forward and sit back and down on your heels.

From the squat position, hold your powerhouse in and begin exhaling after you've come off the floor. Keeping your shins vertical, stand back up. You must keep your heels on the floor throughout the movement.

Perform 3 times.

THE BEAST WITHIN

This exercise is easier to perform on a floor than on a reformer. If not controlled on a reformer, the four springs will catapult you like a flying squirrel. The first time I tried this on the reformer, I broke my right pinky toe (a big manly injury). After two weeks of swelling, bruising, and limping, I again tried this on the reformer and slaughtered my demon: the Russian Squat.

BODY POSITION Stand up tall

THE MIND IN MOTION As you descend to the floor, you must *keep your shins vertical and sit more back than down.* Don't allow your knees to bend over your toes as you squat. In a Pilates studio, you'd perform this exercise on the guillotine, holding handles attached to springs to help counterbalance your body's descent to the floor. As a mat exercise, you must reach forward to counterbalance your weight as you descend. Don't allow your heels to lift up off the floor. If you can not keep your heels on the floor, it means you lack the flexibility in the spine, hips, knees, or legs. Practice sitting down and back onto a chain—while keeping your shins vertical—before attempting a full descent to the floor. You must also *keep your shins vertical* when you ascend from the floor. Men are rarely able to squat this deeply at the beginning. With practice, you'll progressively get lower and lower. If you find it too difficult to squat with a narrow stance, widen your foot stance to allow yourself to go deeper and open your hips; do not place your feet much wider than hip-distance apart. The wider your stance, the more your feet are likely to turn out. This is fine. Unless there is something structurally wrong with your body, you should eventually be able to sit on your heels. It's a natural position for the human body, and it is your birthright to have this level of flexibility! You may also start exhaling as you begin rising from the floor.

CAUTIONS Leave this exercise out if you have hip, knee, ankle, foot, flexibility, or balance problems.

THE ONE-LEGGED RUSSIAN SQUAT

BENEFITS: STRENGTHENS THE LEGS AND POWERHOUSE; INCREASES FLEXIBILITY IN THE SPINE, KNEES, AND HIPS

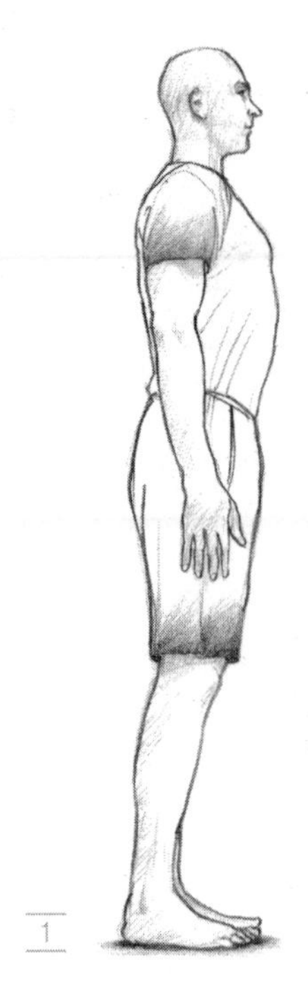

Stand up tall with your feet together.

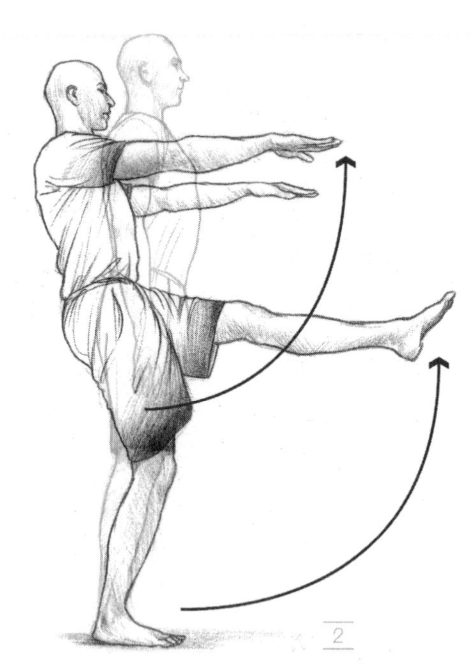

Exhale and lift your arms so that they're parallel to the floor as you lift your left leg up.

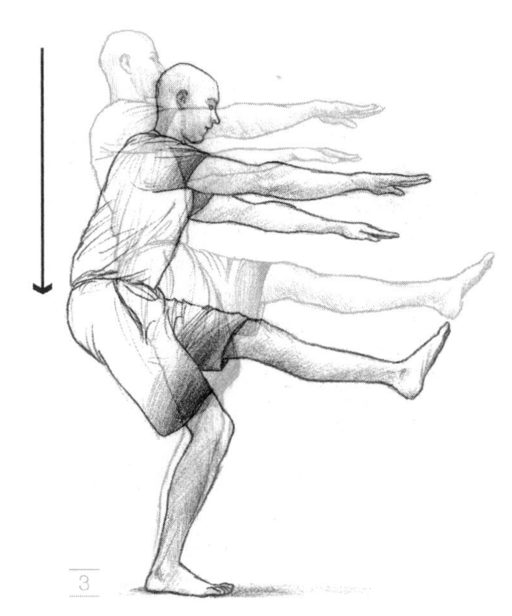

Hold your powerhouse firmly in as you inhale; sit back and down to slightly above the floor. Keep your standing shin as vertical to the floor as possible (it probably won't stay completely vertical; don't lift your heel or let your knee extend past your toes).

Only go as low as you can while maintaining control; keep your standing shin as vertical as possible. Keep your powerhouse strongly engaged.

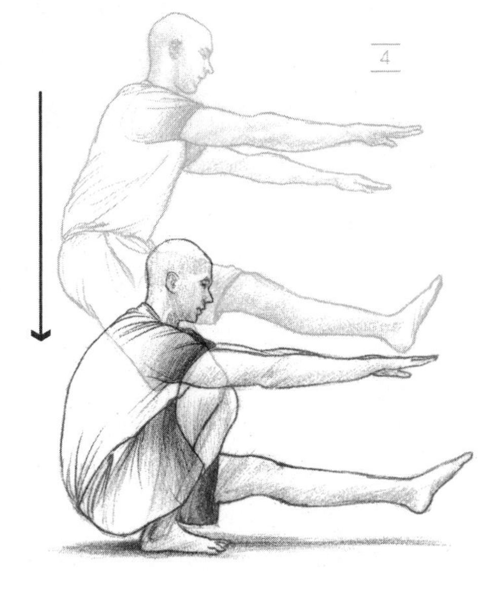

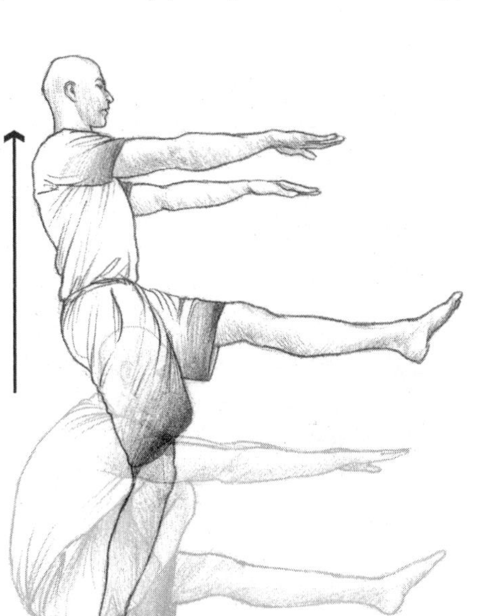

Squeeze your buttocks firmly and press into your grounded foot, especially into your heel as you rise up. Begin slowly exhaling when you're about halfway up. Finish exhaling and stand up as straight as possible.

Perform 3 squats on your right leg, then switch legs and perform 3 squats on your left leg.

THE BEAST WITHIN

BODY POSITION If it's too difficult to hold your leg high, you may lift it only slightly off the floor. Keep your knee on your standing leg aligned with your toes at all times.

THE MIND IN MOTION As you descend to the floor, you must *sit more back than down* and *keep your shins vertical.* Don't allow your knee to bend over your toes as you squat. In a Pilates studio, you'd perform this exercise on the guillotine, holding handles attached to springs to help counterbalance your body's descent to the floor. As a mat exercise, you must reach forward to counterbalance your weight as you descend. Don't allow your heel to lift up off the floor. If you can not keep your heel on the floor, it means you lack the flexibility in the spine, hips, knees, or legs that this exercise requires. Practice sitting a chair while keeping your shin vertical, before attempting a full descent to the floor. You must also keep your shin vertical when you ascend from the floor. If you want to make it easier on your hip flexors, lift your leg in the air only a few inches off the floor and turn this raised leg out from your hip. If your hip flexors cramp, stop the exercise, lie down, and massage them. With practice you'll progressively get lower and lower. Breathing properly is important in this exercise. Hold your breath as you begin to rise off the floor. If you need to exhale as you lift off the floor, start by releasing a small amount of air. Try to begin slowly exhaling after you're about halfway up. Another breathing pattern for this exercise is to exhale on the way down, inhale at the bottom, and exhale after you're about halfway up.

CAUTIONS Leave this exercise out if you have hip, knee, ankle, foot, flexibility, or balance problems.

PART IV

ROUTINES FOR INJURIES

You should always receive your physician's approval before beginning or changing your exercise regiment—especially if you have an injury. If a medical professional suggests an X-ray or M.R.I., then be responsible with your body and follow through. Take every possible step to know the state of your body before resuming or beginning any exercise program.

The following routines are provided as general guidelines. Since every *body* is different, these are not rigid rules. If an exercise hurts or aggravates a condition, then *leave it out!* As your body begins to heal, add exercises back into your workout, starting with the easier ones that develop a stabilized box—such as the Roll Up (see page 33). Make any of the recommended modifications to accommodate your body. If you are unsure about what to add back into your workout, simply consider yourself a beginner and follow the suggested routine in the traditional mat curriculum (see page 25). Consult the cautions at the end of each exercise, and be sure to skip anything that causes you pain or is not recommended for your given condition. After you add exercises that work within the box and strengthen your powerhouse, add additional exercises that demand more powerhouse control—incorporating such movements as rolling, twisting, arching, lying on your stomach, bringing your legs overhead, and balancing.

Also keep to your Pilates level. If you were a beginner before you were injured, perform only the beginner exercises within the respective guidelines for that injury. Likewise, if you were at an intermediate level before you were injured, perform only the beginner and intermediate exercises. Advanced Pilates practitioners may try all the exercises within the suggested guidelines. Regardless of your Pilates level, work intelligently and leave out anything that causes discomfort and/or pain.

When you have taken the necessary steps and are ready to begin working out, start slowly. Listen to your body before, during, and after the workout. You are likely to heal more quickly if you apply a qualitative and methodical approach to your workout; do not fixate on the quantity of workouts or exercises. On occasion, I still strain my body by not listening to it and push too hard. The lesson I've learned from these minor setbacks is the following. Every day your body is different, and you must honor your body's particular condition each time you workout. For example, if your body is functioning at about eighty percent, modify your workout accordingly; if your body feels stronger than usual, step your workout up a notch. Be in the moment, recognize your level of conditioning, and respect yourself. This is the secret to the most satisfying and effective workouts.

Shoulders, neck, back, knee, wrist, hand, elbow, foot, and ankle injuries are among the most common. For these conditions, perform at your Pilates level and simply leave out anything that hurts. For problematic hands and wrists, leave out any weight-bearing exercises—for example, the Leg Pull Front/Back or the Push-up. Eventually, as your hand or wrist heals, try weight-bearing exercises on the first two knuckles of your fists. (This is how martial artists strengthen their wrists.) Apply the same principle to problematic ankles and feet, leave out all weight-bearing exercises until the injury heals. Hips are tricky. For hip injuries or replacements, I recommend that you take some private lessons in a studio because you may need a trained eye to align, modify, and structure your movement.

While certain types of injuries may be common, each injury is an individual experience. For example, two people may have the same neck injury but experience different degrees of pain and ranges of motions. Treat your injury as an event specific to you and your unique body and exercise accordingly. Do not exacerbate the injury by ignoring the tell-tale signs of discomfort or pain. If it does not heal within a reasonable time frame, seek medical help. If your injury is more than minor, do not work out on your own. Find trained professionals to assist you. Be intelligent and responsible.

Unless otherwise stated, perform the exercises in the following suggested routines as originally instructed. Again, listen to your body. Work intelligent. Healing takes time. Be patient with yourself. You have everything to gain.

WORKOUT GUIDELINES FOR AN INJURED OR WEAK NECK AND SHOULDER

With an injured or weak neck/shoulder region, do not perform any exercises that involve rolling, arching, twisting, lifting your body overhead, or lying on your stomach. If necessary, place a small pillow under your head for comfort.

1. The Hundred: Use a small range of motion when you pump your arms up and down. Support your head with a pillow. If your neck or shoulders hurt, stop this exercise and leave it out completely. Perform fewer sets than usual.

2. The Roll Up: Perform with bent knees and keep your ankles under straps or secure your feet under a sturdy, comfortable piece of furniture. Do not reach your arms overhead. Simply walk your hands up and down the back of your legs as you roll up and down.

4. Single Leg Circles: Place a pillow under your head.

6. Single Leg Stretch: Keep your head down on a pillow instead of bringing your chin to your chest. Make sure you don't shrug up your shoulders; keep them down and away from your ears.

8. Single Straight Leg Stretch: Keep your head down on a pillow. If you find it difficult to reach your hands high on your legs with your head down, it's fine to hold them as far down as your hamstrings.

9. Double Straight Leg Stretch: Keep your hands under your bottom instead of interlaced behind your head. Do not lift your head off the floor; keep it down and—if necessary—on a pillow. Do not press into the back of your head. Lower your legs with total control within a smaller range of motion.

11. Spine Stretch Forward: Sit up tall and slide your hands out on the floor in front of you instead of holding them in the air.

13. Corkscrew: People tend to push into the back of their heads during the Corkscrew, incorrectly creating tension in the neck and shoulders. If you perform this exercise, you may try placing a small pillow under your head, use a small range of motion, and keep your buttocks on the floor. Do not bring your legs overhead. Draw small imaginary circles on the ceiling with your legs, keeping your tailbone on the mat.

24. Sidekicks: Do not prop your head up on a supporting hand. Instead, straighten your lower arm onto the floor and lay your head down on your bicep.

WORKOUTS GUIDELINES FOR AN INJURED OR WEAK BACK

With an injured or weak back, do not perform any exercises that involve rolling, arching, twisting, lying on your stomach, or bringing your body weight overhead. For the most part, stick to a "flat and square" workout.

1. The Hundred: Perform with your knees bent and your feet flat on the floor. As you improve, progress to performing the Hundred with bent knees in the air, then finally with straight legs in the air.

2. The Roll Up: Perform with bent knees and ankles under straps or with your feet secured under a sturdy, comfortable piece of furniture. Do not reach your arms overhead. Simply walk your hands up and down the back of your legs as you roll up and down.

4. Single Leg Circles: Perform *small* leg circles with the knee of the circling leg bent. If necessary, also bend the knee of your supporting leg and place that foot flat on the floor.

6. Single Leg Stretch: Attempt this exercise slowly.

8. Single Straight Leg Stretch: Attempt this exercise slowly with slightly bent knees and a small range of motion.

11. Spine Stretch Forward: Start with a small range of motion and gradually increase it as the condition of your back improves.

WORKOUT GUIDELINES FOR INJURED OR WEAK KNEES

With injured or weak knees, do not perform exercises that involve kneeling, lying on your stomach, or constricting your ankles with anything like a strap or a piece of furniture. Try to work your body evenly, making certain that your knees line up (or track) over your toes. This will help to heal and protect your knees. There is some controversy within the Pilates world concerning whether or not you should keep your knees "soft" or "locked" when exercising with injured or weak knees. In the recent past, when I've injured my knees, I have exercised using both the soft and locked knee variations to strengthen them. If the illustrated exercise calls for straight legs or locked knees, I recommend that you try working first with soft knees and then locked knees to determine which version feels better for your condition.

1. The Hundred: Keep your knees soft or locked.
2. The Roll Up: Keep your knees soft or locked.

3. Roll Over: Keep your knees soft or locked.

4. Single Leg Circles: Keep your knees soft or locked.

5. Rolling like a Ball: Hold your hands underneath your legs on the hamstrings so that there is less flexion (bend) of the knee.

6. Single Leg Stretch: Try holding your hands underneath your leg on the hamstring muscle when you bring your leg in. The straight leg may be soft or locked.

7. Double Leg Stretch: Hold your hands underneath your legs on the hamstring muscle.

8. Single Straight Leg Stretch: Keep your knees soft or locked, and pull from the hamstring with your hands.

9. Double Straight Leg Stretch: Keep your knees soft or locked.

10. Crisscross: Only bend your knees slightly. You may keep your extended leg either soft or locked.

11. Spine Stretch Forward: Keep your knees soft or locked.

12. Open Leg Rocker: Keep your knees soft or locked.

13. Corkscrew: Keep your knees soft or locked.

14. The Saw: Keep your knees soft or locked.

18. Neck Pull: Do not use ankle straps. If you cannot keep your lower body in place, without having your ankles held down, leave this exercise out. Otherwise, keep your knees soft or locked.

19. Scissors: Keep your knees soft or locked.

22. The Spine Twist: Keep your knees soft or locked.

23. Jackknife: Keep your knees soft or locked.

24. Sidekicks: Keep your knees soft or locked.

25. Teaser I: Keep your knees slightly bent.

26. Teaser II: Keep your knees slightly bent.

27. Teaser III: Keep your knees slightly bent.

29. Hip Circles: Keep your knees soft or locked.

40. Push up: Do not perform on your knees. As with all of the above, only include this exercise if it's painless.

THE FINAL CUT

Now that you are armed with *The Complete Book of Pilates for Men,* I hope you will let it serve as a continual source of motivation and guidance, setting you on course for a lifetime of incredible fitness. As you can see, Pilates offers a vast terrain of possibility for men, allowing you to strive toward higher levels of physical conditioning. But remember, the challenge begins with you. Using all the guidelines that this book has laid out for you, move intelligently and use your inner strength to cultivate your physical strength.

The mat work that you perform will yield results to match the levels of focus, control, and intelligence that you bring to it. If you rest well, eat well, and challenge your body with caution, you *will* make tremendous progress and perform optimally in all aspects of your life. By contrast, if you sleep poorly, eat poorly, fail to challenge yourself, or push yourself too hard and too quickly, you'll undermine your efforts. As a man who has practiced many types of physical training over the years, I have found that none is more continually satisfying than Pilates. I still participate in many other physical activities, but Pilates is the foundation that integrates everything.

To have your health and a strong, powerful, resilient body (not to mention killer abs) to meet the demands of your chosen lifestyle is worth more than any king's ransom. Just be safe, listen daily to what your body is telling you, and have a damn good time mastering the Pilates mat work!

—DANIEL LYON

GLOSSARY

ANCHOR A verbal cue used to communicate the idea of firmly affixing a section of the body to the floor or mat.

ALIGNMENT The arrangement and proper positioning of the body's parts in relation to each other in a given position—such as standing, lying down, or kneeling.

ARTICULATE A term used within the Pilates method to convey the feeling of moving the vertebrae of the spine in a distinctly singular and sequential fashion.

BOX The visual image of a box or rectangle connecting the shoulders and hip bones to one another.

CHIN TO CHEST The physical gesture of slightly nodding or firmly affixing your chin to or near the hollow of your throat or chest; this movement will elongate your cervical spine (the neck).

CONTROLOGY The name given to Pilates by its founder, Joseph H. Pilates. He sometimes referred to it as the "Pilates Method of Physical Conditioning" as well.

DIAPHRAGM A body partition of muscle and connective tissue separating the chest and abdominal cavities in mammals.[9]

HAMSTRING MUSCLE Any of the three muscles at the back of the thigh that function to extend the thigh when the leg is flexed.[10]

HIP FLEXORS Two muscles, iliacus and psoas major, which together are commonly known as iliopsoas or the hip flexors. This composite muscle is the strongest flexor of the thigh at the hip joint. The iliopsoas muscles are also important antigravity postural muscles.[11]

IMBALANCE A disparity among body parts in relation to strength, flexibility, or alignment.

PELVIC FLOOR A term used to describe the structure and specific musculature of the pelvis.

PELVIC GIRDLE A bony or cartilaginous arch that supports the hind limbs of a vertebrate.[12]

PELVIS A basin-shaped structure in the skeleton of many vertebrates that is formed by the pelvic girdle and the adjoining bones of the spine.[13]

PILATES STANCE (1) A position for the feet in the Pilates method where the heels are placed together and the toes are slightly to moderately separated by a turn out from the hips. (2) The general term for standing in the Pilates method with the heels together and toes apart.

POWERHOUSE Joseph Pilates's term for the abdominal muscles, hips, lower back muscles, and buttocks.

NOTES

[1] Paul C. Bragg and Patricia Bragg, *The Miracle of Fasting: Proven Throughout History for Physical, Mental, and Spiritual Rejuvenation,* 49th ed. (California: Health Science, Year not listed in book), page 242.

[2] Joseph H. Pilates and William John Miller, *Pilates' Return to Life Through Contrology,* copyright 1998 Presentation Dynamics Inc., page 43

[3] George B. Russell, "Keep fit? Ape the Animals says Gym Master, 83," *Sunday News,* May 26, 1963, New York City.

[4] John Briley, "Oldest Living Disciple of Joseph Pilates Tells All," *The Washington Post,* Washington, D.C., March 11, 2003.

[5] John Briley, "Oldest Living Disciple of Joseph Pilates Tells All," *The Washington Post,* Washington, D.C., March 11, 2003.

[6] Doug Tsuruoka, "Learn to Analyze Details: A Swordsman's Wisdom," *Investors Business Daily,* California, June 2, 2003.

[7] Joseph H. Pilates and William John Miller, *Pilates' Return to Life Through Contrology,* copyright 1998 Presentation Dynamics Inc., page 13.

[8] Joseph H. Pilates and William John Miller, *Pilates' Return to Life Through Contrology,* copyright 1998 Presentation Dynamics Inc., page 16.

[9] Webster's New Collegiate Dictionary, copyright 1976 by G&C Merriam & Co., page 315.

[10] Webster's New Collegiate Dictionary, copyright 1976 by G&C Merriam & Co., page 519.

[11] Keith L. Moore, *Clinically Oriented Anatomy,* 3rd ed. (Philadelphia: Lippincott Williams & Williams), pages 385–386.

[12] Webster's New Collegiate Dictionary, copyright 1976 by G&C Merriam & Co., page 846.

[13] Webster's New Collegiate Dictionary, copyright 1976 by G&C Merriam & Co., page 846.

ACKNOWLEDGMENTS

Special thanks to the following people for all they have done and continue to contribute: Judith Regan, Cassie Jones, Jason Puris, Anna Bliss, Dan Green, Simon Green, the vivacious and ever wonderful Romana Kryzanowska, Sari Pace, Drago Mehanzic and everyone at Drago's gymnasium, Alycea Ungaro and everyone at reaLPilates @ Tribeca Bodyworks, William Arbizu, Yvonne Engelmann, Michael Johnson, Ersilia Nikpalj, Fred Blumlein, all my clients, friends, and of course my mother and family most of all.